The 150
Healthiest
Comfort Foods
on Earth

The 150 Healthiest Comfort Foods on Earth

The Surprising, Unbiased Truth about How You Can Make Over Your Diet and Lose Weight While Still Enjoying the Foods You Love and Crave

Jonny Bowden, Ph.D., C.N.S., and Jeannette Bessinger, C.H.H.C.

First published in the USA in 2011 by
Fair Winds Press, a member of
Quayside Publishing Group
100 Cummings Center
Suite 406-L
Beverly, MA 01915-6101
www.fairwindspress.com

15 14 13 12   2 3 4 5

ISBN-13: 978-1-59233-482-7
ISBN-10: 1-59233-482-2

Digital edition published in 2011
eISBN: 978-1-61058-136-3

Library of Congress Cataloging-in-Publication Data available

Photography by Bill Bettencourt

Printed and bound in Singapore

The information in this book is for educational purposes only. It is not intended to replace the advice of a physician or medical practitioner. Please see your health care provider before beginning any new health program.

From Jonny:

To two extraordinary women:

    Taryn Sena Dunivant

    Shannon Janelle Bolin

who bring comfort food to my soul … and joy to my life

and to Amber Linder …

… whose magical smile warms my heart …

From Jeannette:

I dedicate this book to my clients and program participants: beautiful, powerful women, seekers, and foodies from all walks of life, on a quest for the sweetness and joys in living … you are my inspiration. May you be blessed on your journey with the great health and deep pleasures that are your birthright.

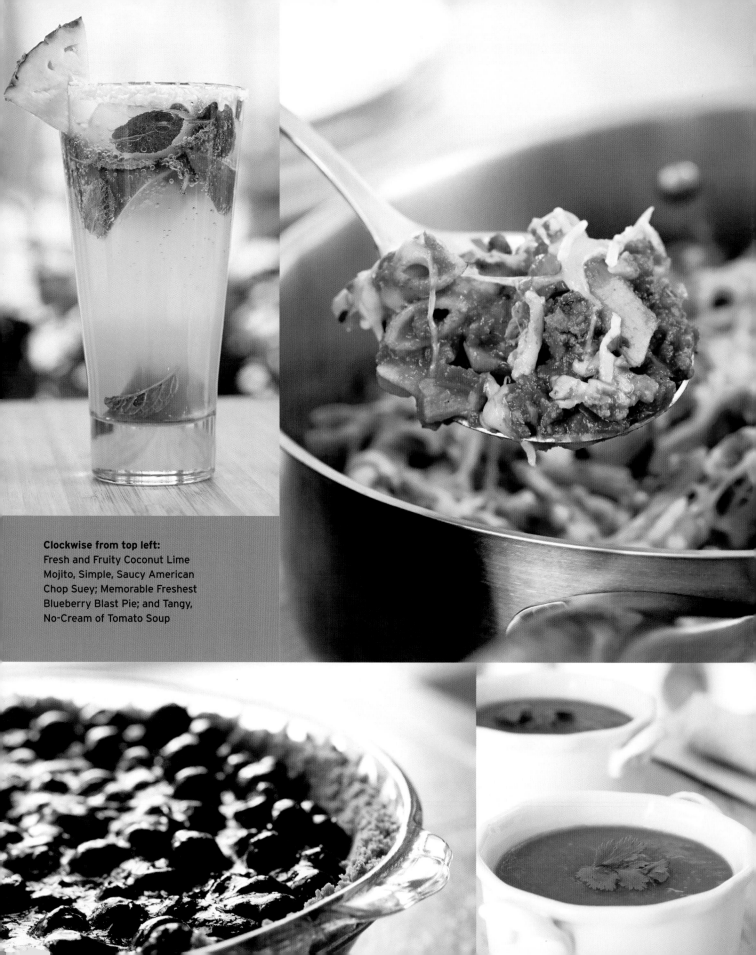

Clockwise from top left:
Fresh and Fruity Coconut Lime
Mojito, Simple, Saucy American
Chop Suey; Memorable Freshest
Blueberry Blast Pie; and Tangy,
No-Cream of Tomato Soup

CONTENTS

2 | Side Dishes

3 | Desserts

4 | Breakfasts

5 | Appetizers, Snacks, and Drinks

Appetizers

Snacks/Drinks

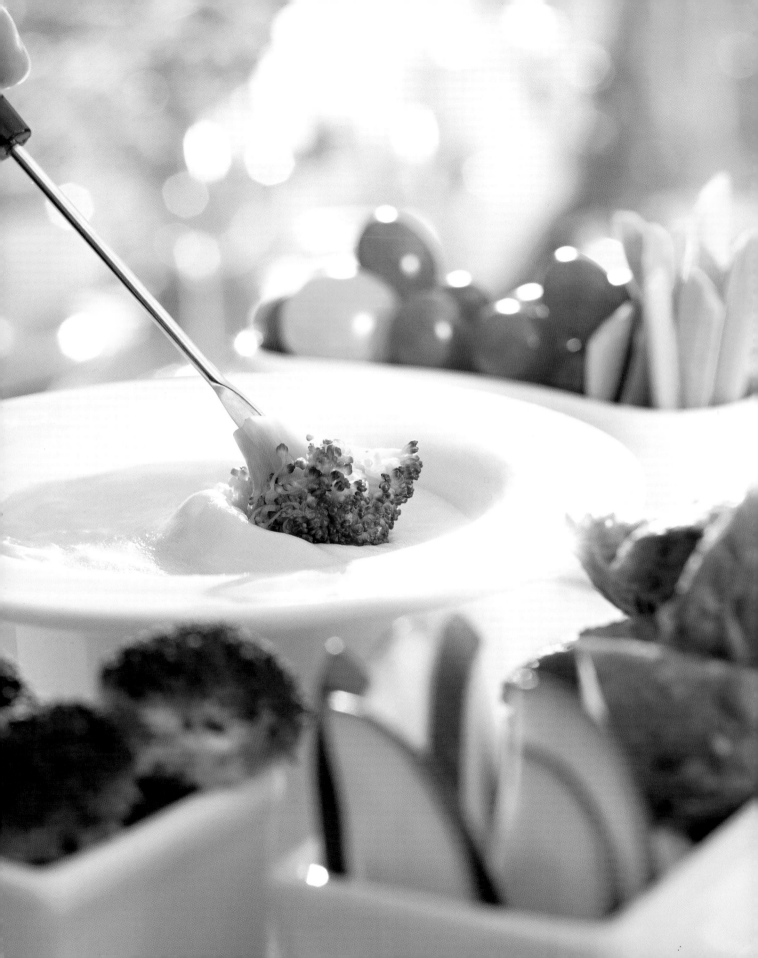

Introduction

I haven't had an ice cream cone in twenty-three years.

Now don't misunderstand me. I've had ice cream. Tons of it. In every incarnation you can imagine: ice cream, ice milk, frozen yogurt, sorbet, gelato, you name it, in every flavor from cookie dough to Cherry Garcia and back again.

But an ice cream cone—as in Jughead and Veronica comic books, as in "ye old sweet shoppe," as in Stewart's Ice Cream or even Dairy Queen, Mr. Softee, or Good Humor, nope.

Nada. Zilch.

Which, after all, is the point of this story.

Recently, my girlfriend, Michelle, and I spent a few nights in a terrific "all-inclusive" resort in Cabo San Lucas, Mexico. If, like me, you've never been to an all-inclusive resort, it has a humongous amount of food of every style, nationality, shape, flavor, and texture available twenty-four hours a day. And one of the things it had available all the time, mind you, was an ice cream cone station.

So I had one. My first in twenty-three years.

All of a sudden I was transported back to my childhood. I remembered family vacations every August at Deerpark Farm in Cuddebackville, New York, and trips into town to Dairy Queen, and walking through the streets of Woodstock, New York, with a cake cone dripping with vanilla fudge ice cream, and I was suddenly and surprisingly flooded with feelings and memories from another time.

All from a stupid ice cream cone.

And finally—profoundly, I might say—I understood all at once what comfort food was all about.

Not to put too fine a point on it, but the sensation of eating that food transported me to a different time. The experience of eating that ice cream cone took me back to the time when I was fourteen, and reminded me that even though decades had passed and I had hopefully changed and grown in many ways in the ensuing years, in some small but important way I had reconnected with the person I was when I was fourteen and pining for adorable, curly-headed Carol Zemsky in the summer camp at Sacks Lodge in Woodstock.

In a world that's increasingly fragmented and digitalized, the ice cream cone offered some small measure of integrity in the truest sense. Like a small, warm pocket of water that you occasionally encounter in the cold ocean, it was a safe haven, a reminder of who I was, a reminder of a happy time when life was less complicated, a reminder that some things never change.

Quite comforting, actually.

Which brings me to the subject of this book.

Having devoted my life to preaching the gospel of health, how do I reconcile my belief in the healing powers of whole, natural foods with the very real and competing need of us humans to have the kind of experience I had with the ice cream cone? That comforting, warm, memory-rich experience of savoring foods so often associated with good times, good friends, and a less-complicated existence?

After all, what pleasure would there be in life if we couldn't occasionally indulge in something that might not be the best thing in the world for us but sure is fun?

So we decided to tackle this project not with the mindset of a food scold (who likes the food police anyway?) but rather with a fellow-traveler mentality, one that asks the simple question, "How can we make food that really isn't all that good for us into food that is—if nothing else— less bad?"

In keeping the taste as close to the original as possible, the calorie counts in certain recipes might still be high for some readers. That's why we suggest that certain comfort foods, such as the brownie pie, not be the mainstay of your diet, but rather an occasional indulgence. Here are some of the ways we found we could improve the overall health value of these favorite dishes while still preserving the familiar flavors and textures (and memories!).

Higher-quality fat. Although many people think fat is bad, the whole question of fat requires a far more detailed discussion than belongs in this cookbook, and it's one I've addressed in several other books. Suffice it to say for now that the only really bad fats are trans fats and damaged fats. By "damaged" I mean the kinds of fats that become transformed by heating and reheating, which is what happens in all fast-food restaurants and many "regular" restaurants where oil is generally used for a week before being tossed. So instead of frying, we baked or braised. Instead of using cheap, highly refined oils, we used cold-pressed or organic ones. You won't find any trans fats or "damaged" fats in this book and there's no need to be frightened of the fat that remains.

Reduction of total fat. Let me be clear: We did this not because fat is bad but because many comfort foods have an awful lot of it and an awful lot of fat, even the very best kind, means an awful lot of calories. You can make almost any comfort food a lot better by just reducing the calories somewhat, and that's exactly why we cut back on fat in general. But we did it in a way that really doesn't compromise taste, substituting, for example, low-fat dairy for full fat or using evaporated skim milk instead of cream.

Reduced sodium. There's pretty good evidence that most Americans consume far more sodium than we need, and that for many people is a real problem. We handled it in these recipes in two simple ways. One, we used less salt. (Not that much less that you'd notice, mind you, but enough so that it'll make a difference!) Second, we used better-quality salts. There's considerable controversy in the nutrition world about salt, but just about everyone agrees that the processed white salt you get from the typical salt shaker is the worst of the bunch because all traces of minerals and nutrients have been removed. We used unrefined sea salt, and sometimes liquid aminos, which provide the same taste we crave from salt but with less sodium and a nice little smattering of nutrients.

Lower glycemic load. This is a biggie. One thing that makes the American diet such a nightmare from a health point of view is the impact most of the foods we eat have on our blood sugar. This impact is measured in something called the "glycemic index" and measured even more accurately in the "glycemic load." You don't need to know what those terms mean technically to understand the basic concept, which is this: When you eat foods, your blood sugar goes up. How high it goes up, and how long it stays there, are important. A rapid rise in blood sugar brings on a rapid rise in the fat-storage hormone known as insulin. Foods that raise blood sugar quickly and keep it up there for a long time have a deleterious effect on health, and in some people can set the stage for pre-diabetes or even full-blown diabetes. One of the best things we can do for our health is to lower the glycemic (sugar) impact of the foods we eat. One of the ways to do this is by adding more fiber (see below) and another way is to trade some of the more heavily processed carbs (extremely high-glycemic impact) for carbs with less of a glycemic impact, such as whole grains and low-sugar fruits. When we talk about "lower glycemic impact" in many of these recipe introductions, you should know that that's a great improvement on the old standbys.

Increased fiber. Periodically you'll read some newspaper report claiming that fiber doesn't really matter and we've been sold a bill of goods and it doesn't prevent any disease. Don't believe it. Although we may not have perfect evidence that more fiber in the diet prevents a specific disease, we have a ton of evidence that high-fiber diets in general are associated with lower rates of cancer, heart disease, and diabetes. In addition to doing intestinal housecleaning work, fiber also slows the entrance of sugars into the bloodstream, thus blunting that "blood sugar roller coaster" that can lead to all kinds of health complications. Fiber's good for you. Period. We tried to up the fiber whenever possible. A gram here, a couple grams there—it won't interfere with your enjoyment of the foods, and it may help you enjoy a longer life!

Increased protein. Now here's something near and dear to my heart. As I've written many times, the word *protein* comes from the Greek, meaning "of prime importance." In addition to providing nutrients that are absolutely essential to the creation of almost everything in your body (from hormones to bones and from neurotransmitters to muscles), protein is very important from a weight-management point of view. Higher-protein diets are more satiating (meaning they make you full—and thus less likely to overeat!). When possible we gently pushed the protein quotient up a bit, which, if anything, usually resulted in improved taste!

Increased nutrients. This one was easy and reminds me of an old trick I used to use to get my stepson to eat broccoli. I'd simply make some homemade juice in the juicer using carrots and apples as a base, and then throw in a stick of broccoli. No teenager alive will notice it, and will respond instead to the overall sweetness created by the apples and carrots. Same thing here—by throwing in some small amounts of what we call "invisible" nutrient boosters (like puréed sweet veggies or even beans), you can make even the most decadent comfort food into something that is no longer nutritionally empty!

Reduced sugar and healthier sweeteners. This is the area where I almost always get into trouble with my readers. They'll look at some of the recipes we've done in the last few books (and I'm sure in this one as well) and write to me saying some version of "how could you?" Usually the "how could you?" refers to the use of sugar or agave nectar syrup, or some other sweetener that I've railed against in my writings, newsletters, columns, and books. So let me answer that very reasonable question: We use sugar (or sweeteners) because this is the real world, because we're trying to create foods and recipes that people will actually eat (and like!), and because—especially in the case of this book—we're simply trying to improve on classic recipes for foods that aren't usually that healthy to begin with.

We're not trying to change the world here, just trying to make comforting foods a bit better for you. So our compromise was to use as little sugar (or sweeteners such as agave) as possible, just enough to make the taste palatable but not enough to send you into a diabetic coma! And by the way—according to my partner Chef Jeannette, who I have absolutely no reason to doubt on this matter, especially because she has two kids to test everything out on—you can safely remove between one-fourth and one-third of white sugar from virtually any baked goods recipe without any discernible change in taste or texture. Seriously. We also tried using natural foods such as applesauce as sweeteners (and as "fat replacements") whenever possible. We're pretty sure you'll like the results.

So while we made some "real-world" compromises with elements including sweeteners, there were some things on which we didn't budge. Our complete hatred of trans fats, for example. You will not find one single drop of hydrogenated oils (including margarines) or any other trans fat–containing food in any recipe in this book. You'll find no high-fructose corn syrup. You'll find no chemicals, artificial colorings, fake foods, or preservatives. You'll find no use of packaged products known to have high levels of MSG.

That may not seem like a lot of stuff to eliminate, but it's the worst of the bunch, and when you eat these fabulous comfort food recipes you can be pretty sure that the mere elimination of these items makes them a whole lot better for you.

Our mission in this book was to create the taste, texture, and feel of the old favorites yet—whenever possible—to replace some of the worst ingredients with ones that made more sense nutritionally. To our delight we found, as we think you will too, that taste never had to suffer. These improved versions of the old standbys from comfort-food land actually taste just as good or better than the originals.

We hope you enjoy making them—and especially eating them—as much as we did.

Enjoy the journey!

—Jonny Bowden

A Note from Chef Jeannette

I have one more word to add to Dr. Jonny's elegant introduction: balance. The essence of a healthy diet lies in high-quality foods, but the soul of skillful eating lies in finding a balance between those recipes that serve our bodies, minds, and energy best, and those that may not dwell at the top of the nutrient scale, but give us deep pleasure and comfort.

What does finding balance look like in action?

If you're eating a heavy-calorie comfort food dish, such as twice-baked potatoes, don't add the cheese puffs and finish it off with a piece of pumpkin pie at the same sitting. Use these recipes skillfully, as rich, nourishing, food-for-the-soul highpoints to a healthy, balanced meal. If you have a hankering for a hot, creamy twice-baked potato, fill the rest of your plate with steamed broccoli in a little lemon and finish it with a big salad. If you want a killer dessert, such as carrot cake with cream cheese frosting, then go for it! But eat a light meal that night, such as a fish and veggie soup.

Balancing calorie-heavy dishes with calorie-light dishes is an almost instinctive act among people I call "natural eaters." People who intuitively eat in a balanced, healthy way enjoy rich, indulgent dishes as much as everyone else does. That thin woman's secret to eating the chocolate fudge pie is that she will stop when she feels satisfied (long before her stomach is stuffed!), and will likely eat lightly for the rest of that meal, and possibly the rest of that day to balance out the extra calories.

As Jonny shared with us, enjoying these foods is part of the deep pleasure of living life to its fullest. We can have our cake and eat it too, as long as we are mindful of what goes into these recipes and how we utilize them in our ongoing daily diets.

I hope you enjoy them as part of a rich, full life.

Blessings on you and yours.

—Jeannette Bessinger

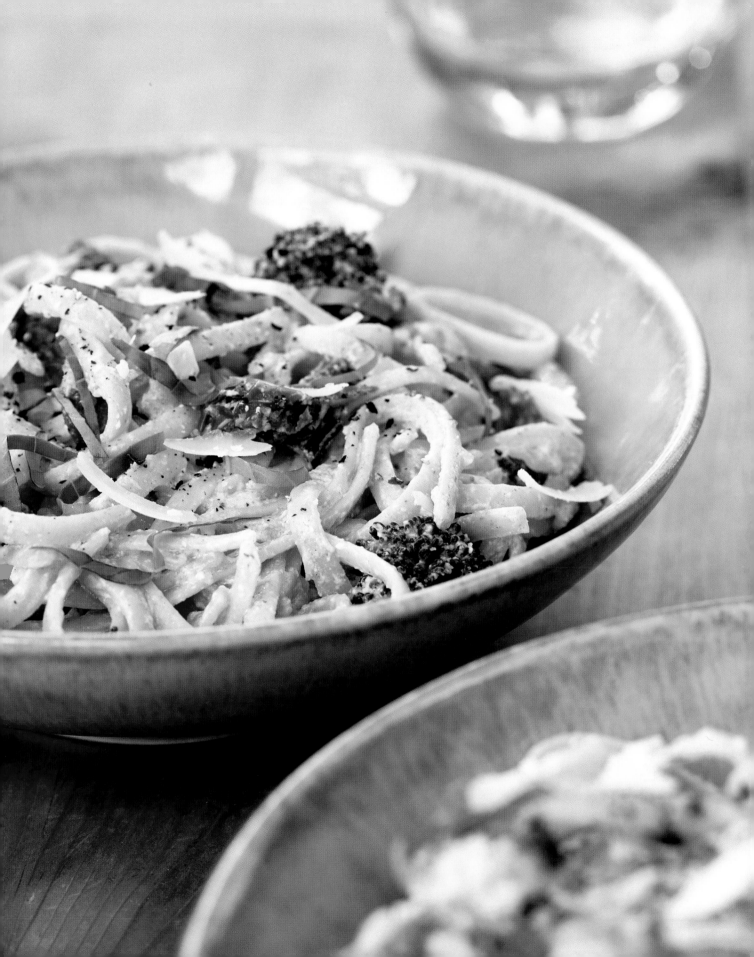

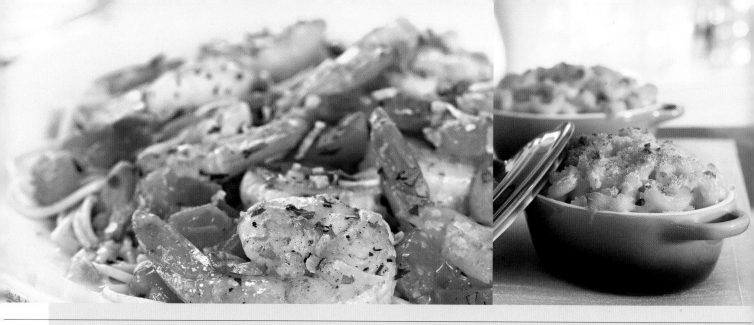

The Mains

Whatever main course you serve, be selective about what protein you choose. Purchase free-range poultry whenever possible, and if you buy deli meat, try to get it fresh (less sodium) and nitrate-free! I recommend only grass-fed beef, which is free of antibiotics, steroids, and hormones and has a better nutritional profile than the factory-farmed kind. And while all fish provides protein and vitamins, cold-water fish (such as salmon) are also a world-class source of the valuable omega-3 fats that contribute to heart health, brain health, and joint health. The meatless dishes in this section will work for both meat-eaters and confirmed vegetarians. Even meat-eaters can enjoy the occasional vegetarian dish—in fact, both Chef Jeannette and I recommend it!

POULTRY

Capsaicin-Rich Jamaican Jerk Chicken

Flavorful Faux Fried Chicken

Flavorful, Fiber-Full, Crispy Chicken Nuggets

Fresh Phyllo Chicken Pot Pie

Better-Than-Mom's Low-Salt Chicken Soup

Not-So-Sweet and Sour Chicken

Light and Tangy Vitamin-C Orange Chicken

Sumptuous White Meat Chicken Cacciatore

Skinny Stuffed Chicken with Zucchini Pappardelle "Pasta"

Lean and Light Curried Chicken Casserole

Light and Lemony Garlic Roasted Chicken

Smoky, Lower-Sugar Barbecue Drumsticks

Zippy Chicken Enchiladas: Protein Aplenty

Tasty Turkey Tetrazzini with Whole-Wheat Egg Noodles

Savory Slow Cooker Tender Turkey Drumsticks

Smoky Lower-Fat Bacon Turkey Burgers

Hearty Spinach and Mushroom Lasagna with Lower-Fat Meat Sauce

Lean and Tasty Sloppy Jonny

Healthy Holidays Dinner: Free-Range Citrus-Stuffed Herbed Turkey; Higher-Fiber Apple-Corn Bread Stuffing; Autumnal Antioxidants: Cranberry-Orange Relish

MEAT

Iron-Man Slow Cooker Beef Stew

In-a-Pinch Spaghetti Bolognese

Lean and Mean Marinated Flank Steak Tostadas

Grass-Fed Italian Feta Meatballs in Tomato Sauce

Lighter-but-Luscious Portobello Beef Stroganoff

Good-for-You Guacamole Grass-Fed Burger

Free-Range Ketchup-Mustard-Relish Sliders

Rich, Muscle-Building Meatloaf

Sinless and Savory Slow Cooker Cabbage Rolls

Lean and Savory Sauced Pot Roast

Grass-Fed Ground Beef Burritos with Cilantro-Orange Salsa

Lemon Cinna-Mint-Spiked Lean Lamb Stew

Simple, Saucy Antioxidant American Chop Suey

Savory Souped-Up Shepherd's Pie

Rack of Lean Lamb with Herbs and Roasted Shallots

SEAFOOD

Less-Butter Baked Scallops and Savory Shiitakes

Zesty Calcium-Stuffed Salmon

Tempting Tuned-Up Tuna Casserole

Protein-Packed, Apple-Glazed Wild-Caught Alaskan Salmon

Tempting Four-Flavors Shrimp Pad Thai

Backyard New England Clambake: Bounty of the Sea

Fresh and Fiber-Full Fish Fingers

Luscious Low-Carb Lobster Rolls

Creamy, Lower-Fat New England Clam Chowder

All-in-One Spicy Shrimp and Brown Rice Jambalaya

Savory, Protein-Rich Chicken and Shrimp Paella

Superfresh and Lemony Olive Oil-Rich Shrimp Scampi

MEATLESS

Higher-Protein, Lower-Cal Creamy Fettuccini Alfredo

Madeover Mac and Cheese—a Calcium and

Vitamin D Bonanza

Chuck's Healthy Eggplant Parm

Tangy, No-Cream of Tomato Soup

Pork-Free Fresh Pea Soup

Smoky Bean Baked Nachos

Lower-Oil Spicy Sesame Peanut Noodles

Tender Greens Pesto with Protein-Packed Pasta

Whole-Grain Home-Grilled Pizza

Rich Cheesy Crudités Fondue

Smoky Hot Whole Grains and Beans Chili

Ingredients

6 shallots, coarsely chopped (or 1 small
    white onion)

1 jalapeño pepper, coarsely chopped
    (remove the seeds to reduce the heat)

1/3 cup (80 ml) low-sodium tamari

Juice of 2 limes

3 tablespoons (45 ml) apple cider vinegar

3 cloves garlic, crushed

2 tablespoons (12 g) finely chopped fresh
    ginger

1 1/2 tablespoons (23 g) Sucanat or brown
    sugar

1/2 teaspoon cinnamon

1/2 teaspoon nutmeg

1/2 teaspoon ground cloves

1/2 teaspoon allspice

2 tablespoons (28 g) coconut oil,
    melted but not hot

4 skinless, boneless chicken breasts

From Chef Jeannette

To Complete the Meal: Serve this chicken over a bed of fresh spring greens or in a whole-grain wrap with alfalfa sprouts and shredded lettuce.

Capsaicin-Rich Jamaican Jerk Chicken

From Dr. Jonny: I always wondered about the origins of the term "jerk chicken," so I did a little digging. Turns out it all started with the Maroons—powerful, escaped ex-slaves who settled in the mountains of Jamaica where they promptly introduced African meat-cooking techniques to the natives of this Caribbean island. The Jamaicans took the technique, which involved smoking the meat for a long time, and spiced it up with local ingredients. The actual term "jerk" probably derived from the Spanish word *charqui*, used to describe dried meat, and has come to mean the practice of poking holes in the meat to fill with spices prior to cooking. (Now you can safely go on *Jeopardy* and choose "Esoteric Cooking Information for 200, Alex.") Anyway. Traditional jerk chicken is usually made with a lot of oil and sugar, but our version goes light on both ingredients. We also used white breast meat to cut down on calories, though you can totally use chicken thighs with great results (and not a whole lot more calories). Marinate the breasts overnight; new research shows it helps protect the meat and reduces the formation of cancer-causing compounds called HCAs (heterocyclic amines). You'll never miss the extra calories with this flavorful marinade. Fun fact: Capsaicin is the compound in peppers that makes them hot, but it also has profound effects on pain. It works by depleting or interfering with substance P, a chemical involved in transmitting pain impulses to the brain. Capsaicin, usually extracted from hot peppers, is also found in a lot of creams used to treat the pain of arthritis and fibromyalgia.

In a food processor or blender, combine the shallots, jalapeño, tamari, lime juice, vinegar, garlic, ginger, Sucanat, cinnamon, nutmeg, cloves, and allspice and process until the vegetables are well puréed, scraping down the sides as necessary. Drizzle in the oil as you are processing to combine.

Lay the chicken out in a shallow glass storage container and cover with the marinade. Flip the chicken pieces to thoroughly coat. Cover and marinate overnight, turning occasionally.

Preheat a grill to medium. Remove the chicken from the marinade, scraping off any excess, and grill for 3 to 5 minutes, flip, and grill for 3 to 5 minutes more, or until cooked through but still juicy.

Yield: 4 servings

Per Serving: 348.6 calories; 3.3 g fat (11% calories from fat); 58.5 g protein; 16.3 g carbohydrate; 0.2 g dietary fiber; 141.5 mg cholesterol; 171.9 mg sodium

Flavorful Faux Fried Chicken

Ingredients

Olive oil cooking spray plus bottled olive oil,
for drizzling

1½ cups (345 g) plain low-fat yogurt

3 or 4 cloves garlic, minced, to taste

½ cup (50 g) finely chopped scallions

1 tablespoon (15 ml) lemon juice, preferably
fresh-squeezed, optional

½ teaspoon each salt and fresh-ground
black pepper

1½ cups (75 g) whole-wheat panko bread
crumbs

2 teaspoons (1.4 g) dried basil

1 teaspoon dried oregano

4 or 5 chicken drumsticks (about
1¼ pounds, or 565 g), skinned

4 or 5 skinless chicken thighs
(about 1 pound, or 455 g)

From Dr. Jonny: How do you improve on deep-fried chicken? Easy. First get rid of the extra calories from the frying oil. While you're at it, remove the skin (more calories you don't need). Add ingredients that are rich in nutrients, such as yogurt (for probiotics and calcium) and garlic (which helps reduce blood pressure and strengthens immunity). The result? Something that's as flavorful and satisfying as deep-fried chicken but is ten times better for you! Enjoy.

Preheat the oven to 375°F (190°C, or gas mark 5). Spray a light coating of olive oil on a large baking sheet and set aside.

In a shallow bowl, combine the yogurt, garlic, scallions, lemon juice, salt, and pepper, and mix well.

In another shallow bowl, combine the panko crumbs, basil, and oregano, and toss lightly to mix.

Dip each piece of chicken first into the yogurt mixture and roll to coat. Then roll in the panko mixture to coat. Lay the coated pieces on the baking sheet with space between each one. Bake for 40 to 45 minutes, until chicken is cooked through (should read 165°F [74°C] on an instant-read thermometer).

Yield: 4 or 5 servings (about 2 pieces each)

Per Serving: 397.5 calories; 15 g fat (34% calories from fat); 46.2 g protein; 17.5 g carbohydrate; 2.1 g dietary fiber; 171.2 mg cholesterol; 472.6 mg sodium

From Chef Jeannette

Keep your chicken chilled until the last possible moment. After skinning them, put the drumsticks into the freezer for a few minutes while you coat the thighs. The yogurt will adhere better to very cold skinless chicken.

To skin the drumsticks, grab the skin at the top of the meatiest part of the leg and pull it downward toward the thinner section. It will peel downward easily to the bone at the bottom. Because this is slippery work, use a knife to pin the skin to a cutting board and then pull the chicken leg away from it to separate.

Time-Saver Tip: Skip the fresh garlic, scallions, and lemon juice, and just mix 4 teaspoons (12 g) high-quality organic ranch dressing mix (omit the salt and pepper) or 2 teaspoons (6 g) each of garlic and onion powder (keep the salt and pepper) into the yogurt. You can also use preseasoned Italian whole-wheat bread crumbs in place of the panko and herbs.

Ingredients

High-heat cooking spray

1¹/₂ cups (120 g) organic, no-added-sugar cornflakes (we like Nature's Path)

¹/₄ cup (40 g) shaved Parmesan cheese

1 tablespoon (6.5 g) ground flaxseed

¹/₄ teaspoon garlic powder

¹/₄ teaspoon onion powder

¹/₄ teaspoon fresh-ground black pepper

¹/₄ teaspoon cayenne pepper, optional

¹/₂ teaspoon salt, divided

1 egg

1¹/₂ pounds (680 g) chicken tenders or chicken breast, cut into 2-inch (5-cm) strips

Dip

1 tablespoon (20 g) no-added-sugar apricot jam (we like Polaner's)

2 tablespoons (30 g) Dijon mustard

¹/₄ cup (60 g) plain low-fat yogurt

From Chef Jeannette

Your children won't have any idea that these nuggets are both high in fiber and trans fat-free! If your family prefers to dip their nuggets, try serving them with applesauce, a high-quality, low-sugar barbecue sauce (see our recipe for homemade sauce on page 36), or honey mustard.

Flavorful, Fiber-Full, Crispy Chicken Nuggets

From Dr. Jonny: Let me ask you a question: What part of the chicken is a nugget? And where on the planet is a natural chicken nugget? I've never seen one and I doubt you have, either. A healthy fast food nugget is an oxymoron. They're a terrific comfort food, but they're usually deep-fried in reused vegetable oil, and coated in a batter that contains sugar, white flour, and artificial flavors and colors that come from a test tube. But, and this is a big but, they sure do taste great. And who wouldn't love to have all that taste without the negatives? Well, your wait is over. This recipe is lower in calories than the "classic" nuggets, it's baked instead of fried, and it's much higher in fiber, due to the flaxseeds (which also contain valuable cancer-fighting lignans as opposed to cancer-causing chemicals!). Chef Jeannette has coated them with cornflakes to keep this dish a crispy crowd-pleaser. Your family will love them as much as I do.

Preheat the oven to 400°F (200°C, or gas mark 6). Spray a baking sheet with a light coating of high-heat oil.

Combine the cornflakes, cheese, flax seed, garlic powder, onion powder, peppers, and ¼ teaspoon of the salt in a food processor or blender, and pulse or grind until it's crumbly. (You can also crush with a rolling pin in a gallon-size resealable bag.) Pour into a shallow bowl.

In another shallow bowl, lightly beat the egg and remaining ¼ teaspoon salt together. Dip each tender into the egg to thoroughly coat, and then roll it in the cornflake mixture until it's thoroughly covered.

Lay the tenders out uniformly on the prepared baking sheet and bake for about 12 minutes, or until the coating is crisp and the chicken is cooked through.

To make the dip: While the chicken is cooking, in a small bowl whisk together jam, Dijon, and yogurt and serve on the side as a dipping sauce for the warm tenders.

Yield: 4 servings (about 12 tenders)

Per Serving: 413.6 calories; 6.9 g fat (17% calories from fat); 49.4 g protein; 32.12 g carbohydrate; 2.8 g dietary fiber; 164.5 mg cholesterol; 823.7 mg sodium

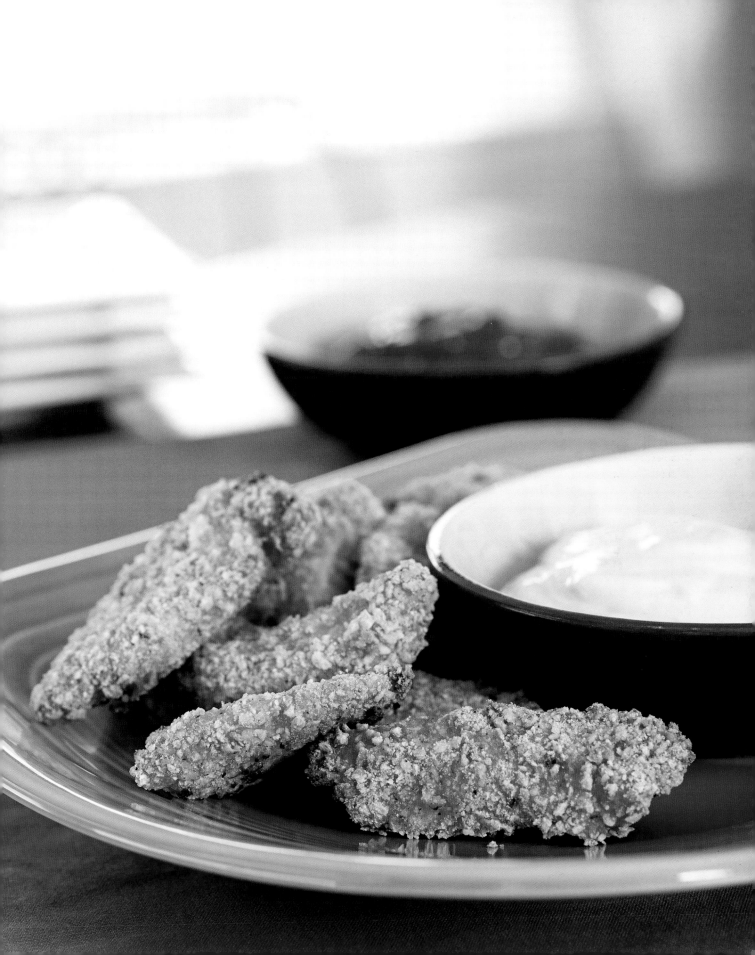

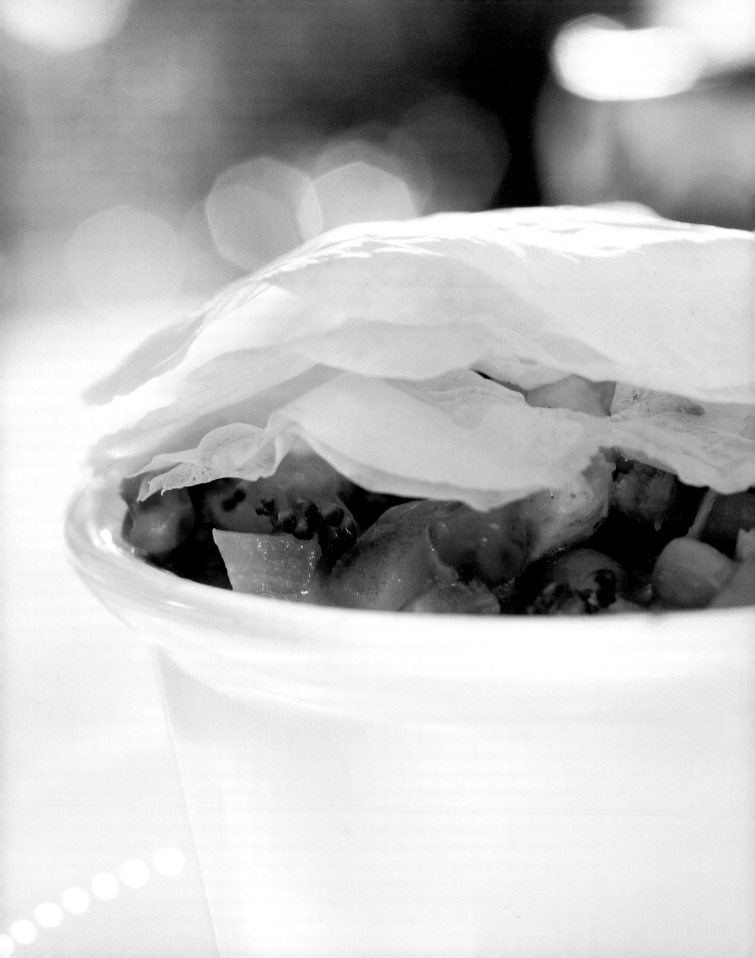

Fresh Phyllo Chicken Pot Pie

Ingredients

Olive oil cooking spray
2½ tablespoons (37 ml) olive oil, divided
3 boneless, skinless chicken breasts, cut
    into bite-size pieces
Salt and fresh-ground black pepper, to taste
1 medium leek, chopped
1 large carrot, peeled and chopped
1 stalk celery, peeled and chopped
2 medium Yukon gold potatoes, unpeeled
    and cut into bite-size chunks
2 cups (142 g) small broccoli florets
2 cloves garlic, minced
½ cup (64 g) flour
2 cups (475 ml) chicken broth
1 cup (235 ml) evaporated skim milk
½ teaspoon salt
¼ teaspoon white pepper
1 short fresh sprig rosemary (about
    3 inches, or 7.5 cm)
2 sprigs fresh thyme
1½ cups (195 g) frozen baby peas, thawed
4 sheets phyllo dough, thawed

From Chef Jeannette

Time-Saver Tip: To save peeling and chopping time, replace the carrot, celery, broccoli, and peas with a frozen medley of similar vegetables. Try pearl onions, carrots, green beans, broccoli, corn, and so on. Choose about 3 cups (390 g) assorted veggies, thaw, and add when you add the chicken.

From Dr. Jonny: I don't want to name names, but Pepperidge Farm Original Flaky Crust Chicken Pot Pie contains 510 calories per serving. Which, if you read the label, is half a small pie. So for any normal person, a single serving of that dish is more than 1,000 calories. And while no particular manufacturer is more guilty of this than the rest, most of them make the prepared pies with a whole lot of trans fats in the crust. Add heavy fatty gravy and a bunch of salt and . . . well, you get the picture. We rescue the beloved chicken pot pie from its nutritional toxic waste pile by using light layers of phyllo dough, which both preserves the pie feeling and lightens up on the calories. Oh, and it completely eliminates the trans fats. Replacing heavy cream with evaporated skim milk goes a long way toward cutting back on calories. We also use all white-meat chicken and a plethora of fresh, nutrient-rich veggies: broccoli with its cancer-fighting indoles; celery with vitamin A, potassium, and vitamin K; and leeks with even more vitamin K plus beta-carotene, calcium, iron, and potassium. Now that's a chicken pot pie you can believe in!

Preheat the oven to 350°F (180°C, or gas mark 4). Spray a 9 x 9-inch (23 x 23-cm) baking dish with olive oil and set aside.

Heat 1 teaspoon of the olive oil over medium-high heat and add the chicken. Sprinkle with salt and pepper to taste. Cook for a couple of minutes or until just lightly browned. Remove the chicken and set aside.

Add 2 teaspoons (10 ml) of the olive oil to the hot pan and add the leek, carrot, and celery and cook for 3 minutes, stirring frequently. Add the potatoes, broccoli, and garlic and cook for a minute or two longer.

In a small bowl, whisk the flour into the chicken broth and pour it over the vegetables. Add the evaporated milk, salt, white pepper, rosemary, and thyme. Bring the mixture to a boil, stirring constantly. Reduce the heat to a low simmer and cook, covered, for 7 to 9 minutes, or until the mixture thickens. Remove the rosemary and thyme sprigs and discard. Add the chicken and peas and stir to combine. Pour the mixture into the prepared baking dish.

Trim the phyllo dough sheets to 9 x 9 inches (23 x 23 cm). Place one sheet of the phyllo over the mixture to fit just inside the baking dish and brush very lightly with the remaining olive oil. Repeat with all four sheets. Place the dish on a foil-lined baking sheet (to catch any drips) and bake for 30 minutes or until filling is bubbling and phyllo is nicely browned.

Yield: 6 servings
Per Serving: 370.9 calories; 8.3 g fat (22% calories from fat); 38.6 g protein; 34.3 g carbohydrate; 3.6 g dietary fiber; 72.5 mg cholesterol; 700.7 mg sodium

Ingredients

1 large turnip, quartered

4 large carrots, peeled and sliced

1 medium parsnip, peeled and sliced into
   ¼-inch (6-mm) rounds

2 stalks celery, sliced

1 leek, ends trimmed and coarsely chopped
   (wash well to remove all grit)

2 cups (60 g) stemmed and coarsely
   chopped kale

4 cloves garlic, minced

1 fresh rosemary stem (4 to 6 inches, or
   10 to 15 cm) (or ½ teaspoon dried)

2 tablespoons (4.8 g) chopped fresh thyme
   (or 1 teaspoon dried)

1 bay leaf

½ teaspoon each salt and fresh-ground
   black pepper

1 broiler chicken (3 to 4 pounds, or 1.4 to
   1.8 kg), neck and giblets removed

8 cups (1.9 L) water or enough to cover
   chicken and vegetables

2 tablespoons (28 ml) tarragon vinegar
   (or sherry or red wine vinegar)

¼ cup (15 g) chopped fresh parsley,
   optional

Better-Than-Mom's Low-Salt Chicken Soup

From Dr. Jonny: In an earlier book, *The Most Effective Natural Cures on Earth*, I devoted a number of words to one of the most well-known "natural cures" in the world: chicken soup. Why? Because it actually works, and there's now scientific research to support that (not that my Jewish grandmothers needed any proof!). Generations upon generations have found chicken soup to be among the most comforting foods in the world, especially when you're sick. Try our version with high-quality free-range chicken. We removed nearly all the excess fat calories simply by chilling the soup first and then skimming off the solids (good thinking, Chef Jeannette!). But that does mean you need to prepare it at least a day before eating. We think it's worth it to lighten the load. Besides, who makes one serving of chicken soup anyway? It freezes beautifully for later, so the little extra time to remove all those unnecessary calories more than pays off. We kept the salt to a bare minimum, skipped the empty-calorie white noodles, and loaded it up with great root veggies like carrots, turnips, leeks, and parsnips. You'll absolutely love this soup! Fun fact: Parsnip is thought of as a winter vegetable because its real flavor doesn't completely reveal itself until the roots have been exposed to freezing or near-freezing temperatures for between two and four weeks in the fall and early winter. The starch in the parsnip changes into sugar, giving it its utterly unique (and very sweet) taste.

Add the turnip, carrots, parsnip, cerlery, leek, and kale to a large slow cooker. Top with the garlic, rosemary, thyme, bay leaf, salt, and pepper. Place the chicken on top and add water to cover. Sprinkle in the vinegar and cook on low for 7 to 8 hours or on high for 4 to 5 hours.

Remove the turnip, rosemary stem, and bay leaf and discard. Taste the soup and adjust the seasonings, if necessary. Remove the chicken, and refrigerate the chicken and the soup separately overnight. When the soup has chilled, carefully remove all the congealed fat from the surface. Debone the chicken and remove all the skin and cartilage.

Discard the bones, skin, and cartilage, and add the chicken meat to the soup. Heat in a large pot for about 15 minutes over medium heat, or until hot. Stir in the parsley and serve.

Yield: about 10 servings

Per Serving: 212.5 calories; 1.5 g fat (9% calories from fat); 34.7 g protein; 12.1 g carbohydrate; 3.2 g dietary fiber; 84 mg cholesterol; 267 mg sodium

Ingredients

1 can (15 ounces, or 425 g) pineapple chunks
   in water or juice (not syrup!), drained
   and liquid reserved
2 tablespoons (28 ml) low-sodium tamari
2 tablespoons (32 g) tomato paste
1 to 2 tablespoons (20 to 40 g) honey, or to
   taste (for more or less sweet)
1 tablespoon (15 ml) apple cider vinegar, or
   to taste (for more or less sour)
¼ teaspoon red pepper flakes
2 teaspoons (10 ml) peanut oil
1¼ pounds (567 g) chicken tenders, halved
6 ounces (170 g) prepared sliced red and
   yellow bell peppers with onions
   (or 1 large red pepper and
   ½ large onion, chopped)
1 cup (75 g) stringless snow peas
¼ cup (4 g) fresh chopped cilantro,
   optional

From Chef Jeannette

To Complete the Meal: Serve it with
sweet, steamed Vidalia onions. Peel and
slice two Vidalias across the center. Place
them into a microwave-safe glass dish
with 2 tablespoons (28 ml) water and
cover. Cook for about 4 minutes, turning
the dish once halfway through, or until
soft. Garnish each half with a thin slice of
butter and a sprinkling of garlic salt.

Not-So-Sweet and Sour Chicken

From Dr. Jonny: Hey, here's something to put on the list of things
you never want to think about too carefully: How does sweet and sour
chicken from the Chinese takeout get that bright red color? (Yep, that
one's right up there with "how do sausages get made?") Nutritionally,
our version of the old favorite is head and shoulders above the nasty
red concoction we're all used to, but without any loss of taste! We've
dumped the artificial additives (including whatever God-awful red dye
they use in the original), the MSG, and most of the sugar. What's more,
we've bumped up the nutrition with lean chicken (hopefully free-range),
vitamin C (from the peppers and pineapples), sulfur for your skin (from
the onions), plus heart-healthy potassium and fiber from the snow peas.
(Full disclosure: This recipe was so quick, easy, and delicious that we
actually borrowed it from our *150 Healthiest 15-Minute Recipes on Earth*
and gave it an encore presentation in this book. If you missed it the
first time, you'll understand why we reprinted it here when you whip
it up.)

In a small bowl, whisk together 3 tablespoons (45 ml) of the reserved
pineapple juice, tamari, tomato paste, honey, cider vinegar, and red pepper
flakes. Set aside.

Heat the oil in a large skillet or Dutch oven over medium-high heat. Add
the chicken and cook for 1 minute on each side. Reduce the heat to medium
and add the peppers, onions, and snow peas, sautéing for 2 minutes. Pour
in the sauce, mix, and cook, stirring frequently, for about 3 minutes, or until
the veggies have started to soften. Stir in the pineapple and cook for 1 to
2 minutes, or until the pineapple is hot and the chicken is cooked through.
Top with the cilantro.

Yield: 4 servings
Per Serving: 508.1 calories; 24.9 g fat (44% calories from fat); 23.8 g
protein; 48 g carbohydrate; 4.7 g dietary fiber; 58.1 mg cholesterol;
1,057 mg sodium

Ingredients

Chicken

2 tablespoons (28 ml) low-sodium tamari (or low-sodium soy sauce)

¾ cup (175 ml) fresh-squeezed orange juice (from about 3 large navel oranges, or use 100 percent juice, not from concentrate)

2 tablespoons (40 g) honey

1¼ pounds (565 g) chicken tenders

2 teaspoons (10 ml) sesame oil

Orange Sauce

1 cup (235 ml) orange juice (from about 4 large navel oranges, or use 100 percent juice, not from concentrate)

1 tablespoon (15 ml) low-sodium tamari

2 tablespoons (28 ml) 100 percent maple syrup

1 tablespoon (15 ml) rice vinegar

1 tablespoon (8 g) finely grated ginger

½ teaspoon dry mustard

2 teaspoons (4 g) orange zest

Broccoli

12 ounces (340 g) broccoli florets

1 tablespoon (8 g) toasted sesame seeds, optional

Light and Tangy Vitamin-C Orange Chicken

From Dr. Jonny: Orange chicken is a Chinese takeout favorite everywhere, but it's unfortunately one of the worst offenders in the fat and sugar department. It's typically breaded (unnecessary processed carbs) and deep-fried in who-knows-what kind of oil. (Speaking of frying oils, recent investigations show that take-out restaurants typically reuse oil for up to a week, creating absolutely horrendous chemical compounds you're better off not asking about!) You wind up with a dish that's slathered in a thick syrup (somewhat disgusting when you really think about it) that might have a hint of orange flavor (probably from a chemical) but very little of the nutrients found in a real orange. If all this makes you disgusted with the idea of orange chicken, don't be! Our version is rich, warm, and sweet, and it has both calcium and vitamin C (one of the most powerful antioxidants on the planet) from the pure orange juice (not canned orange flavor), plus it's sweetened with real maple syrup. (We use grade B because it has more minerals.) And . . . our chicken is grilled. No unnecessary breading, no damaged disgusting reused oil! Best of all, it tastes great—light and tangy.

To make the chicken: In a shallow glass dish, whisk together the tamari, orange juice, and honey. Add the chicken tenders, turning to coat, and marinate, covered, in the refrigerator, for 30 minutes to overnight (longer marinating time creates stronger flavors). Drain the chicken well in a double-mesh sieve.

Heat the oil in a large skillet or Dutch oven over medium-high heat. Place the chicken in the pan and cook for 1 to 3 minutes per side, or until nearly no pink remains. Remove the chicken with tongs and set aside.

To make the orange sauce: Add the orange juice, tamari, syrup, vinegar, ginger, and dry mustard to the pan and whisk to combine well. Simmer for about 10 minutes, or until the mixture thickens into a glaze. Return the chicken to the pan, add the zest, and cook for a couple of minutes, or until hot and cooked through but still juicy.

To make the broccoli: While the sauce is cooking, steam the broccoli in a large steamer pot for about 3 minutes, or until tender-crisp. Fold the broccoli into the chicken mixture and garnish with the sesame seeds.

Yield: 4 servings

Per Serving: 588 calories; 28.9 g fat (44% calories from fat); 27.5 g protein; 57.7 g carbohydrate; 2.5 g dietary fiber; 62.2 mg cholesterol; 1,180.6 mg sodium

From Chef Jeannette

Serving Suggestion: This dish is delicious served over hot brown rice. If you want to save time at dinner, buy a few packages of precooked, frozen brown rice to get a steaming grain on the table in just a couple of minutes.

Time-Saver Tip: Skip the marinating step and just use leftover or prepared grilled chicken strips. Add cooked chicken to the pan for the last 3 minutes of cooking time to heat and serve. You could also use slices of prebaked tofu or vegan "faux" chicken for a no-cholesterol vegetarian dish.

Want to skip the thickening time on the sauce? Mix 1½ tablespoons (12 g) kudzu with 1½ tablespoons (25 ml) orange juice until dissolved and add it to the simmering sauce. Cook for 1 to 2 minutes or until thickened.

Variation: For an additional antioxidant boost, replace the broccoli with two sliced and lightly sautéed red bell peppers.

Ingredients

2 teaspoons (10 ml) olive oil

4 skinless chicken breast halves, bone in

Salt and fresh-ground black pepper, to taste

1 yellow onion, thinly sliced

½ zucchini, julienned (or coarsely grated, to save time)

8 ounces (225 g) sliced cremini mushrooms

2 cloves garlic, minced

⅓ cup (80 ml) dry white wine

2 large, ripe heirloom tomatoes

¼ cup (60 ml) chicken broth or water, optional if more liquid is needed

¾ teaspoon oregano

1 tablespoon (8.6 g) capers

¼ cup (10 g) slivered fresh basil, optional

From Chef Jeannette

Time-Saver Tip: Replace the fresh tomatoes and broth with a can (14.5 ounces, or 410 g) of whole or diced tomatoes, undrained.

Sumptuous White Meat Chicken Cacciatore

From Dr. Jonny: Have you been asking yourself, "Where does the word 'cacciatore' come from, anyway?" No? Well, I didn't really think so, but I'll tell you anyway: It means "hunter" in Italian, and in cuisine, anything called alla cacciatore means a meal that's served "hunter-style," typically with the same basic go-to ingredients you're likely to find in an omelet: tomatoes, onions, bell pepper, and mushrooms. Plus herbs, and—once in a while—wine. But I digress. We improved on the classic version of chicken cacciatore (which uses the whole chicken) by sticking to white meat and slightly reducing the overall oil content. Both "fixes" lower the calorie count, as does removing the skin. Meanwhile, we left the bone in for more succulence and juiciness. What's not to like? Bonus nutritional points for the mushrooms, a frequently underrated food that actually contains quite a bit of nutrition for its vanishingly low-calorie count: potassium, fiber, choline (for the brain), and even a bit of folate. Not to mention plant chemicals such as beta-glucans, which have been found to be helpful adjuncts in the fight against cancer.

Heat the oil over medium-high heat in a large skillet or Dutch oven. Add the chicken and sprinkle lightly with salt and pepper. Cook until lightly browned (about 4 to 5 minutes) and then flip, season the other sides lightly with salt and pepper, and brown (about 3 to 4 minutes). Remove the chicken and set aside.

Add the onion and zucchini and cook for 3 minutes, stirring frequently. Reduce the heat to medium, add the mushrooms, and cook, stirring occasionally, until the mushrooms release their juices and begin to brown, about 8 to 10 minutes. Add the garlic and wine and cook for a few minutes until the wine has reduced by half. Add the tomatoes, and if the mixture is not very juicy, add the broth, oregano, and capers.

Return the chicken to the pan, stir gently, cover, and simmer, turning the chicken pieces occasionally, until the chicken is cooked through and very tender, about 20 to 25 minutes. Add additional broth or water if the mixture becomes too dry. Remove from the heat, stir in the basil, and serve.

Yield: 4 servings

Per Serving: 373.4 calories; 4.3 g fat (11% calories from fat); 35.3 g protein; 50.2 g carbohydrate; 8.3 g dietary fiber; 70.8 mg cholesterol; 208.2 mg sodium

Skinny Stuffed Chicken with Zucchini Pappardelle "Pasta"

From Dr. Jonny: Think "stuffed chicken" and you're likely to conjure up some multithousand-calorie concoction of oozy cream and cheese with a low-quality, fried breading to boot. Not so fast, grasshopper. Our high-quality version is a low-cal, protein-packed main dish with a light, tangy filling and a bit-o-crunch baked topping that's made from crispy whole-wheat panko bread crumbs mixed with ground almonds. Yogurt—rich in beneficial bacteria called probiotics—helps with digestion and immunity, while spinach provides iron, calcium, and two nutrients extremely helpful for eye health: lutein and zeaxanthin. Zucchini cleverly replaces actual pasta for incredibly low-cal, low-carb broad, thin pappardelle "noodles" (with nice hits of vitamins A and C to boot!) that will fill you up without weighing you down.

Ingredients

Chicken

Olive oil cooking spray

4 chicken breast halves (5 ounces, or 140 g each)

½ teaspoon each salt and fresh-ground black pepper

¾ cup (175 g) plain low-fat Greek yogurt, divided

⅓ cup (40 g) crumbled feta cheese

3 cloves garlic, minced (or 2 teaspoons, or 6 g, prepared minced garlic)

1¼ teaspoons oregano, divided

1 cup (130 g) chopped frozen spinach, thawed and squeezed against a double-mesh sieve to remove excess moisture

1 tablespoon (15 ml) fresh-squeezed lemon juice

2 tablespoons (6 g) whole-wheat panko bread crumbs

1 tablespoon (9 g) almond meal, optional (we like Bob's Red Mill)

Zucchini Noodles

4 medium zucchini, ends trimmed

1 tablespoon (15 ml) olive oil

¼ teaspoon each salt and fresh-ground black pepper

To make the chicken: Preheat the oven to 350°F (180°C, or gas mark 4). Spray an 11 x 7-inch (28 x 18-cm) baking dish lightly with olive oil and set aside.

Place the chicken breasts between two sheets of waxed paper and pound with a mallet until they are about ⅛ inch (3 mm) thick. Sprinkle evenly with salt and pepper.

In a small bowl, combine ½ cup (115 g) of the yogurt, feta, garlic, ¾ teaspoon of the oregano, spinach, and lemon juice. Spread one-fourth of the spinach filling down the center of each piece of chicken. Roll the chicken up, tucking in the ends, and pin them together with toothpicks that have been soaked in water. Place them seam-side down in the prepared baking dish. In a small bowl, toss together the remaining ½ teaspoon oregano, panko crumbs, and almond meal. Spread 1 tablespoon (15 g) of the remaining yogurt onto each piece of chicken, and sprinkle the crumb topping evenly over all four pieces. Bake, uncovered, for 20 to 25 minutes, until the chicken is cooked through. Remove the toothpicks before serving.

To make the zucchini noodles: While the chicken is baking, using a mandolin, slice the zucchini lengthwise into long, thin ribbons (for "stronger" noodles, do this on three or four sides and discard the central core of seeds). Heat the oil in a large skillet over medium heat. Lay the zucchini slices gently in the pan and sprinkle lightly with salt and pepper. Cover and cook, turning gently a few times for even cooking (tongs work best for this), for about 9 minutes, or until very tender but not falling apart. Serve one stuffed chicken breast over one-fourth of the zucchini noodles.

Yield: 4 servings

Per Serving: 285.4 calories; 8.3 g fat (28% calories from fat); 36.3 g protein; 16.4 g carbohydrate; 4.1 g dietary fiber; 82.3 mg cholesterol; 805.7 mg sodium

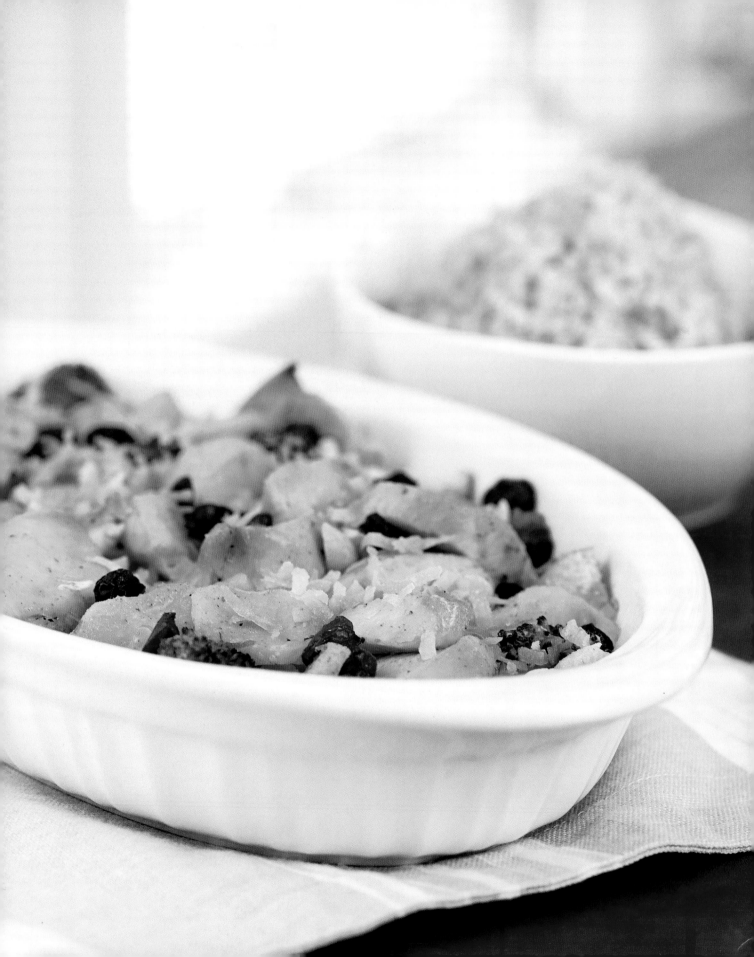

Lean and Light Curried Chicken Casserole

Ingredients

1/2 lemon

3 chicken breasts (about 11/4 pounds, or 565 g)

Salt and fresh-ground black pepper, to taste

4 to 6 cups (946 to 1420 ml) water (see page 34)

1 cup (190 g) dried brown basmati rice

1 can (12 ounces, or 355 ml) evaporated skim milk

1/3 cup (77 g) plain low-fat Greek yogurt

1/2 cup (113 g) all-natural mayonnaise (or vegan mayonnaise for fewer calories)

2 teaspoons (10 g) organic chicken Better Than Bouillon

2 tablespoons (28 ml) fresh-squeezed lemon juice

21/2 tablespoons (16 g) high-quality curry powder, or to taste

4 cups (about 12 ounces, or 340 g) large fresh broccoli florets

1 can (8 ounces, or 225 g) sliced water chestnuts, drained

1/3 cup (48 g) roasted unsalted peanuts

1/4 cup (22 g) flaked or shaved unsweetened dried coconut

1/3 cup (50 g) raisins

From Dr. Jonny: Unlike some of the other dishes in this book, we didn't have to do a lot to make curried casserole into a healthy comfort food. Curry gets its yellow color from a spice called turmeric, which is as close to a superfood as anything in the spice kingdom could possibly be. (I gave it a star in my book *The 150 Healthiest Foods on Earth*, meaning it is a standout among standouts!) Turmeric contains curcuminoids, some of the healthiest compounds in the world, which have demonstrated both anticancer and anti-inflammatory activity. We put together a simple, mild, and creamy casserole that's designed to hit the spot when you're looking for something soothing with just a hint of heat. And it may be simple, but it's far from empty, nutritionally speaking. Its creamy base comes from a mix of high-protein Greek yogurt and evaporated skim milk (for extra calcium), a small amount of natural mayo, and a hint of lemon to enrich and deepen the already spectacular flavors. Fresh broccoli adds color and a ton of plant compounds called indoles, which can help prevent cancer. The water chestnuts add a surprising and delightful crunchy texture. Note: Use the organic version of evaporated milk—because the milk is concentrated, it's all the more important that it be "clean."

Preheat the broiler. Squeeze the lemon all over the chicken breasts, front and back, and sprinkle lightly with salt and pepper. Place on the broiler rack and broil for 5 minutes, then turn and broil for 2 to 3 minutes, or until the chicken is almost cooked through, with a little pink remaining. Remove from the heat, cool briefly, and slice into 2-inch (5-cm) strips.

While the chicken is cooking, bring at least 4 cups (946 ml) of water (more if the water level isn't at least 2 inches [5 cm] high in your pot) to a rolling boil in a large pot.

While the water is heating, rinse and drain the basmati rice well. Add the rice to the boiling water and stir it to prevent sticking or clumping. Let it boil for 30 minutes, uncovered, and drain it through a sieve for 10 seconds. Return the rice to the empty cooking pot, off the heat, and cover it with a tight-fitting lid. Allow it to sit and steam for 10 minutes, uncover, and fluff to serve.

(continued on page 34)

From Chef Jeannette

This method of cooking the brown rice is adapted from an article in issue 11 of *SAVEUR* magazine (www.saveur.com) called "Perfect Brown Rice." Cooking the rice in extra water like pasta and then steaming it in its own moisture turns out tender grains that don't clump together. I still religiously use my beloved rice cooker for ease, but this is a great, reliable stovetop technique that works equally well for all types of brown rice.

This recipe runs on the juicy side, so it's good to use rice to soak up all the flavors. If you'd prefer to go dairy-free, you can also swap out the evaporated milk for a 12-ounce (340 g) block of firm silken tofu. Blend or whisk the tofu until very creamy and follow the rest of the recipe directions. It will separate a bit, but the flavor is great!

Time-Saver Tip: To shorten the prep time, use leftover or prepared cooked chicken breast and prepared chopped broccoli florets, then follow the recipe directions as usual. You can also use prepared frozen brown rice in place of regular—just heat and eat!

While the rice is cooking, preheat the oven to 375°F (190°C, or gas mark 5).

In a large bowl, add the evaporated milk, yogurt, mayonnaise, bouillon, lemon juice, and curry powder and whisk until well combined. Add the cooked chicken pieces, broccoli, and water chestnuts, and toss gently to combine. Spoon the mixture into a 9 x 13-inch (23 x 33-cm) baking pan and bake for 20 to 25 minutes, or until the broccoli is tender-crisp.

Serve over the rice with sprinkles of peanuts, coconut, and raisins.

Yield: about 6 servings
Per Serving: 595.1 calories; 24.4 g fat (37% calories from fat); 41.9 g protein; 55.7 g carbohydrate; 6.6 g dietary fiber; 78.9 mg cholesterol; 494.7 mg sodium

Light and Lemony Garlic Roasted Chicken

Ingredients

2 onions, peeled and roughly chopped

3 carrots, peeled and roughly chopped

3 stalks celery, roughly chopped

1 roasting chicken (3½ to 4 pounds, or 1.6 to 1.8 kg), giblets removed

2 large lemons

4 cloves garlic, minced or mashed

1 teaspoon butter, softened

1 teaspoon olive oil

2 teaspoons (12 g) salt

1 teaspoon fresh-ground black pepper, or to taste

From Dr. Jonny: One of the most disturbing revelations of Dr. David Kessler's excellent book, *The End of Overeating*, was how much sugar is in restaurant food, even the stuff you'd never expect to have sugar in it—like the breaded coatings for fried chicken, or the sauces, glazes, and dressings on almost anything that comes out of the kitchen. These layers of fat, salt, and sugar are artfully and purposefully created to make you crave the food put in front of you—after all, restaurants are in business to sell more (not less) food! This goes for baked chicken as well, which is often covered in more butter, oil, and salt than you really need or want. Ours uses tiny amounts of each and replaces the rest with a tasty garlic paste. Hints of lemon and garlic really pop up the richness in this bird! And remember, you can up the nutritional value of this dish by choosing free-range chicken; look for labels that say "no hormones," or "antibiotic free"—there's nothing "comforting" about drugs in your comfort food!

Preheat the oven to 425°F (220°C, or gas mark 7).

Place the onions, carrots, and celery in a layer in the bottom of a roasting pan.

Rinse the chicken and pat well with paper towels to dry the skin as much as possible. Allow it to rest for about 20 minutes to get rid of some of the chill in the meat before roasting. Roll the lemons hard under the heel of your hand to break up the fibers (or heat for 10 seconds in the microwave). Slice them in half, squeeze them slightly over the skin and into the cavity of the chicken, and then pack all four halves inside.

In a small bowl, mash the garlic, butter, olive oil, and salt together into a paste and smear it evenly all over the chicken. Sprinkle to taste with fresh-ground pepper. Place the chicken on top of the vegetables, breast up (or use a clay pot as directed). Bake the chicken for about 1 hour and 15 minutes, or until cooked through (juice from a pierced thigh should run clear, not pink, and the temperature at the meaty part of the leg should reach about 160°F [71°C] on an instant-read thermometer). Remove from the oven and let rest under a tent of aluminum foil for 10 to 15 minutes to finish cooking. Slice the chicken and serve with the vegetables.

Yield: 6 servings

Per Serving: 355.9 calories; 8.9 g fat (22% calories from fat); 55.8 g protein; 13.1 g carbohydrate; 4 g dietary fiber; 175 mg cholesterol; 1,024.4 mg sodium

Ingredients

1 tablespoon (15 ml) olive oil

¼ cup (40 g) finely chopped sweet onion

2 large cloves garlic, minced (or 1 teaspoon prepared minced garlic)

1 cup (245 g) tomato sauce (or low-sugar organic ketchup—organic to avoid high-fructose corn syrup)

¼ cup (60 ml) apple cider, apple juice, or applesauce

¼ cup (60 ml) cider vinegar

2 tablespoons (26 g) Sucanat, sugar, or xylitol, or to taste

1 teaspoon dry mustard

½ to 1 teaspoon chipotle chile pepper, to taste (start with less and increase for more heat and smoke)

¼ teaspoon salt

8 to 10 chicken drumsticks (about 2 pounds, or 905 g)

From Chef Jeannette

Even Healthier: To reduce the calories and saturated fat in this dish, skin the chicken legs before scoring and grilling them. Grab the skin at the top of the meatiest part of the leg and pull it downward toward the thinner section. It will peel downward easily to the bone at the bottom. Because this is slippery work, it will help to use a knife to pin the skin to a cutting board and then pull the chicken leg away from it to separate.

Smoky, Lower-Sugar Barbecue Drumsticks

From Dr. Jonny: One reason we get addicted to food is added sugar. Barbeque sauce is an excellent case in point. It's absolutely loaded with sugar, making it much easier to eat than you bargained for. Our version is just as flavorful as any you've ever tasted, but with less than half the typical amount of added sugar. Listen, we all love chicken legs—they're classic comfort food, taking us back to those halcyon days of summer picnics and family reunions. (Okay, maybe the wonderful family reunions weren't always so wonderful, but still.) Hint: Feel free to use the dark meat: the benefits of white meat over dark have been overstated. There are only about 30 calories of difference between 4 ounces (115 g) of white and 4 ounces (115 g) of dark meat, plus they have the same amount of protein, so enjoy!

Heat the oil in a cast-iron skillet over medium heat. Add the onion and cook for 3 to 4 minutes, or until just beginning to brown. Add the garlic and cook for 1 minute. Reduce the heat to medium-low and add the tomato sauce, cider, vinegar, Sucanat, dry mustard, chile pepper, and salt, whisking gently to combine well. Keep just at a simmer (reduce the heat to low, if necessary) and cook, stirring occasionally, for about 20 minutes (and up to 40 minutes over low heat—flavor will deepen with longer cooking time). Adjust the seasonings, if necessary, and remove from the heat. Purée until smooth in a blender (use caution: it's hot) or using an immersion blender (place sauce in a deep bowl to prevent splattering).

While the sauce is cooking, preheat the grill to medium (or preheat the broiler). Make two deep diagonal cuts across the meaty part of each drumstick. Place the drumsticks on a lightly oiled grill or broiler pan and cook for 15 to 20 minutes (depending on plumpness), or until cooked through. Remove from the heat, baste with the barbecue sauce to taste, and serve.

Yield: 4 servings

Per Serving: 442.8 calories; 23.3 g fat (47% calories from fat); 44.9 g protein; 10.6 g carbohydrate; 1.2 g dietary fiber; 183.7 mg cholesterol; 657.4 mg sodium

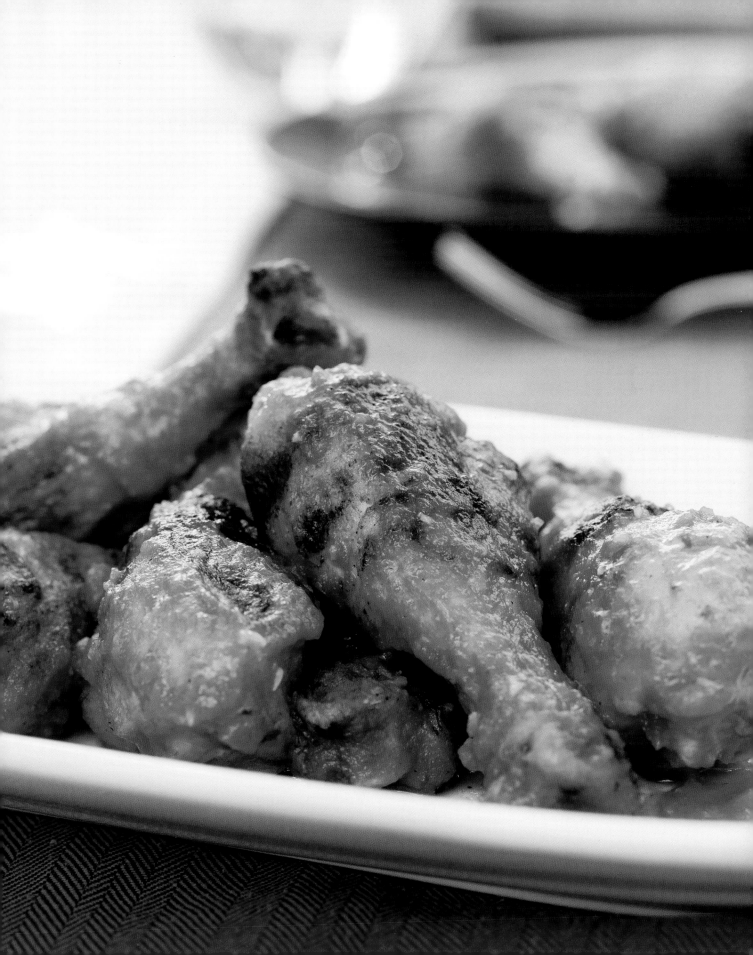

Ingredients

Olive oil cooking spray

1½ tablespoons (25 ml) olive oil

1 small yellow onion, chopped

2 cloves garlic, minced

1 can (14.5 ounces, or 410 g) fire-roasted diced tomatoes, undrained

¼ cup (65 g) tomato paste

¼ cup (60 ml) low-sodium vegetable broth or water

1 tablespoon (7.5 g) chili powder

½ teaspoon cumin

½ teaspoon oregano

½ teaspoon salt

½ teaspoon Sucanat, sugar, or xylitol

1½ cups (338 g) cooked shredded chicken breast

1 cup (256 g) cooked black beans (drained and rinsed, if using canned)

2 cups (60 g) loosely packed baby spinach, optional

Four 8-inch (20-cm) whole-grain wraps or soft corn tortillas (e.g., whole-grain Wrap-Itz by Tamxico's)

1¼ cups (145 g) shredded Monterey Jack or sharp Cheddar cheese, divided

From Chef Jeannette

Time-Saver Tip: If you're in a hurry, use a high-quality prepared enchilada sauce instead of making your own from scratch.

Zippy Chicken Enchiladas: Protein Aplenty

From Dr. Jonny: Enchiladas are classic Mexican-American comfort food. Problem is, they are packed with calories, and—sorry to say—without a lot going for them in the nutrition department. A few tweaks to the recipe and they're no longer a guilty pleasure. Our version uses lean white chicken meat, more beans for extra protein, and a good dose of fiber. We lose the white flour wraps, replace them with more flavorful whole-grain ones, and boost the nutrition even further with spinach (which contains iron, vitamin C, and the superstars of eye nutrition, lutein and zeaxanthin) and onion (a great source of the anti-inflammatory flavonoid quercetin). Use a lighter hand on the cheese and you'll still get all the flavor you love with a serious reduction in calories and a big boost in the nutritional benefits!

Preheat the oven to 350°F (180°C, or gas mark 4). Spray a 7 x 11-inch (18 x 28-cm) Pyrex (or other tempered glass) baking dish lightly with olive oil and set aside.

Heat the oil in a large skillet over medium heat. Add the onion and cook for about 4 minutes, or until it begins to soften. Add the garlic and cook for 1 minute. Add the diced tomatoes, tomato paste, broth, chili powder, cumin, oregano, salt, and Sucanat, and whisk or mix gently until well combined. Increase the heat to bring to a simmer. Cover, reduce the heat, and simmer for about 10 minutes. Purée the mixture to desired consistency using an immersion blender (pour the sauce into a deep bowl first to prevent splattering), or carefully in your blender. Adjust the seasonings if necessary.

In a medium bowl, gently mix the chicken, beans, spinach, and 1 cup (235 ml) of the sauce.

Set up your enchilada station: Pour a little of the remaining sauce into the bottom of the prepared baking dish and spread it evenly to form a thin layer. Lay your wraps and half the cheese out near your oven. Evenly divide the chicken and bean mixture among the middle of the four wraps and top each with a sprinkling of cheese. Fold the far edge of the wrap toward you, up and over the filling. Tuck in the two sides and fold the final edge away from you to close the wrap. Lay the wrap seam-side down on the sauce in the prepared baking pan, nestling the wraps together. Pour the remainder of the sauce evenly over the enchiladas and top with the remaining cheese. Bake for 30 minutes.

Yield: 4 servings

Per Serving: 607.9 calories; 21.2 g fat (31% calories from fat); 47.6 g protein; 56.9 g carbohydrate; 15.4 g dietary fiber; 104.1 mg cholesterol; 869.5 mg sodium

Tasty Turkey Tetrazzini with Whole-Wheat Egg Noodles

Ingredients

Olive oil cooking spray

8 ounces (225 g) whole-wheat egg noodles

2 teaspoons (9 g) butter

2 teaspoons (10 ml) olive oil

1 small yellow or white onion, chopped

8 ounces (225 g) sliced fresh mushrooms (wild mushrooms work well, if available)

2 cloves garlic, minced

2 tablespoons (28 ml) dry white wine

¼ teaspoon tarragon

2 cups (475 ml) low-sodium chicken broth

3 tablespoons (27 g) powdered arrowroot (or cornstarch)

1 can (12 ounces, or 355 ml) evaporated skim milk

½ teaspoon each salt and fresh-ground black pepper

½ teaspoon paprika (smoked or sweet)

3 cups (420 g) diced or shredded cooked turkey breast (or chicken)

2 tablespoons (14 g) toasted wheat germ

3 tablespoons (15 g) shredded Parmesan cheese

From Chef Jeannette

In a pinch you can use two cans (each 4 ounces, or 115 g) of high-quality sliced mushrooms, drained, in place of the fresh.

From Dr. Jonny: How do you preserve the creamy, satisfying texture of turkey tetrazzini and lose the least-healthy parts of this traditional recipe, like the canned cream of mushroom soup (way too high in sodium) and the nutritionally empty white noodles? Easy. First, we used our old standby, evaporated skim milk, which not only keeps things creamy but also lowers the calories substantially. Next, we replaced those dumb white noodles with whole-wheat egg noodles—they're thick, chewy, and satisfying and they have more fiber to boot. (Which, come to think about it, is exactly why they're more chewy and satisfying. Duh!) Turkey remains a great source of reasonably low-calorie protein—3 ounces (85 g) of meat gives you nearly 20 grams of protein plus a nice smattering of important minerals such as potassium and the cancer-fighting selenium.

Preheat the oven to 350°F (180°C, or gas mark 4). Spray a medium casserole dish lightly with olive oil and set aside.

Cook the noodles until al dente according to package directions.

In a large skillet, heat the butter and oil over medium heat. Add the onion and cook for 3 minutes. Add the mushrooms and cook until their juices have evaporated. Add the garlic and cook for 30 seconds. Add the wine and tarragon and cook until the wine is nearly evaporated.

Pour the broth into a medium bowl and whisk in the arrowroot until dissolved. Pour the broth mixture over the onion and mushrooms and bring to a boil. Simmer for about 2 minutes, or until thickened. Reduce the heat to low, stir in the milk, salt, pepper, and paprika, and cook for about 3 minutes.

In a large bowl, combine the hot mixture, turkey, and noodles and mix gently until well combined. Pour the mixture into the prepared baking dish and cover with aluminum foil.

Bake for 20 minutes. Remove the foil and top with the wheat germ and Parmesan. Bake for 5 to 10 minutes more, until hot throughout.

Yield: about 6 servings

Per Serving: 268.9 calories; 5.1 g fat (16% calories from fat); 28.3 g protein; 27.5 g carbohydrate; 2.6 g dietary fiber; 51.4 mg cholesterol; 383.5 mg sodium

Savory Slow Cooker Tender Turkey Drumsticks

Ingredients

3 turkey drumsticks

1 tablespoon (15 ml) olive oil

Salt and fresh-ground black pepper, to taste

1 large Vidalia onion, chopped

3 large carrots, peeled and sliced into thin coins

2 large cloves garlic, minced

½ teaspoon crumbled dried sage

2 tablespoons (8 g) chopped fresh parsley

1 tablespoon (2.4 g) chopped fresh thyme (or 1 teaspoon dried)

1 lemon, halved

From Dr. Jonny: Turkey is a great, healthy source of protein (more than 20 grams per 3-ounce serving), and turkey drumsticks are always a favorite. And you don't have to wait till the holidays to enjoy them. This recipe is supereasy and superfast, and when you use the slow cooker it cooks to a delicious tenderness in its own juices, with no added fat calories. Yum. Seriously. Perfectly healthy fat replaces the conventional gravy or commercial cream of mushroom soup that generally smothers a dish like this. (Note: A can of commercial cream of mushroom soup has an astonishing 1,995 mg of sodium. Need I say more?) Onions are a rich source of sulfur, so good for the skin, not to mention that they are one of the richest sources of a flavonoid called quercetin, which is one of the most anti-inflammatory plant compounds on the planet. (Quercetin has also been shown to have significant anticancer properties.) Something to remember: Turkeys are frequently raised under horrific factory-farmed conditions, so if possible, get the free-range variety. They're almost always better for you anyway.

Coat the bottom of the slow cooker and the drumsticks with olive oil. Sprinkle the drumsticks liberally with salt and pepper. Place the onion and carrots in the bottom of the cooker and top with the prepared drumsticks.

In a small bowl, mix the garlic, sage, parsley, and thyme together and sprinkle evenly over the drumsticks. Gently squeeze the lemon halves to release their juices into the vegetables and nestle them in the bottom of the pot.

Cook on low for 8 to 10 hours, or high for 4 to 5 hours, or until the meat is cooked through and the veggies are very tender.

Yield: 4 servings

Per Serving: 292.8 calories; 15.6 g fat (49% calories from fat); 27 g protein; 12.4 g carbohydrate; 3.7 g dietary fiber; 97.2 mg cholesterol; 141.5 mg sodium

Smoky Lower-Fat Bacon Turkey Burgers

Ingredients

4 strips turkey bacon, nitrate-free

1¼ pounds (567 g) leanest ground turkey

⅓ cup (27 g) whole rolled oats

1 teaspoon dry mustard

1 teaspoon cumin

½ teaspoon each salt and fresh-ground black pepper

¼ teaspoon cayenne pepper, optional

2 teaspoons (10 g) low-sugar ketchup

2 teaspoons (10 ml) Worcestershire sauce (organic to avoid high-fructose corn syrup)

1 teaspoon 100 percent maple syrup

1 teaspoon apple cider vinegar

¼ cup (25 g) minced scallion, optional

4 whole-grain sandwich thins

2 to 4 teaspoons (10 to 20 g) country Dijon mustard, low-sugar ketchup, or low-sugar barbecue sauce, to taste

4 red lettuce leaves

8 thin slices ripe avocado

4 thick slices tomato

From Dr. Jonny: A bacon cheeseburger is as American as apple pie, but unfortunately not exactly a nutritional bonanza, mostly because of the quality of the meat (poor to horrible) and the amount of fat and calories. Our turkey burger version is naturally lower in fat, and you can reduce the calories even more by using delicious, leaner ground turkey. With the turkey bacon you save a couple of grams of fat and calories, but do try to find one without nitrates. (While nitrates per se are not necessarily dangerous, they can metabolize into some nasty compounds that can be dangerous. If you can't get nitrate-free meat, at least take some vitamin C along with it, as vitamin C tends to neutralize the damaging effects of the nitrate metabolites.) Avocado, a superstar in the food kingdom, plus slices of fat, juicy tomatoes and red onions complete the dish. Delicious and satisfying and way better for you than the usual restaurant fare. Fun fact: Many people don't know this, but avocado (which is technically a fruit, not a vegetable) is actually a very high-fiber food. One California avocado contains 9 grams of fiber, and one Florida avocado contains an almost unbelievable 17 grams, slightly more than a full cup of the highest-fiber beans on Earth.

Cook the bacon to crispy in a dry skillet over medium heat according to package directions, break in half, and set aside on paper towels.

Preheat the grill to medium heat.

In a large bowl, gently mix together the turkey, oats, dry mustard, cumin, salt, peppers, ketchup, Worcestershire, syrup, vinegar, and scallion until just combined. Do not overhandle or the burgers will be tough.

Form 4 loose patties and gently indent the centers of each one for more even cooking. Grill for about 4 to 6 minutes, flip, and grill for another 4 to 6 minutes, or until cooked to desired doneness.

Toast the sandwich thins for the last 30 seconds of cooking time and coat with your condiment of choice. Serve each burger stacked with 2 bacon strip halves, 1 lettuce leaf, 2 slices of avocado, and 1 slice of tomato.

Yield: 4 burgers

Per Serving: 536.8 calories; 27 g fat (44% calories from fat); 34.9 g protein; 81.9 g carbohydrate; 7.7 g dietary fiber; 124.4 mg cholesterol; 979.8 mg sodium

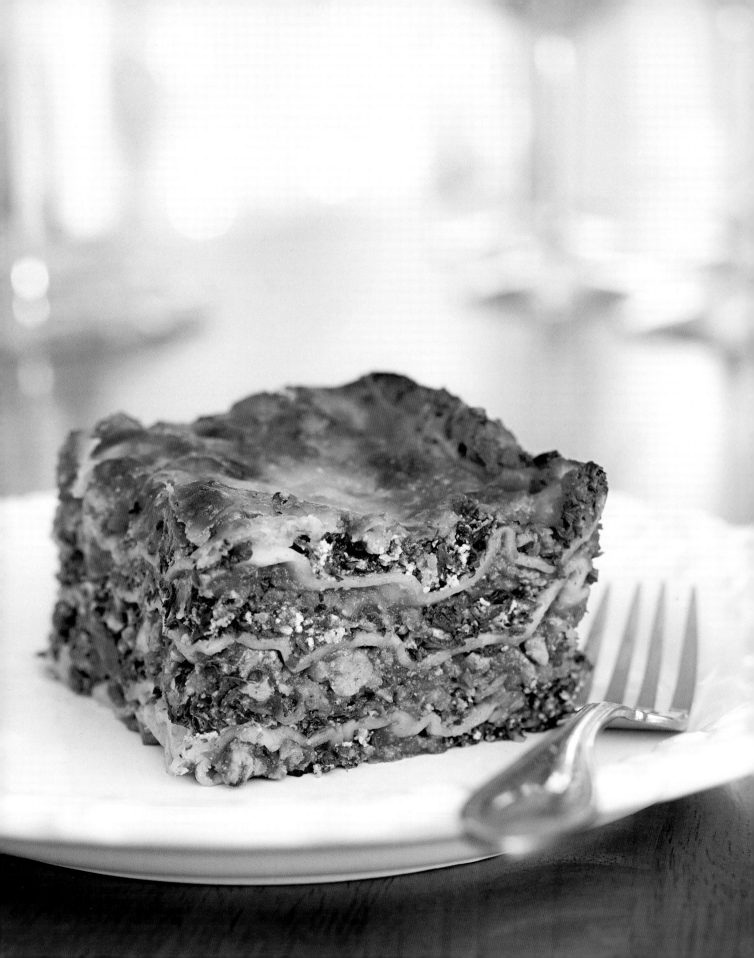

Hearty Spinach and Mushroom Lasagna with Lower-Fat Meat Sauce

Ingredients

2 teaspoons (10 ml) olive oil

1 yellow onion, diced fine

8 ounces (225 g) prepared sliced cremini mushrooms

6 cloves garlic, minced (or 1 tablespoon, or 10 g, prepared minced garlic)

1 pound (455 g) leanest ground turkey

1/2 teaspoon each salt and fresh-ground black pepper

1 pound (455 g) part-skim ricotta cheese

1 egg

3/4 cup (60 g) shredded Parmesan cheese (or Asiago), divided

15 ounces (425 g) frozen chopped spinach, thawed and well drained (squeezed or pressed against a double-mesh sieve to remove as much liquid as possible)

1 can (6 ounces, or 170 g) tomato paste

2/3 cup (155 ml) hot water

1 can (28 ounces, or 795 g) crushed tomatoes

1 tablespoon (1.3 g) dried parsley

1 teaspoon Sucanat, sugar, or xylitol

1 teaspoon salt

1 teaspoon granulated garlic

1 teaspoon basil

1 teaspoon oregano

1/2 teaspoon red pepper flakes, optional

8 ounces (225 g) no-cook lasagna noodles

2 cups (230 g) shredded part-skim mozzarella cheese

From Dr. Jonny: You can make lasagna a heck of a lot better by simply using lean turkey, part-skim ricotta, and a light hand with the mozzarella. What could be simpler? Restaurant lasagna is swimming in grease and is mostly cheese and full-fat hamburger or sausage, and we're not talking the highest quality meat to begin with. These easy fixes make a tasty—and far better for you—version of the old comfort food fave. Punch up the flavors with some calcium-rich (and lower-calorie) Parmesan and as many herbs and spices as you like. And punch up the nutrients with fresh onion, mushrooms, and spinach. The onion's loaded with sulfur for the skin and anti-inflammatory agents for everything else, the almost-zero-calorie mushrooms have a surprising amount of potassium, and spinach—well, they don't call it the super-star of leafy greens for nothing: high calcium, fiber, potassium, folate, vitamin A, and a whopping 888 mcg of bone-building heart-healthy vitamin K in every cup!

Preheat the oven to 350°F (180°C, or gas mark 4).

In a large skillet or Dutch oven, heat the oil over medium-high. Add the onion and cook for 3 minutes or until it starts to soften. Add the mushrooms and cook for 3 minutes. Add the garlic and cook for 30 seconds. Add the turkey and break it up. Sprinkle the salt and pepper over all and cook, turning frequently, for 5 to 7 minutes or until the turkey is cooked through (no pink remaining) and the vegetables have softened. Remove the pan from heat, drain any excess fat, and set aside.

While the turkey is cooking, combine the ricotta, egg, 1/2 cup (40 g) of the Parmesan, and the spinach in a mixer and beat on low until well combined. Set aside.

In a large bowl, combine the tomato paste and water and whisk until smooth. Add the crushed tomatoes, parsley, Sucanat, salt, garlic, basil, oregano, and red pepper flakes, if using, and whisk until well combined. Add the turkey-mushroom mixture to the sauce and stir well to combine. Spread a thin layer of sauce on the bottom of a 9 x 13-inch (23 x 33-cm)

(continued on page 44)

From Chef Jeannette

This lasagna can also be assembled up to 2 days ahead of time and stored in the refrigerator until you are ready to bake. Add 15 minutes of cooking time before removing the foil. You can also freeze it uncooked for up to 2 months: Seal it with microwave-safe plastic wrap, cover with foil, and snap on a rubber lid (if using Pyrex or a similar storage dish). When you are ready to prepare it, thaw in the refrigerator for 36 hours, remove the plastic, replace the foil, and bake as directed for chilled lasagna. It doesn't actually take a lot more time to double this recipe, so I always make two lasagnas and freeze one for later or to share with a friend.

Even Healthier: To boost the fiber in this dish, cook up whole-wheat noodles to use in place of the no-cook white ones: Follow package directions for al dente noodles minus 1 minute of cooking time. Drain and use like the no-cook noodles, but no need to leave spaces in between.

For more nutrients and antioxidants, sauté extra seasonal vegetables in a bit of olive oil with sprinkles of salt and fresh-ground pepper to add to the sauce with the turkey and mushrooms. I like diced colored bell peppers, thin-sliced zucchini or yellow squash, shredded carrots, and chopped broccolini (baby broccoli).

pan. Place one row of lasagna noodles in the pan, leaving a little space between for expansion. Cover with one-third of the ricotta mixture, one-third of the sauce, and one-third of the mozzarella. Repeat the layers, ending with mozzarella on the top. Sprinkle the remaining ¼ cup (20 g) Parmesan cheese evenly over the top of the lasagna. Cover tightly with aluminum foil and bake for 1 hour, or until noodles are tender and sauce is bubbly. Remove the foil and bake for another 10 minutes or until cheese is melted.

Let sit for 15 minutes before slicing.

Yield: 10 servings
Per Serving: 429.3 calories; 15.2 g fat (31% calories from fat); 29.7 g protein; 47.5 g carbohydrate; 6.1 g dietary fiber; 91.2 mg cholesterol; 867 mg sodium

Lean and Tasty Sloppy Jonny

From Dr. Jonny: One of my most vivid memories of sleep-away camp—besides being subjected to the camp version of fraternity hazing—was the big, juicy sloppy Joe we used to get served every Tuesday night. Delicious? Sure. Comforting? Of course. Nutritious? Not so much. Enter this scrumptious version, which is made with ultra-lean ground turkey and a sauce so flavorful you won't believe it's actually good for you. Chef Jeannette offers a variety of serving options, all of them good, none of them featuring the disgusting soggy white buns that traditionally accompany this dish. Serve with whole-grain sandwich thins or hollowed-out veggies. And the addition of beans ups the fiber content, making this high-protein dish even more of a nutritional bargain. Note: Cooked tomato sauce is a terrific source of the cancer-fighting antioxidant lycopene!

Ingredients

2 teaspoons (10 ml) olive oil

1 sweet onion, diced

1 red bell pepper, seeded and diced

2 cloves garlic, minced

1 pound (455 g) lean ground turkey
(or leanest ground beef)

1/2 teaspoon each salt and fresh-ground
black pepper

1 can (14 ounces, or 400 g) tomato sauce

2 tablespoons (30 g) Dijon mustard

2 tablespoons (28 ml) Worcestershire sauce
(choose organic to avoid high-fructose
corn syrup)

1 tablespoon (15 ml) 100 percent maple
syrup

1 tablespoon (7.5 g) chili powder

1 can (15 ounces, or 425 g) black or kidney
beans, drained and rinsed

Heat the oil in a large skillet over medium-high heat. Add the onion and bell pepper and sauté for 3 to 4 minutes. Add the garlic and sauté for 1 minute. Add the turkey, salt, and pepper, stirring to break up the meat and combine it with the veggies. Cook for 5 to 6 minutes or until all of the pink is gone.

While the turkey is cooking, in a small bowl whisk together the tomato sauce, mustard, Worcestershire, syrup, and chili powder. Drain any excess oil from the cooked turkey and reduce the heat to medium-low. Gently stir in the beans and tomato sauce mixture, and cook for 5 to 7 minutes, until hot throughout.

Yield: 4 servings

Per Serving: 401.2 calories; 13.2 g fat (29% calories from fat); 32 g protein; 40.7 g carbohydrate; 12.8 g dietary fiber; 89.9 mg cholesterol; 1,285.4 mg sodium

From Chef Jeannette

Serving Suggestions: This Joe mix is hearty enough to stand on its own, naked and bunless, as a main dish. I personally love sloppy Joe mix served over a huge bed of fresh, crisp lettuce with a chopped tomato garnish for a nice, light meal. If you'd like to contain the "sloppiness," serve on whole-grain sandwich thins instead of refined, bulky, high-carb hamburger buns. Or better yet, serve it scooped into fresh veggies for a low-cal micronutrient blast. Try seeded cucumber halves, hollowed-out tomatoes, or, my favorite: Remove the tops of 4 red, yellow, or orange bell peppers, scoop out the seeds, cook for about 7 minutes in boiling water until tender, drain well, and stuff to the brims with Joe mix.

Time-Saver Tip: For a superquick, low-cal, vegetarian alternative, substitute a frozen package (12 ounces, or 340 g) of vegan "beef" crumbles for the ground meat and skip the meat sauté step, reducing the heat to medium-low and adding the sauce and beans right away.

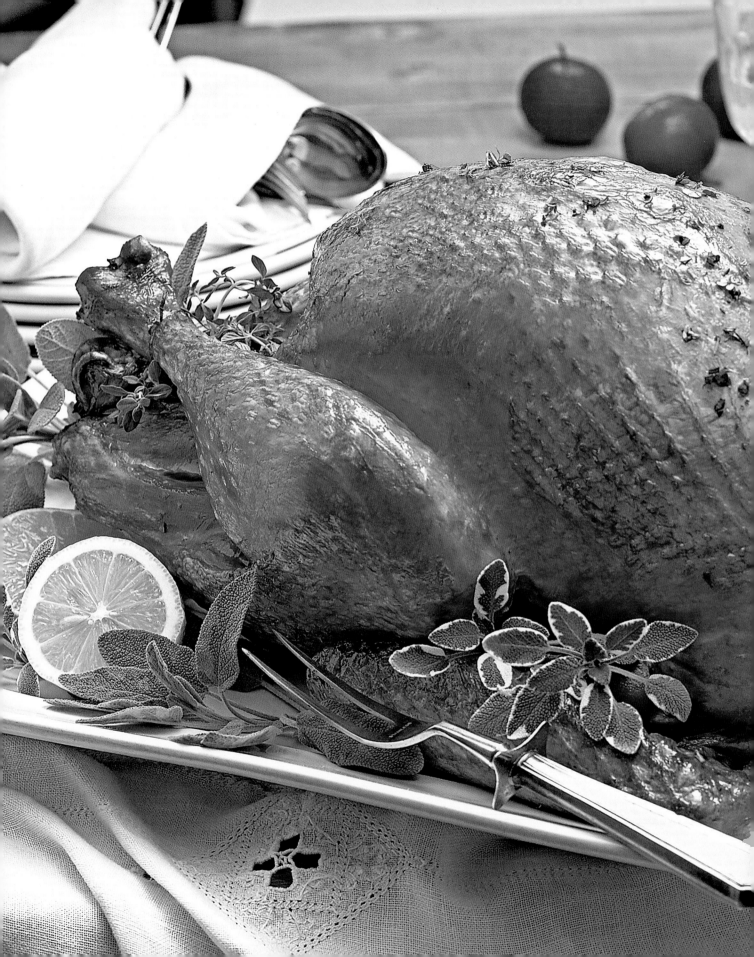

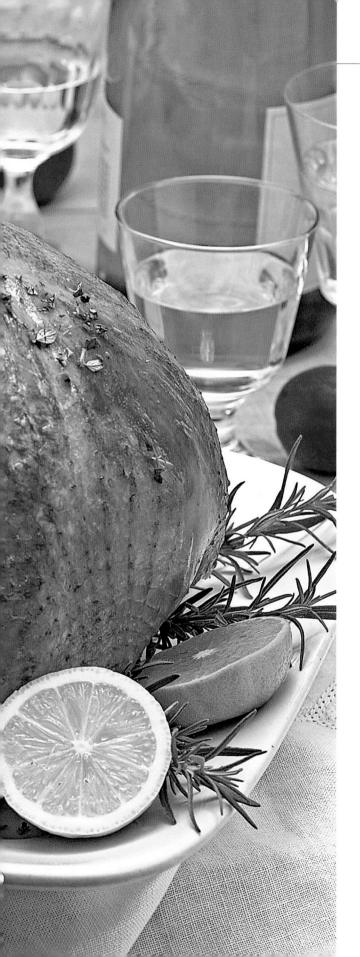

HEALTHY HOLIDAYS DINNER: Free-Range Citrus-Stuffed Herbed Turkey, Higher-Fiber Apple-Corn Bread Stuffing, and Autumnal Antioxidants: Cranberry-Orange Relish

From Dr. Jonny: The holidays don't have to be a time when you stop eating healthy foods; you can still enjoy many of the fabulous comforting offerings the season provides in abundance. Here's a tremendous and traditional holiday meal for you that won't leave you feeling one bit deprived. The turkey and cranberry-orange sauce are borrowed from *The Healthiest Meals on Earth*—one of our most popular recipes—but the dressing is all new. It's a remake of a comfort food staple, which—although classic—is usually a high-glycemic, low-nutrient affair that can wreak havoc with your waistline. Our version is way better and just as tasty.

Ingredients

Brining Solution

3 gallons (12 L) water

3 cups (900 g) salt

1½ cups (510 g) raw honey

2 tablespoons (12 g) finely grated lemon peel, optional

2 tablespoons (12 g) grated orange peel, optional

1½ tablespoons (7.5 g) cardamom pods, optional

1 tablespoon (4.3 g) dried thyme, optional

Turkey

1 turkey (18 to 20 pounds, or 8.2 to 9.1 kg), free-range, not self-basting

8 sprigs each of fresh rosemary (young and tender, not woody), sage, and thyme (or other herbs of your choice), rinsed and lightly dried (should total about 1¼ to 1½ cups, or 55 to 90 g, when coarsely chopped)

2 shallots

1 whole head garlic

1 lemon

1 orange

4 tablespoons (½ stick, or 55 g) butter, softened

2 tablespoons (28 ml) olive oil

Salt and fresh-ground black pepper, to taste

½ cup (120 ml) sherry

Free-Range Citrus-Stuffed Herbed Turkey

From Dr. Jonny: We made the turkey "sans gravy" and stuffed it with a flavor-rich combo of herbs and citrus for a juicy and aromatic bird. (Free-range turkey only, please! You don't need the added hormones and steroids!) Traditionally, this type of a whole-bird preparation calls for at least one stick of butter, but we reduced it and mixed it with olive oil, giving you a nice mix of heart-healthy fat and valuable olive phenols. (To get all the "good stuff," use extra-virgin olive oil.) Fun fact: Contrary to popular belief, most of the fat in butter is actually monounsaturated fat, the same healthy fat found in olive oil!

To make the brining solution: Combine all the ingredients, stirring until the salt and honey are dissolved.

To make the turkey: Rinse the turkey and pat it dry. Place the turkey in a lobster pot or large stockpot. Pour in the brining solution to cover the turkey completely. Place the turkey in the refrigerator for 12 to 24 hours. Remove the turkey from the brine, rinse very well under running water, and dry thoroughly, including the cavity. If you want crisper skin, brine and rinse the turkey the day before and place it, breast-side up and uncovered in the basting pan, in the refrigerator overnight to allow excess moisture to evaporate.

Preheat the oven to 400°F (200°C, or gas mark 6).

Stem and coarsely chop the herbs, setting aside about three-quarters of them (about ⅔ to 1 cup, or 40 to 60 g). Mince the remaining one-fourth (about ½ cup, or 30 g) of the herb mixture and put into a medium bowl.

Peel the shallots and garlic. Cut the shallots in half, crush the garlic cloves, and add to the herbs. Quarter but do not peel the lemon and orange and squeeze them gently to make a little juice, tossing the fruit and juice together with the herb mixture.

Using your hands, mix the softened butter with olive oil in a small bowl until creamy.

Moving carefully so as not to puncture the skin, work your hand between the turkey skin and the breast as far as you can go to create a pocket over both breasts. Smear half of the butter/olive oil mixture over the breasts, covering as much meat as you can.

From Chef Jeannette

If you are working with a large turkey (that will take a longer cooking time) or desire a milder herb flavoring, use the whole herb stems (without chopping) under the skin. Just remove the large pieces when the cooking is complete and use as a garnish.

If you don't own a V rack, try using two miniature loaf pans (4 x 3 inches or 5 x 3 inches, or 10 x 7.5 cm or 13 x 7.5 cm), facedown and set on either side of your roasting pan (in the middle, lengthwise). If using the loaf pans, there is no need for foil.

Place half of the reserved coarsely chopped herbs in each pocket (on top of each breast). Do this carefully, and when complete, gently reshape (from the outside) the herb "pouches" above each breast to look rounded and smooth. Season both cavities with salt and pepper and stuff them with the fruit-herb mixture. Tuck the wings behind the back, tuck the skin folds over the cavities to close, and truss the legs. Smear the entire bird with the remaining butter/olive oil mixture, then season with salt and pepper. Slowly pour the sherry inside the breast pockets, working it around to the leg joints.

Place a V rack inside a roasting pan and cover with aluminum foil. Poke about 15 holes into the foil. Place the turkey on the V rack, breast-side down. Bake for 45 minutes, then reduce the oven temperature to 325°F (170°C, or gas mark 3). Turn the turkey breast-side up, baste (you can supplement juices with a few tablespoons of sherry if you wish), cover with foil, and continue to cook for 2½ to 3 hours more, depending on the size of the turkey.

Remove the foil to brown the breast and continue to cook for another 30 to 40 minutes, or until the thickest part of the breast and innermost parts of the thighs and wings register at least 165°F (74°C) on a meat thermometer. When the turkey is done, the legs should roll loosely on the joint and the leg juices should run clear.

Let the turkey rest on a cutting board for about 20 minutes before carving it.

Yield: 36 servings
Per Serving: 330.9 calories; 13.1 g fat (35% calories from fat); 40.5 g protein; 10.4 g carbohydrate; 1 g dietary fiber; 166.6 mg cholesterol; 2,539 mg sodium

Ingredients

1 tablespoon (15 ml) olive oil

2 links (4 ounces, or 115 g each) organic chicken-apple sausage

1 green apple, unpeeled, cored, and finely diced

1 large Vidalia onion, finely chopped

2 stalks celery, finely sliced

1/2 teaspoon salt

One 8 x 8-inch (20 x 20-cm) pan prepared high-fiber corn bread, cut or broken into bite-size chunks

1/2 cup (55 g) toasted sliced or slivered almonds or toasted pine nuts

1/4 cup (12 g) finely chopped chives, optional

1 1/2 tablespoons (2.6 g) minced fresh rosemary (or 1 teaspoon dried and crumbled)

1 cup (235 ml) low-sodium chicken broth

1/3 cup (80 ml) apple cider

2 tablespoons (14 g) toasted wheat germ (or ground flaxseed), optional, for more fiber

From Chef Jeannette

For the corn bread: Alternatively, use our recipe for Zingy Whole-Grain Broccoli Corn Bread (page 113) in this book, but omit the jalapeños. To save time, use a high-quality (whole-grain, low-to-no-sugar) prepared corn bread mix, such as Hodgson Mill Cornbread and Muffin Mix, instead of preparing it from scratch. It's fine to make the corn bread a day or two ahead of time.

Higher-Fiber Apple-Corn Bread Stuffing

From Dr. Jonny: Holiday stuffing not only "stuffs" the turkey, it also stuffs your belly. And let's face it, that doesn't really feel that good now, does it? The usual ingredients are the usual suspects—dried white bread (ugh) and, if you use a prepared mix, very high sodium and very high-glycemic impact (meaning it does stuff to your blood sugar that you don't want!). Simple fixes make this a far healthier choice. High-fiber corn bread replaces the white stuff, and the added treats like onion, tart green apples, almonds or pine nuts, and wheat germ add a host of nutrients rarely found in conventional stuffing: sulfur for the skin, fiber and phytochemicals from the apples, monounsaturated fat and minerals from the nuts, and vitamin E from the wheat germ. No butter used here, just a scant tablespoon of extra-virgin olive oil. The flavor quotient goes through the roof with just two links of low-cal chicken-apple sausage, fresh chives, and that old favorite, rosemary. Chef Jeannette asked me to pass on to you the fact that it's safer to bake the dressing separately instead of baking it inside the turkey. Fun fact: In ancient China, rosemary was used for headaches and topically for baldness.

Preheat the oven to 325°F (170°C, or gas mark 3).

Heat the oil in a large Dutch oven over medium heat. Remove the sausage links from their casings and crumble into small pieces into the pan. Cook until lightly browned, stirring frequently, about 6 minutes. Add the apple, onion, celery, and salt, stirring to combine, and continue to cook for 8 to 10 minutes, or until the fruit and veggies are tender, stirring occasionally. Remove the Dutch oven from the heat and gently stir in the corn bread, nuts, chives, and rosemary until well combined.

In a small bowl, whisk the broth and cider together and pour gently over the dressing mix a little at a time, folding gently in between, until desired moistness is reached. Do not soak the corn bread—the mixture shouldn't be soggy. Sprinkle with the wheat germ, cover the Dutch oven lightly with aluminum foil, and bake until hot throughout, 20 to 25 minutes.

Yield: about 10 servings

Per Serving: 275.6 calories; 12.3 g fat (39% calories from fat); 9.8 g protein; 32.6 g carbohydrate; 1.8 g dietary fiber; 44.2 mg cholesterol; 687.9 mg sodium

Ingredients

4 cups (440 g) fresh cranberries, or 2 bags (each 8 ounces, or 225 g) frozen, unsweetened cranberries, thawed and rinsed

2 oranges, peeled and halved

1/2 cup (170 g) raw honey, or to taste

From Chef Jeannette

Substitution Tip: If you can't find fresh cranberries, substitute 4 cups (440 g) dried whole cranberries, but use 4 small oranges and omit the honey. Dried cranberries are almost always heavily sweetened, so this version doesn't have the crisp tartness of the fresh, but it is still better for you than the stuff in a can! Look for juice-sweetened only, not the sugar-sweetened varieties.

Autumnal Antioxidants: Cranberry-Orange Relish

From Dr. Jonny: This tangy orange-cranberry relish is made with fresh cranberries, not canned, and less than half the sugar of conventional canned relish. You may not realize it, but cranberries are one of the healthiest foods on Earth. They have one of the highest antioxidant ratings and are loaded with plant compounds known as flavonoids, which may reduce the risk of atherosclerosis. Emerging research also indicates that they may help protect brain cells. In any case, they taste great, and this fabulous relish is a perfect complement to the heady, herb-infused turkey!

In a blender or food processor, blend together the cranberries, oranges, and honey until a juicy relish is formed.

Yield: 12 to 14 servings

Per Serving: 63.7 calories; 0.1 g fat (1% calories from fat); 0.4 g protein; 16.9 g carbohydrate; 2.1 g dietary fiber; 0 mg cholesterol; 1.1 mg sodium

Ingredients

1 pound (455 g) baby carrots

1 pound (455 g) small new potatoes, unpeeled, halved (or 2½ cups, or 565 g,
prepared peeled and chopped butternut
squash chunks for less starch)

2 large yellow onions, quartered

1½ pounds (680 g) cubed beef stew meat
(about 2-inch, or 5-cm, pieces)

1 can (14 ounces, or 400 g) diced tomatoes,
undrained

⅓ cup beef broth (or ⅓ cup, or 80 ml,
water plus 1 teaspoon organic beef
Better Than Bouillon)

¾ cup (175 ml) burgundy wine (or dark
beer)

4 cloves garlic, crushed and chopped

1 teaspoon oregano

1 teaspoon marjoram

1 teaspoon thyme

½ teaspoon each salt and fresh-ground
black pepper, or to taste

1 bay leaf

⅓ cup (20 g) sundried tomato strips
(dried or in oil, well drained), optional

¼ cup (15 g) chopped flat-leaf parsley,
optional

From Chef Jeannette

For additional green-veggie minerals such
as iron, calcium, and magnesium, add
2 cups (110 g) of chopped fresh kale at the
start of the cooking time, or a 10-ounce
(285-g) box of frozen chopped spinach,
peas, or green beans for the last 10
minutes of cooking time.

Iron-Man Slow Cooker Beef Stew

From Dr. Jonny: Few foods offer hearty comfort as well as a hot,
tasty, well-made beef stew does. Here's a way to make it healthy as
well: Choose lean, grass-fed beef. Most restaurant beef stew is made
with fatty, low-quality factory-farmed beef, complete with a nice (un-
wanted) helping of antibiotics, steroids, and hormones. Not so with
grass-fed. You'll get everything you need from beef—iron, B$_{12}$, and the
highest quality protein—without any of the "ingredients" you don't
want. And speaking of iron, we need it—badly. (Especially growing
kids!) There are actually two kinds of iron in our diet—heme iron and
nonheme iron. The heme kind is far more absorbable but is only found
in animal products. Chef Jeannette actually chose vegetables for this
stew with an eye to increasing the absorbability of the iron—vitamin
C–rich tomatoes, for example, plus sundried tomatoes, and the potatoes with skin! This stew is as easy as pie to prepare—you assemble
the ingredients in a flash in the morning and return home to a rich,
warm, fragrant dish that is sure to satisfy on any chilly night!

In a large slow cooker (at least 3.5 quarts or 3.3 L), scatter the carrots,
potatoes, and onions. Lay the beef cubes on top.

In a medium bowl, combine the tomatoes, broth, wine, garlic, oregano,
marjoram, thyme, salt, and pepper and mix gently to combine. Pour evenly
over the meat and vegetables and add the bay leaf. Cook on high for about
4 hours, or on low for 6 to 7 hours, or until the vegetables are tender and
the meat is cooked through but not overdone. Add the sundried tomatoes
during the last 10 minutes of cooking time (during the last 5 if using oil-
packed tomatoes), and stir in the parsley just before serving.

Yield: about 6 servings
Per Serving: 397.6 calories; 8.6 g fat (19% calories from fat); 43.7 g
protein; 30.8 g carbohydrate; 5.6 g dietary fiber; 96.4 mg cholesterol;
370.5 mg sodium

In-a-Pinch Spaghetti Bolognese

From Dr. Jonny: Classic Italian Bolognese sauce is full of different rich and fatty meats, such as sausage and ground pork. It takes several hours of cook time and, though divine, we think it's possible to mimic the effect of that rich, comforting meaty sauce with far fewer calories (and a lot less time). Our version uses the leanest, grass-fed ground beef and adds mushrooms for additional heartiness and nutrients that include polysaccharides, plant compounds with both anti-tumor and immunostimulating properties. We threw in the trifecta of mirepoix veggies (carrots, onion, and celery) to give it a more complex flavor base. (For those who might be interested, *mirepoix* is the French name for this traditional trio of veggies which, taken together, provide nice amounts of beta-carotene, vitamin A, vitamin K, anti-inflammatory agents such as quercetin, and a host of other minerals, vitamins, and phytochemicals.) And we use whole-grain pasta, as always, to boost the fiber content. *Mangia!*

Ingredients

1½ tablespoons (25 ml) olive oil
1 small yellow onion, chopped
1 stalk celery, finely chopped
1 medium carrot, finely chopped
8 ounces (225 g) sliced fresh mushrooms
1 pound (455 g) leanest ground beef
Salt and fresh-ground black pepper, to taste
⅓ cup (80 ml) dry red wine
1 can (28 ounces, or 795 g) crushed
    tomatoes
3 tablespoons (48 g) tomato paste
½ teaspoon oregano
½ teaspoon basil
½ teaspoon garlic powder
Pinch of Sucanat or sugar
12 ounces (340 g) whole-grain spaghetti
    (we like Barilla Plus)
Fresh-grated Parmesan cheese,
    optional, to taste

Heat the oil in a large skillet over medium heat. Add the onion, celery, and carrot and cook for 5 minutes. Add the mushrooms and cook for 2 minutes. Add the beef, stirring to break it up, and cook for about 10 minutes, or until no pink remains. Drain off any excess oils.

Lightly season the beef with salt and pepper, then add the wine and cook for 1 minute. Add the tomatoes, tomato paste, oregano, basil, garlic powder, and Sucanat and stir to mix well. Reduce the heat to low, cover, and simmer for 35 to 45 minutes, stirring occasionally. Adjust the seasonings, if necessary.

At the end of the sauce cooking time, cook the spaghetti according to package directions.

Serve the spaghetti topped with the sauce, to taste, and a few sprinkles of Parmesan.

Yield: 4 servings
Per Serving: 621.3 calories; 12.8 g fat (18% calories from fat); 42.9 g protein; 88.1 g carbohydrate; 6.2 g dietary fiber; 70.3 mg cholesterol; 465.3 mg sodium.

Ingredients

Juice of 3 limes, divided

½ yellow onion, minced

1 serrano chile, seeded and chopped

3 large cloves garlic, minced

1 large bunch cilantro, chopped, divided

½ teaspoon chili powder

½ teaspoon cumin

Pinch of Sucanat or sugar

¼ cup (60 ml) olive oil

1¼ pounds (567 g) flank steak

¼ cup (60 g) plain low-fat Greek yogurt, optional, for garnish

¼ teaspoon salt, optional

Salt and fresh-ground black pepper, to taste

8 fresh 6-inch (15-cm) corn tortillas (organic, sprouted corn for the highest quality, such as Food for Life)

Drizzle of olive oil

4 cups (280 g) shredded lettuce

2 heirloom tomatoes, thickly sliced

1 Hass avocado, sliced, optional

1 cup (260 g) prepared salsa (or use fresh; see our recipe for All-Natural Spicy Salsa Guacamole [page 229] for a salsa-guacamole combo)

Lean and Mean Marinated Flank Steak Tostadas

From Dr. Jonny: I'm new to Mexican food, in part because I'm a relative newcomer to Southern California, where Mexican food is available on every corner. Also, the Mexican food I sampled when I lived back East tended to be filled with artificial ingredients, made with white flour, and generally not all that appetizing. Here's what we did to make our version: First, we upgraded the tacos to tostados, an immediate improvement on the dry, tasteless taco shells that are boxed for months at a time and loaded with preservatives. Second, we made them with high-quality soft tortillas containing all-natural ingredients without a hint of chemicals. Use the finest quality grass-fed beef for its array of omega-3 fats and for its complete absence of hormones, steroids, and antibiotics. Skip the cheese altogether, and swap the sour cream for high-protein, low-calorie Greek yogurt. Marinate and grill lean flank steak for a high-flavor, low-fat centerpiece. Now that's a healthy dish!

Set aside 2 teaspoons (10 ml) of the lime juice.

In a large glass baking dish, mix together the remaining lime juice, onion, serrano, garlic, about ¾ cup (12 g) of the cilantro, chili powder, cumin, Sucanat, and olive oil until well combined. Lay the steak(s) in the dish and turn to coat. Cover and marinate for 1 to 3 hours in the refrigerator, turning occasionally. Just before grilling the meat, prep your veggies and salsa, if making fresh. In a small bowl, whisk together the yogurt, reserved lime juice, salt, and remaining cilantro (up to ⅓ cup, or 5 g), and set aside.

Preheat the oven to broil.

To cook the marinated meat, heat the grill to medium, wipe off any excess vegetables from the marinade, sprinkle the meat lightly with salt and pepper to taste, and grill to medium-rare (or desired doneness), flipping once halfway through the cooking time, about 4 minutes per side for 1-inch (2.5 cm) thickness (thick pieces will take longer than thinner cuts). Thinly slice the cooked meat across the grain.

While the meat is cooking, using a basting brush, lightly paint the tortillas with a drizzle of olive oil, arrange on a broiling sheet, and broil in batches for 1 to 2 minutes until lightly toasted.

To make the tostadas, lay them out, cover with equal amounts of shredded lettuce, tomato slices, avocado slices, and steak slices, and top with salsa, to taste, and a dollop of the yogurt garnish.

Yield: 4 servings

Per Serving: 617.9 calories; 34 g fat (48% calories from fat); 38 g protein; 45.6 g carbohydrate; 10.4 g dietary fiber; 59 mg cholesterol; 661.3 mg sodium

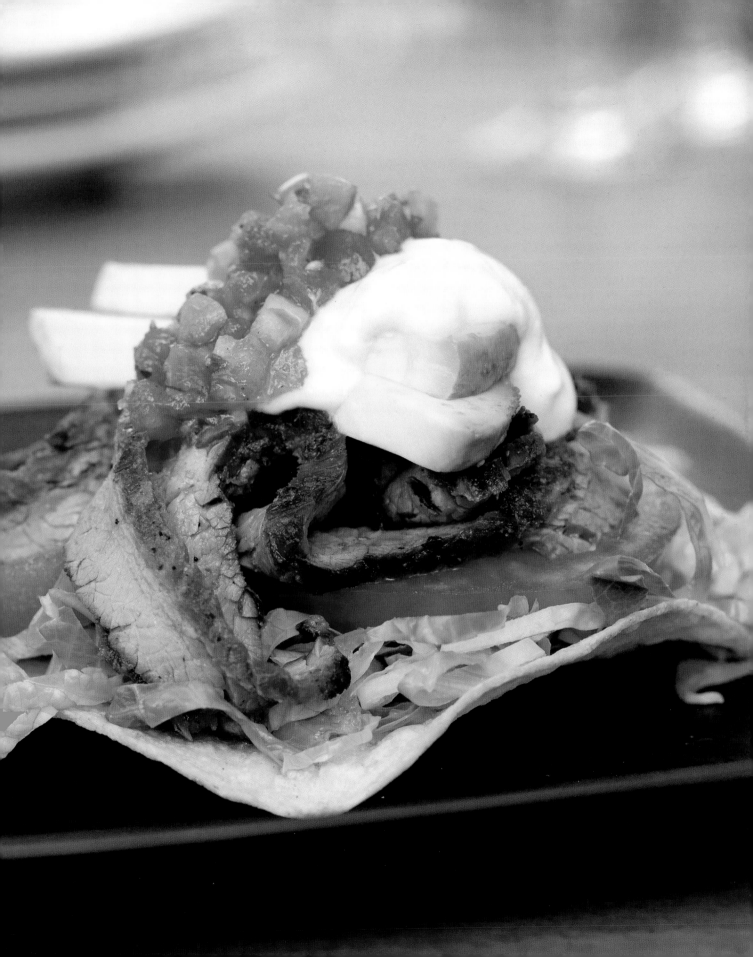

Grass-Fed Italian Feta Meatballs in Tomato Sauce

Ingredients

1 egg

⅓ cup (50 g) feta cheese

1 pound (455 g) grass-fed leanest ground beef

¼ cup (30 g) whole-wheat bread crumbs

¼ cup (40 g) minced onion

1 tablespoon (6.5 g) ground flaxseed

½ teaspoon salt

¼ teaspoon fresh-ground black pepper

1½ teaspoons (1.5 g) oregano, divided

1 teaspoon basil, divided

2 teaspoons (10 ml) olive oil

3 cloves garlic, minced

1 can (14.5 ounces, or 410 g) crushed tomatoes

Pinch of Sucanat or sugar

¼ teaspoon red pepper flakes

1 tablespoon (15 ml) red wine vinegar

From Dr. Jonny: Meatballs can be the "Spam" of the beef world—you never know what's in them. Sadly, for most generic examples it's anything from ground pork to full-fat ground beef to mystery sausage, and I can guarantee you none of it is high quality. Our meatballs are made with grass-fed beef for all the usual reasons: higher concentration of heart- and brain-healthy omega-3 fatty acids; no antibiotics, steroids, or growth hormones; natural leanness; and a full, rich flavor that's hard to beat. Grass-fed beef is a hard act to improve on, but to make the classic meatball we rolled it up with whole-wheat bread crumbs and used nature's most perfect food—the egg—plus ground flaxseed for fiber, omegas, and cancer-fighting lignans. And wait, there's more! A little feta cheese for tartness and richness and a virtual medley of Italian seasonings really make these meatballs worthy of a four-star restaurant.

Preheat the oven to 400°F (200°C, or gas mark 6).

In a large bowl, whisk or beat the egg together with the feta until it is mostly smooth. Add the beef, bread crumbs, onion, flaxseed, salt, pepper, 1 teaspoon of the oregano, and ½ teaspoon of the basil and mix with your hands until well combined. (Don't overdo it as overmixing the meat will make your meatballs tough.) Form into about 25 small (about 1-inch, or 2.5-cm) meatballs.

In a Dutch oven, heat the oil over medium heat and cook the meatballs, rolling them around to brown all sides, until almost cooked through, 7 to 10 minutes. Drain any excess oil (if using lean grass-fed, you should have no excess). Add the garlic and cook for 1 minute. Add the tomatoes, remaining ½ teaspoon each of oregano and basil, 2 pinches of sugar, red pepper flakes, and red wine vinegar, stirring gently to combine. Reduce the heat and cook for 10 to 15 minutes more, covered, or until the meatballs are cooked through.

Yield: 4 to 6 servings

Per Serving: 196.1 calories; 8.8 g fat (40% calories from fat); 20.2 g protein; 8.5 g carbohydrate; 1.7 g dietary fiber; 89.7 mg cholesterol; 389.8 mg sodium

Lighter-but-Luscious Portobello Beef Stroganoff

Ingredients

8 ounces (225 g) whole-wheat egg noodles

2 tablespoons (28 g) butter, divided

1 pound (455 g) top sirloin, thinly sliced into 2-inch (5-cm) strips

Salt and fresh-ground black pepper, to taste

1 tablespoon (15 ml) olive oil

4 shallots, chopped

6 ounces (170 g) sliced portobello mushroom caps

2 tablespoons (4.8 g) chopped fresh thyme (or 1 teaspoon dried)

2 large cloves garlic, minced

¼ cup (60 ml) red wine

1 cup (230 g) plain low-fat Greek yogurt

¾ teaspoon paprika (smoked or sweet)

½ teaspoon each salt and fresh-ground black pepper

1 cup (130 g) frozen peas, thawed

From Dr. Jonny: Last time I sampled beef Stroganoff at a restaurant I thought to myself, Man, this stuff tastes great! Unfortunately, that thought was followed by, But what about this junky meat and the high-calorie sour cream? Luckily, you can still have your beef Stroganoff. Use better meat, dump the sour cream, and voilà, you've got a healthier version of an old favorite. By using grass-fed meat you immediately lose the hormones, antibiotics, and steroids that make factory-farmed meat such a nutritional nightmare, yet you keep all the good things about beef that you never hear about—its high-quality protein, vitamin B$_{12}$, absorbable iron, and a cancer-fighting fat called CLA that is just about absent in "regular" beef. We also dumped the nutritionally empty white noodles for whole-wheat egg noodles, which, for my money, taste better anyway. We also reduced the total amount of butter by about two-thirds and replaced some of it with heart-healthy olive oil, simply to get a nicer mix of different kinds of fats and to goose up the nutritional value with some of those really healthy phenols (plant compounds) found in virgin olive oil. And by substituting high-protein Greek yogurt for the sour cream, the texture stays the same. Rich and delicious, this wonderful Stroganoff really hits the spot!

Prepare the egg noodles according to package directions. While the noodles cook, heat 1 tablespoon (14 g) of the butter in a large skillet over medium-high heat. Add the beef in a single layer (might take 2 batches), sprinkle lightly with salt and pepper, and cook, turning to brown both sides, to desired doneness. Remove the cooked slices with tongs and set aside. Reduce the heat to medium, remove the pan from the heat, and wait 1 or 2 minutes for the temperature to decrease. Return the pan to the heat, add the olive oil, shallots, mushrooms, and thyme, and cook until the mushrooms begin to soften, about 5 minutes. Add the garlic and wine and cook, stirring frequently, until most of the liquid has cooked off. When the wine is almost gone and the mushrooms are tender, remove the pan from the heat and stir in the yogurt, paprika, salt, and pepper, and mix well. Stir in the beef and peas. Heat over a new burner set to low for 2 minutes or until just heated through. Use caution, as high temperatures will cause the yogurt to separate. Adjust the seasonings and serve over the egg noodles.

Yield: 4 or 5 servings

Per Serving: 618.5 calories; 22.6 g fat (33% calories from fat); 32.5 g protein; 75 g carbohydrate; 3.9 g dietary fiber; 75.8 mg cholesterol; 416.7 mg sodium

Ingredients

1 ripe Hass avocado, peeled, pitted, and
    coarsely chopped

2 tablespoons (30 g) plain low-fat Greek
    yogurt

¼ cup (4 g) chopped fresh cilantro

1 tablespoon (15 ml) fresh-squeezed lime
    juice

1 small clove garlic, minced

¾ teaspoon salt, divided

⅓ cup (33 g) diced scallion

¾ cup sweet heirloom cherry tomatoes
    (Sungold or Yellow Teardrop, if you can
    find them), chopped

1 pound (455 g) grass-fed ground beef (or
    organic, 96 percent lean)

¼ to ½ teaspoon chipotle chile pepper (or
    cayenne or fresh-ground black)

4 whole-grain sandwich thins

8 crisp green lettuce leaves, optional

Good-for-You Guacamole Grass-Fed Burger

From Dr. Jonny: So here's the thing: Meat isn't bad for you. What? Yep. What's bad for you—and it's really, really bad—is the stuff that's in factory-farmed meat: steroids, antibiotics, hormones, pesticides, and a terrible balance of omega-6 to omega-3 fats. You can avoid all this by eating grass-fed meat, which comes from happy cows raised on their natural diet of pasture and is distinctly absent of any of the above-mentioned chemicals, which are in all likelihood responsible for all the bad things you've heard about meat. Grass-fed meat is also a good source of both omega-3 fats and a fat you haven't heard much about—conjugated linolenic acid, or CLA, which has known anticancer activity and also helps combat obesity. And the flavor of grass-fed is superb: juicy and succulent. Ditch the monster-size burgers to save on calories; 1 pound (455 g) is easily enough for four single-serving patties. We've skipped the cheese and replaced it with a yogurt-based guacamole of Greek yogurt (high in protein), avocado, and garlic. We've deliberately kept the spices on the simple side to highlight the rich flavor of the beef. Amazing that when the food is really good to begin with you don't need much to improve it!

Preheat the grill (or broiler) to medium and scrub clean.

In a medium bowl, mix together the avocado, yogurt, cilantro, lime juice, garlic, and ¼ teaspoon of the salt, mashing up the avocado with a fork until well incorporated. Fold in the scallions and chopped tomatoes and set aside.

In another medium bowl, gently mix together the beef, remaining ½ teaspoon salt, and pepper, and form 4 loosely packed burgers. To keep burgers juicy, do not overhandle meat or pack patties too tightly. Gently indent the centers of each patty to encourage even cooking.

Grill (or broil) patties for 7 to 9 minutes for medium burgers, or to desired doneness, turning once midway through the cooking time.

Place the sandwich thins facedown on the grill for the last 45 seconds of cooking time to warm and lightly toast. To serve the burgers, stack 2 lettuce leaves and 1 cooked patty on the bottom half of each sandwich thin. Spread with one-fourth of the yogurt guacamole and top with the upper half of each sandwich thin. Serve immediately.

Yield: 4 burgers

Per Serving: 389.1 calories; 15.1 g fat (34% calories from fat); 31.5 g protein; 32.9 g carbohydrate; 6 g dietary fiber; 71 mg cholesterol; 829.7 mg sodium

Ingredients

1 pound (455 g) leanest ground beef

2 tablespoons (32 g) tomato paste

2 tablespoons (32 g) dill pickle relish

1½ tablespoons (23 g) Dijon mustard

1 tablespoon (7 g) onion powder

½ teaspoon garlic granules

½ teaspoon salt

¼ teaspoon lemon pepper

Free-Range Ketchup-Mustard-Relish Sliders

From Dr. Jonny: When I was a teenager coming home from a night of carousing, the sight of a little white distinctly shaped castle was like an oasis in the desert . . . the neon lights blinking "White Castle" meant we had hit the mother lode for late-night food. We'd go in and order a dozen burgers apiece and go through them in less time than it takes for Michael Phelps to do a 100-meter butterfly on a bad day. (Note to trivia buffs: That's about 51 seconds.) I loved the grease-soaked mini-buns those burgers came on, and the pickle, ketchup, and mustard more than made up for the fact that the meat was essentially tasteless. Who even noticed? So when Chef Jeannette decided to come up with a healthy version of my beloved White Castle burgers I was fascinated. After all, isn't the whole point that they're real junk food in the truest sense of the word? Actually, no. Sliders—the generic name for what I grew up knowing as White Castle hamburgers—are usually very fatty mystery meat, heavy on the bun (which is almost always the cheapest and worst kind of white bread). Upgrade with free-range ground beef for its high content of omega-3 fats and its total absence of hormones and steroids. The tomato paste gives the burgers a pinkish tint and a rich flavor (and gives you the health benefits of lycopene, a powerful antioxidant). With the condiments built right in, these "sliders" are really handy at a barbecue. If you want to use buns, at least go for the multigrain sandwich thins over the big white useless hamburger buns. Even better, and especially easy with these mini-burgers, serve them on top of a huge fresh salad with tons of juicy tomatoes. These "sliders" will have your taste buds singing "Kumbaya," and you won't need to feel a bit of guilt for enjoying them!

Preheat the grill to medium-high.

In a large bowl, combine all the ingredients and mix thoroughly, but gently. Do not overhandle beef or your burgers will be tough. Form into 6 mini-patties and using your thumb, gently indent each patty in the middle to ensure more even cooking. Grill for 3 to 4 minutes, flip, and cook for an additional 2 to 3 minutes, or to desired doneness.

Yield: about 4 servings

Per Serving: 184.1 calories; 6 g fat (29% calories from fat); 25.2 g protein; 6.2 g carbohydrate; 0.6 g dietary fiber; 70.5 mg cholesterol; 589.5 mg sodium

From Chef Jeannette

Do not overhandle the meat mixture or your meatloaf will get tough.

Time-Saver Tips: Use prediced onion, preshredded carrots, and prepared minced garlic to save chopping time. You can also grate zucchini and carrots in seconds using the grater attachment on your food processor. Or skip making the sauce and use a prepared high-quality, low-sugar ketchup in its place.

Rich, Muscle-Building Meatloaf

From Dr. Jonny: If there's one thing you need to build muscles it's protein. Pure and simple. The protein in food breaks down to smaller units called amino acids, which in turn are used to build just about everything in your body from hormones to neurotransmitters to bones to . . . you guessed it . . . muscles. No protein in your diet and you're looking like the "before" ads in the back of those muscle-building mags. And why am I telling you this? Because meatloaf is all about protein—pure, unadulterated protein from one of the best sources on the planet—beef. Now my mother, bless her heart, was not the world's greatest cook. Or even the second greatest. (Maybe not even in the top million.) But one thing she did make was meatloaf, which I loved, largely because it was "kid food," stuffed with those nutrient-empty bread crumbs out of a cardboard box, and smothered in low-quality gravy, which by kid standards was just fine. It still had protein, mind you, but you can do better. Chef Jeannette's version has the same rich flavor and complex texture you crave, but with fewer calories and much better ingredients. As always, you're way better off using grass-fed ground beef. Why? Because it has the best fat in the world (omega-3s), contains no hormones, steroids, or antibiotics, and is naturally leaner to boot. (We love the beef from U.S. Wellness Meats, available through a link on my website, www.jonnybowden.com, under "healthy food.") Unlike my mother's meatloaf, this version has added onion, green pepper, and carrots, which ups the nutrition benefit with beta-carotene, vitamin C, and all those fabulous plant chemicals known as flavonoids, which act as antioxidants and anti-inflammatory agents.

Ingredients

Sauce

1 cup (240 g) high-quality, low-sugar
    ketchup
3 tablespoons (45 ml) apple cider vinegar
2 teaspoons (10 ml) Worcestershire sauce
    (choose organic to avoid high-fructose
    corn syrup)
3 tablespoons (60 g) honey
2 cloves garlic, minced (or 1 teaspoon
    granulated garlic)
1/2 teaspoon chili powder

Meatloaf

11/2 tablespoons (25 ml) olive oil
1 yellow onion, finely diced
1 small green bell pepper, seeded and
    finely diced
1 cup (110 g) finely grated carrots
3 large cloves garlic, minced
11/2 pounds (680 g) leanest ground beef
    (or lean ground turkey or half and half)
2 eggs, lightly beaten
2/3 cup (55 g) whole rolled oats
2 tablespoons (14 g) ground flaxseed
1 teaspoon salt
1/2 teaspoon fresh-ground black pepper
2 tablespoons (30 g) prepared horseradish
1 teaspoon dry mustard

To make the sauce: In a small mixing bowl, whisk together the ketchup, vinegar, Worcestershire, honey, garlic, and chili powder until well mixed. Set aside.

To make the meatloaf: Preheat the oven to 350°F (180°C, or gas mark 4).

Heat the oil in a large sauté pan over medium heat. Add the onion, pepper, carrots, and garlic, and cook, stirring occasionally, until the vegetables have softened, 8 to 10 minutes. Remove from the heat.

In a large mixing bowl, add the ground beef, eggs, oats, flaxseed, salt, pepper, horseradish, and mustard, and mix together gently. Fold in the sautéed vegetables and mix until just combined. Spoon the mixture gently into a standard loaf pan and poke about 10 deep holes into the top of the meatloaf using the handle of a wooden spoon. Pour the sauce over the meatloaf, into the holes to allow it to flow into the loaf. Place the loaf pan into a shallow, foil-lined roasting pan (to catch any drips) and bake for about 1 hour, or until completely cooked in the center (it should read 165°F, or 74°C, on an instant-read thermometer).

Yield: about 9 slices

Per Serving: 232 calories; 8.6 g fat (32% calories from fat); 19.4 g protein; 54.4 g carbohydrate; 2.1 g dietary fiber; 93.9 mg cholesterol; 632.6 mg

From Chef Jeannette

Time-Saver Tip: To skip the steaming step for the cabbage, simply freeze the whole cored head, thaw it in the refrigerator, and use the uncooked leaves. The freezing breaks down the tough fibers and makes the leaves tender and pliable. (This trick works with other tough greens such as kale, as well. If you freeze and thaw kale, you can sauté it in just a couple of minutes for a quick, tender plate of nutrient-rich greens.)

Sinless and Savory Slow Cooker Cabbage Rolls

From Dr. Jonny: I'll admit that when I think of comfort food, cabbage rolls aren't the first things that pop into my mind. Or even the second. But they're probably on the top-ten list for people with an Eastern European background (like my paternal grandma, Blanche, for example, who loved them). And they're kind of healthy to begin with (more on that in a moment). But you can make them even better by upgrading to grass-fed beef (giving you more omega-3s and some cancer-fighting fat known as CLA—conjugated linolenic acid—both of which are absent from factory-farmed meat). Replace the white rice with brown for more fiber and B vitamins and you're good to go. Fun fact: Researchers discovered the anticancer compounds in cabbage (known as indoles) while puzzling over the fact that Polish women had such low rates of breast cancer compared to their genetically similar relatives in the United States. They eventually realized that the Eastern Europeans consumed large amounts of cabbage on a regular basis. An analysis of the phytochemicals in cabbage revealed the presence of indoles, which affect hormone metabolism in a positive way, lowering the risk for cancer.

Ingredients

1 small head green cabbage

1 pound (455 g) leanest ground beef

2 cups (330 g) cooked brown basmati rice

½ cup (80 g) minced onion (the food processor will do this quickly)

¼ cup (60 ml) milk (low-fat cow's or plain, unsweetened soy or almond)

1 egg, beaten

4 cloves garlic, minced

1 stalk celery, finely diced

1 teaspoon salt

¾ teaspoon fresh-ground black pepper, or more, to taste

Few dashes hot pepper sauce, to taste

2 cans (each 14.5 ounces, or 410 g) diced tomatoes, undrained

1 can (6 ounces, or 170 g) tomato paste

1 teaspoon Sucanat or sugar

2 tablespoons (28 ml) red wine vinegar

1 tablespoon (15 ml) Worcestershire sauce (organic, to avoid high-fructose corn syrup)

¾ teaspoon garlic powder

¾ teaspoon onion powder

½ teaspoon oregano

¼ teaspoon each salt and fresh-ground black pepper

Core and steam the whole cabbage head in a large steamer pot of boiling water for about 4 minutes, or until the leaves are just tender and pliable. Remove the cabbage, reserving a few cups of the cooking liquid, and separate the leaves, cutting away and discarding any hard ribs. Set aside.

In a large bowl, gently and thoroughly mix together the beef, rice, onion, milk, egg, garlic, celery, salt, pepper, and hot sauce, until well combined.

Line the bottom of a large slow cooker with the small or torn cooked leaves from the cabbage. Using the larger leaves, place a generous ¼ cup (50 g), more for the large leaves, of mixture into each cabbage leaf, folding the bottom up over the mixture, then folding the sides over and rolling from the bottom up. Place the rolls, seam-side down, on top of the cabbage layer in the cooker, nestling them close together, and stacking them when necessary.

Mix the diced tomatoes with the tomato paste, Sucanat, vinegar, Worcestershire, garlic powder, onion powder, oregano, salt, and pepper until well combined, and pour over the top, adding enough reserved cabbage stock to just cover the rolls. Cook on low for 8 to 9 hours, or until the rolls are tender and the beef is cooked through.

Yield: about 6 servings

Per Serving: 250.1 calories; 5.8 g fat (21% calories from fat); 22.1 g protein; 28.4 g carbohydrate; 4.8 g dietary fiber; 83.1 mg cholesterol; 794.3 mg sodium

Ingredients

1 large onion, coarsely chopped

4 medium carrots, peeled and sliced into
    $1/4$-inch (6-mm) rounds (or use a 1-pound,
    or 455-g, bag of mini-baby carrots to
    save time)

2 stalks celery, sliced

$3/4$ pound (340 g) baby new potatoes, halved
    or quartered if large, unpeeled

1 can (14.5 ounces, or 410 g) diced tomatoes
    in sauce, undrained

2 tablespoons (32 g) tomato paste

3 tablespoons (45 ml) red wine vinegar

4 cloves garlic, crushed and chopped

1 tablespoon (15 g) Dijon mustard

1 teaspoon Sucanat, sugar, or xylitol

$1/2$ teaspoon each salt and fresh-ground
    black pepper

$1/2$ teaspoon dried rosemary, crumbled

$1/4$ teaspoon cumin

$1/4$ teaspoon turmeric

$1/8$ teaspoon cayenne pepper

Pinch of allspice

2 to $2^{1}/_{2}$ pounds (905 to 1135 g) boneless
    bottom round roast

From Chef Jeannette

Even Healthier: For a unique flavor twist
with more fiber and vitamin A and less
starch, substitute a large sweet potato or
half a medium butternut squash for the
white potatoes. Peel and dice into $3/4$-inch
(1.9-cm) chunks.

Lean and Savory Sauced Pot Roast

From Dr. Jonny: As a kid, I really liked pot roast even though I had no idea what it actually was. Most pot roast recipes call for "beef chuck," which is basically mystery meat—not to mention extremely fatty. A simple upgrade makes this comfort food healthier: Just choose bottom round, a leaner cut of meat that will give you all the flavor of the original with fewer calories. It'll still cook up nice and tender because Chef Jeannette prepares it in a slow cooker and smothers it in a juicy, flavorful tomato sauce, eliminating the need for high-cal gravy. Leaving the skins on the potatoes adds fiber and vitamins, and using a slow cooker saves calories because you don't need extra "browning" fat. Note: If you really want to make this a healthy dish, choose grass-fed beef!

Scatter the onion evenly in the bottom of a large slow cooker. Add the carrots, celery, and potatoes.

In a medium bowl, mix together the tomatoes, tomato paste, vinegar, garlic, mustard, Sucanat, salt, pepper, rosemary, cumin, turmeric, cayenne, and allspice until well combined.

Place the roast over the vegetables and carefully pour the tomato sauce over all. Cook on low for 6 to 8 hours, or until the meat is tender and cooked through.

Yield: 6 to 7 servings

Per Serving: 382.6 calories; 14.7 g fat (34% calories from fat); 36.4 g protein; 24.5 g carbohydrate; 5.3 g dietary fiber; 108.6 mg cholesterol; 344.4 mg sodium

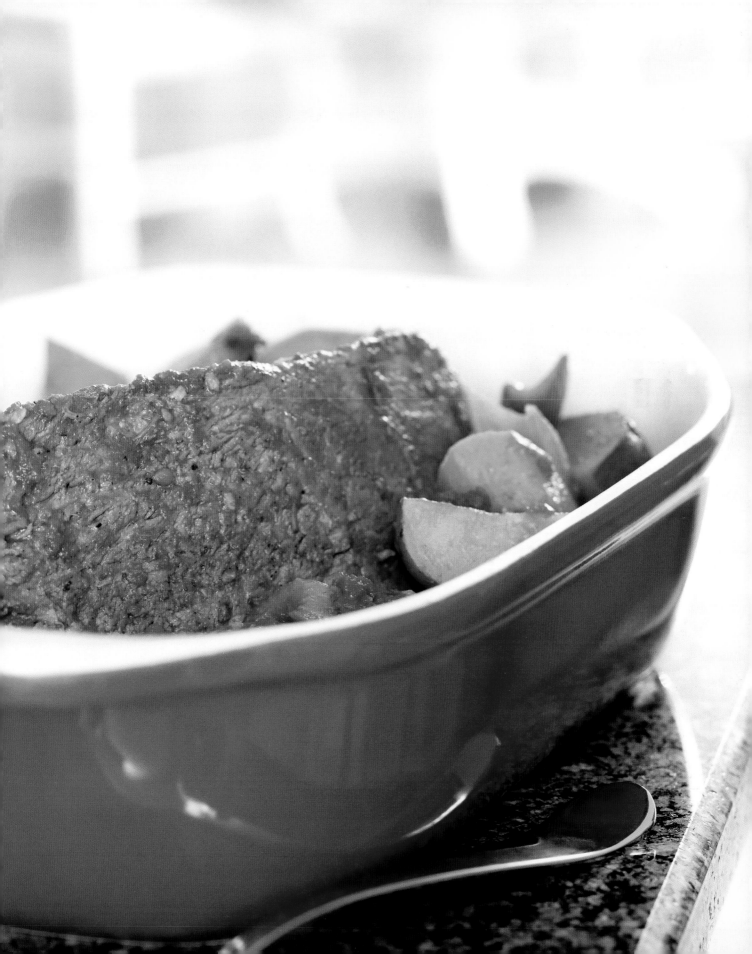

Ingredients

Salsa

1 large, juicy navel orange

1 lime

½ small serrano or jalapeño pepper, seeded and finely chopped (or ¼ cup, or 45 g, finely chopped roasted red pepper, for a milder version)

¼ cup (4 g) chopped fresh cilantro

3 tablespoons (30 g) finely chopped red onion

Pinches of Sucanat, salt, and black pepper, to taste

Burritos

6 (10-inch, or 25-cm) whole-grain tortillas (or wraps)

1 pound (455 g) grass-fed leanest ground beef

½ white onion, quartered

2 large ripe plum tomatoes, quartered

4 cloves garlic, crushed

1 teaspoon cumin

½ teaspoon chili powder

¾ teaspoon salt

½ teaspoon fresh-ground black pepper

¼ teaspoon red pepper flakes

1 can (15 ounces, or 425 g) kidney beans, rinsed and drained

½ cup (50 g) sliced scallion

½ cup (35 g) shredded lettuce

Grass-Fed Ground Beef Burritos with Cilantro-Orange Salsa

From Dr. Jonny: You can improve on the typical fast-food burritos—a comfort food that just about everyone in Southern California loves—with a few simple upgrades. We make ours with Mexi-spiced lean ground beef (grass-fed is best!) and spike the flavor with a delicious and tangy orange salsa instead of high-calorie (and often inferior) cheese. Kidney beans make this a high-fiber dish, and whole-grain wraps replace the flabby white ones used in the typical take-out restaurant. Fun fact: According to the always interesting informative website foodreference.com, the ancient Egyptians worshipped the onion, believing that its spherical shape and concentric rings symbolized eternity. When Egyptian artists created images of vegetables out of precious metals, only the onion was made from gold.

To make the salsa: Using a sharp paring knife, slice away the peels and white pith of the orange and lime. Working over a small bowl to catch any juices, cut the pulp sections free from the central membranes and add to the bowl. Break the sections up into small pieces. Add the pepper, cilantro, and red onion, and stir to combine. Season to taste with Sucanat, salt, and pepper, and set aside to let the flavors combine.

To make the burritos: Preheat the oven to 350°F (180°C, or gas mark 4).

Stack and wrap the tortillas tightly in aluminum foil and heat for 10 minutes just before using to soften (or microwave in a paper towel for 10 seconds).

In a large skillet over medium heat, brown the ground beef until no pink remains, 8 to 10 minutes. Drain any excess oils.

While the meat is cooking, add the white onion, tomatoes, and garlic to a food processor or blender and process until mostly smooth.

After the meat is drained, stir in the cumin, chili powder, salt, black pepper, and red pepper flakes until well combined. Stir in the tomato-onion purée until well mixed. Simmer for 5 to 6 minutes until the mixture is thick and cooked through. Stir in the beans and cook for another 2 minutes until heated. Stir in the scallion, adjust the seasonings if necessary, and remove from the heat. Drain any excess juices. Spread out the warm tortillas on a work surface and place equal amounts of shredded lettuce and the beef and bean mixture in the centers. Fold in the bottom edge, tuck in the sides, and roll toward yourself, leaving the seam-side down. Top each burrito with salsa, to taste, and serve immediately.

Yield: 6 servings

Per Serving: 310.2 calories; 4.3 g fat (14% calories from fat); 25.9 g protein; 43.3 g carbohydrate; 11 g dietary fiber; 46.9 mg cholesterol; 623.3 mg sodium

Lemon Cinna-Mint-Spiked Lean Lamb Stew

From Dr. Jonny: Lamb stew is great, but it can run a little heavy on the fats, making it a higher-calorie dish than it needs to be. Smothering it in white potatoes doesn't help much. We "health it up" by using the leanest cuts from the leg and shoulder and replacing half of the white potatoes with sweet carrots. Bingo. In one fell swoop you lower the calories, increase the fiber, and drop in a nice portion of beta-carotene and vitamin A from the carrots. Tantalizing undertones of lemon, cinnamon, and mint give this rich meaty stew a special twist that will help satisfy your deepest cravings. Fun fact: Cinnamon is an ancient herbal medicine that's mentioned in Chinese texts as long ago as 4,000 years. A 2010 study from the U.S. Department of Agriculture found that cinnamon may help reduce risk factors that are associated with both heart disease and diabetes.

Ingredients

2 teaspoons (10 ml) olive oil
1 pound (455 g) leanest 1½- to 2-inch (3.8- to 5-cm) lamb cubes
Salt and fresh-ground black pepper, to taste
1 large sweet onion, chopped
1 stalk celery, chopped
3 cloves garlic, crushed and chopped
3 large carrots, peeled and diced into small cubes or sliced into thin coins
2 tablespoons (8 g) chopped fresh oregano (or 1½ teaspoons, or 1.5 g, dried)
3 cups (710 ml) low-sodium chicken broth
⅔ cup (160 ml) dry red wine
1 can (15 ounces, or 425 g) tomato sauce
1 tablespoon (16 g) sundried tomato paste (or regular)
Pinch of Sucanat
1 teaspoon lemon zest
½ teaspoon cinnamon
8 golf ball-size new potatoes, unpeeled and quartered
1 small lemon, peeled and finely chopped
3 tablespoons (18 g) chopped fresh spearmint (or peppermint if that's all you can find)

Heat the oil in a large Dutch oven over medium-high heat. Add the lamb cubes and season lightly with salt and pepper. Lightly sear on all sides. Add the onion and celery and cook until the onion starts to soften, about 4 minutes. Add the garlic and cook for 30 seconds. Add the carrots and oregano and cook, stirring constantly, for about 30 seconds. Add the broth, wine, tomato sauce, sundried tomato paste, Sucanat, zest, and cinnamon, and stir to combine. Add the potatoes and lemon, stir, and bring just to a boil. Reduce the heat to low, cover, and simmer until the lamb and veggies are tender, 75 to 90 minutes. Adjust the seasonings if necessary. Sprinkle the mint over the top and serve.

Yield: about 6 servings
Per Serving: 426.2 calories; 13.8 g fat (29% calories from fat); 22.8 g protein; 51.9 g carbohydrate; 8.3 g dietary fiber; 49.9 mg cholesterol; 524.8 mg sodium

Ingredients

8 ounces (225 g) whole-grain pasta (we like Barilla Plus penne, ziti, elbows, or whole-wheat egg noodles)

1 tablespoon (15 ml) olive oil

1 small sweet onion, finely chopped

4 cloves garlic, minced

1 pound (455 g) leanest ground beef

½ teaspoon salt

½ teaspoon fresh-ground black pepper

1 can (28 ounces, or 795 g) crushed tomatoes

1 can (14.5 ounces, or 410 g) tomato sauce

2 tablespoons (32 g) tomato paste

¼ cup (60 ml) red wine

½ teaspoon Sucanat, sugar, or xylitol

1 teaspoon oregano

1 teaspoon basil

½ teaspoon red pepper flakes, optional

¼ cup (30 g) shredded mozzarella cheese

¼ cup (25 g) grated Parmesan cheese

Simple, Saucy Antioxidant American Chop Suey

From Dr. Jonny: Also called macaroni and beef, American chop suey is a classic family comfort food—noodles, beef, and pasta in red sauce with cheese—often made with Hamburger Helper. Yum. At least until you read the ingredients on the box: cornstarch, sugar, monosodium glutamate, dextrose, partially hydrogenated soybean oil (that's trans fats, folks). And we haven't even gotten to the inferior meat part. You can do better. Opt for grass-fed beef for an instant upgrade, use higher-quality noodles (like the higher protein Barilla Plus varieties), and take it easy on the cheese. Presto, you've got this simple but tasty homemade sauce. The result is an American goulash that satisfies better than anything that comes out of a box! Fun fact: Tomatoes, which are featured in three different ways in this recipe, are a major source of a powerful antioxidant called lycopene, which has shown in preliminary research to be protective against several cancers as well as some cardiovascular diseases. And cooking the tomatoes, as in sauce, for example, makes it easier for the body to absorb the lycopene.

Cook the pasta until al dente according to the package directions.

Heat the oil in a large nonstick sauté pan or Dutch oven over medium heat. Add the onion and sauté until softened, 5 to 6 minutes. Add the garlic and stir, cooking for about 1 minute. Add the ground beef, salt, and pepper, and break the meat apart, cooking through until no pink remains, about 7 minutes. Pour off any excess oil. Add the crushed tomatoes and tomato sauce and mix to combine. Stir in the tomato paste, wine, Sucanat, oregano, basil, and red pepper. Increase the heat to medium-high, and bring to a simmer. Cover, lower the heat, and simmer for about 15 minutes. Gently fold in the cooked pasta. Sprinkle the mozzarella and the Parmesan over the top. Cover again for about 3 minutes or until the cheese is melted, and serve warm.

Yield: about 6 servings

Per Serving: 369.7 calories; 9.3 g fat (22% calories from fat); 27.3 g protein; 45.3 g carbohydrate; 5.6 g dietary fiber; 53.9 mg cholesterol; 915.1 mg sodium

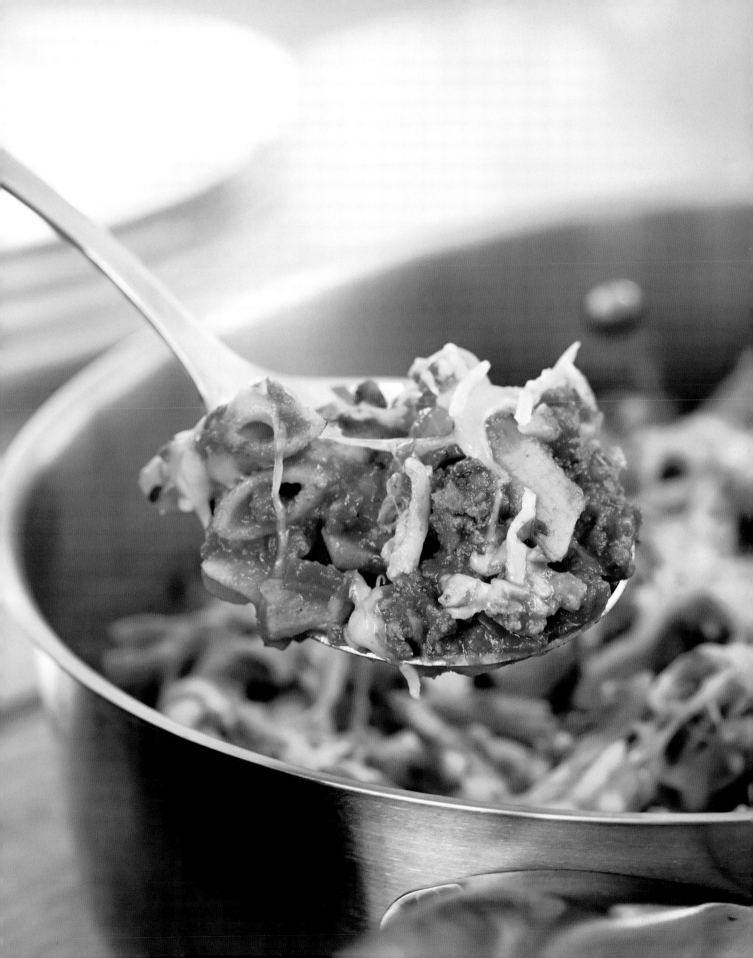

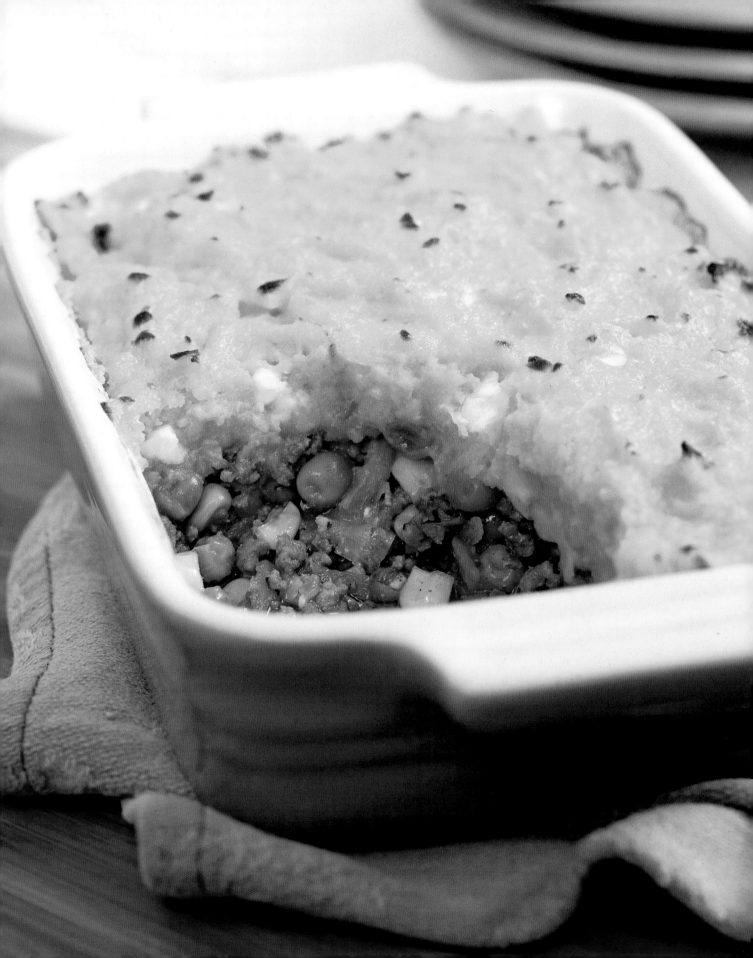

Ingredients

Olive oil cooking spray

2 teaspoons (10 ml) olive oil

1 yellow onion, chopped

½ cup (55 g) grated carrot

2 cloves garlic, minced

1 pound (455 g) leanest ground grass-fed beef

¾ teaspoon salt, divided

½ teaspoon fresh-ground black pepper

1 teaspoon thyme

1 cup (130 g) frozen corn

1 cup (130 g) frozen peas

½ cup (120 ml) beef broth, plus more if necessary

2 packages (each 12 ounces, or 340 g) organic puréed butternut squash, thawed and well drained

¼ cup (38 g) feta cheese, broken into pebble-size crumbs

From Chef Jeannette

Even Healthier: To make the freshest version of this dish, use fresh butternut in place of the frozen. Peel, seed, and cube a butternut squash (1½ to 2 pounds, or 680 to 905 g) or use prepared peeled cubes and boil in lightly salted water for 10 to 15 minutes until very tender. Drain well and beat in the mixer with the feta and salt and proceed as directed. You can also use fresh corn cut from the cob and fresh peas in place of the frozen and follow exactly the same directions.

Savory Souped-Up Shepherd's Pie

From Dr. Jonny: What's the difference between meat pie and shepherd's pie? Glad you asked. Meat pie is exactly what it sounds like—it's basically a pastry crust filled with meat. Shepherd's pie, on the other hand, has no crust and consists of a layer of ground meat, vegetables, and a topping of creamy mashed potatoes. The shepherd's pie is then baked till the top layer of potatoes turns a nice golden brown. So what's not to like? Not much, except that many of these dishes are made with an awful lot of mushy white potatoes, starchy gravy, and (usually) fatty and inferior meat. Chef Jeannette's version lowers the impact on your blood sugar, pumps up the nutritional content substantially, and, as a bonus, saves a lot of prep time. How? Swap out the mashed potato topping for puréed butternut squash—which, by the way, is one of the naturally sweetest veggies on Earth and just as satisfying and creamy as the white stuff. Much lower in calories than potatoes and much richer in nutrients—1 cup (255 g) of squash provides way more potassium than a banana, as well as 84 mg of calcium, 39 mcg of folate, and, like all red or orange veggies and fruits, a ton of vitamin A (22,868 IUs) and beta-carotene (9,368 mcg). Upgrade to grass-fed meat and you've got a comfort food that actually meets my definition of a health food! Fun fact: Butternut squash is rich in a compound that's a lesser-known relative of beta-carotene—it's called beta-cryptoxanthin. Several observational studies suggest that beta-cryptoxanthin could potentially act as a chemopreventive agent against lung cancer.

Preheat the oven to 400°F (200°C, or gas mark 6) and lightly spray a 9 x 13-inch (23 x 33-cm) baking dish with olive oil. Set aside.

In a large skillet, heat the oil over medium heat. Add the onion and carrots and sauté for about 5 minutes, until the onion begins to soften. Add the garlic and cook for 1 minute. Add the beef and break it up. Cook until no pink remains, about 10 minutes, and drain off any excess oils. Sprinkle ½ teaspoon of the salt, pepper, and thyme onto the beef and stir to mix. Reduce the heat to low and stir in the corn, peas, and beef broth. Cook for about 8 minutes, adding more broth if necessary to keep the mixture moist.

While the beef is cooking, in a large bowl add the drained squash, feta, and remaining ¼ teaspoon salt, and stir to mix.

Pour the beef mixture into the prepared baking dish. Spoon the squash mixture evenly over the top of the beef. Bake for about 25 minutes, or until the mixture is bubbling and the squash is heated through.

Yield: about 6 servings

Per Serving: 228 calories; 7.1 g fat (28% calories from fat); 20.9 g protein; 22.1 g carbohydrate; 2.2 g dietary fiber; 52.7 mg cholesterol; 564.7 mg sodium

Rack of Lean Lamb with Herbs and Roasted Shallots

Ingredients

2 racks lamb (each about 8 ribs or 1 pound
   [455 g]), trimmed and frenched
¼ cup (60 ml) olive oil, divided
4 cloves garlic, minced
2 tablespoons (12 g) minced fresh mint
2 tablespoons (3.4 g) minced fresh
   rosemary
1 tablespoon (2.4 g) minced fresh thyme
½ teaspoon coarse-ground pepper
8 shallots, peeled
½ teaspoon salt, or to taste

From Dr. Jonny: For the moment, let's put aside any concerns we might have about eating lamb (and yes, I'm a sucker for these gorgeous creatures, too). But the fact is, lamb is one of the healthiest meats on the planet. Precisely because it's young the animal hasn't had too much time to accumulate toxins. In general, lamb isn't factory farmed, so added antibiotics, steroids, and hormones aren't the problem they are with factory-farmed beef. (And if you really want the best, it's possible to get grass-fed New Zealand lamb at many grocery stores or butchers.) Lamb is high in protein, is relatively low in fat, and contains zinc, niacin, selenium, vitamin B$_3$, and all eight essential amino acids. The frenching process removes the layer of heavy fat, leaving the exposed lean and tasty chops. To bump up the flavors even more, we marinate—overnight, if you can—with a fabulous mix of mint, rosemary, and thyme, all of which really pop the flavor of the already tender meat. Serve it with creamy roasted shallots on the side; it's comfort food at its best! Fun fact: Marinating with herbs such as rosemary before cooking or grilling significantly reduces heterocyclic amines, a potential carcinogen (cancer-causing compound), according to research by J. Scott Smith, Ph.D., at Kansas State University.

Slice each rack in half so you have 4 sections of about 4 ribs each.

In a small bowl, mix together 2 tablespoons (28 ml) of the olive oil, garlic, mint, rosemary, and thyme. Smear the mixture evenly all over the surface of the meat and sprinkle evenly with the pepper. Wrap the meat in plastic and marinate in the refrigerator overnight.

The next evening, preheat the oven to 400°F (200°C, or gas mark 6).

Coat the shallots in a thin coating of olive oil and set aside.

Take out the racks from the refrigerator and peel away the plastic wrap, removing any large pieces of herb. Sprinkle lightly with salt. Heat the remaining 2 tablespoons (28 ml) of oil in a large ovenproof skillet over medium-high heat. Sear the fatty sides until golden brown, about 4 minutes. Flip the racks so they are sitting fat sides up. Arrange the prepared shallots around the lamb racks and place the pan in the oven. Cook for 20 to 25 minutes or until desired doneness—watch the shallots closely. Turn them once and remove if they are getting too browned. Let the racks rest for 10 to 15 minutes before cutting. To serve, slice the racks into chops and serve with a couple of the roasted shallots on the side.

Yield: 4 servings
Per Serving: 414 calories; 34 g fat (77% calories from fat); 16 g protein; 7 g carbohydrate; 0.2 g dietary fiber; 63 mg cholesterol; 68 mg sodium

Less-Butter Baked Scallops and Savory Shiitakes

Ingredients

1¼ pounds (565 g) sea scallops

¾ cup (175 ml) dry sherry

3 tablespoons (45 g) butter, divided

1 tablespoon (15 ml) olive oil

8 ounces (225 g) shiitake (or cremini) mushrooms, thickly sliced

4 shallots, chopped

2 cloves garlic, minced

Pinches of salt and fresh-ground pepper

⅓ cup (40 g) whole-grain bread crumbs

2 tablespoons (10 g) fresh-grated Parmesan cheese

¼ lemon, optional

From Dr. Jonny: The conventional wisdom has it that baked scallops is a healthy dish if only it weren't for all that butter. Well, I don't agree, as I happen to think organic butter is a perfectly fine food. But I do agree that the baked scallop dishes I've seen in restaurants are swimming in the stuff, which presents a problem, not because of the saturated fat, but rather because of the enormous number of calories that so much butter adds to the mix. Our lightened-up version has the scallops marinating in sherry to compensate for the reduced butter content. We also upgraded the bread crumbs to the whole-grain variety for a bit more fiber. Parmesan cheese goes perfectly with this dish, and is way lower in calories than you might think. At only 22 calories per tablespoon it's still got a fair amount of calcium (55 mg per tablespoon) and—for those of you watching your fat—barely more than 1 gram. The mushrooms are high in fiber as well as minerals such as potassium, and scallops are a terrific source of low-calorie protein.

Combine the scallops and sherry in a glass storage container and marinate for 2 hours to overnight. Drain well, reserving ⅓ cup (80 ml) of the marinade.

Preheat the oven to 400°F (200°C, or gas mark 6). Add 2 tablespoons (29 g) of the butter to a 1½-quart (1.4-L) casserole dish and place in the oven for a couple of minutes until the butter is melted. Remove the casserole and set aside.

In a large skillet, melt the remaining 1 tablespoon (15 g) of butter with the olive oil over medium heat. Add the mushrooms in a single layer and cook for about 3 minutes without stirring. Turn them once and cook for a couple more minutes, until they just start to brown. Add the shallots and cook for about 1 minute, or until the shiitakes are lightly browned. Add the garlic, salt, and pepper, and cook for about 30 seconds. Add ⅓ cup (80 ml) of the reserved marinating liquid and cook for about 2 minutes, or until the mushrooms and shallots are fairly tender and much, but not all, of the liquid is cooked off. Add the scallops to the pan and toss gently to combine. Cook for about 3 minutes, turning once.

Pour the mixture into the prepared casserole dish and sprinkle the bread crumbs and cheese over the top. Bake for 10 to 12 minutes, or until the scallops are cooked through but still very tender—their centers should still have a slight pink tinge. Squeeze lemon over all before serving.

Yield: 4 servings

Per Serving: 634.9 calories; 14.6 g fat (20% calories from fat); 36.9 g protein; 83.2 g carbohydrate; 1.6 g dietary fiber; 71.9 mg cholesterol; 390.4 mg sodium

Zesty Calcium-Stuffed Salmon

From Dr. Jonny: If you've read any of my previous books or any of my monthly columns for *Clean Eating* or *Better Nutrition*, or in fact, if you've read anything I've written in the last decade, you know that I am an unabashed fan of wild Alaskan salmon. Actually, "fan" is too mild a word—I'm absolutely nuts about wild Alaskan salmon. Unlike its farm-raised brethren, wild Alaskan salmon is a "cleaner" fish with far less contamination from PCBs than the farm-raised kind, and with higher levels of the potent antioxidant astaxanthin. Then, of course, there are the omega-3s, possibly one of the most important components of a healthy diet ever discovered—wild salmon is just teeming with these "wellness molecules." For stuffing, Chef Jeannette has chosen Neufchâtel cheese, which not only has the same creamy texture and rich flavor as cream cheese but is also high in calcium and magnesium and has only about two-thirds the fat (saving you some unnecessary calories without sacrificing taste!). Add olives and olive oil and the piquant zing of fresh lemon and capers and you're good to go! What a dish!

Ingredients

Olive oil cooking spray
⅓ cup (77 g) Neufchâtel cheese, softened
1 teaspoon lemon zest
2 teaspoons (10 ml) fresh-squeezed lemon juice
2 tablespoons (12 g) minced scallion
2 teaspoons (2.6 g) minced fresh parsley
2 tablespoons (13 g) finely chopped pitted kalamata olives, optional
1 to 2 teaspoons capers, optional, to taste (rinse to remove some of the saltiness, if desired)
4 skinless salmon fillets (each 4 to 6 ounces, or 115 to 170 g, about 1 inch, or 2.5 cm, thick)
Olive oil, for drizzling
Salt and fresh-ground black pepper, to taste
8 thin slices lemon cut widthwise "around the equator" (⅛ inch, or 3 mm, thick)
½ lemon, optional

Preheat the oven to 350°F (180°C, or gas mark 4). Lightly spray an 11 x 7-inch (28 x 18-cm) glass baking dish with olive oil and set aside.

In a small bowl, combine the cheese, zest, lemon juice, scallion, parsley, and olives, and mix well (an immersion blender or rubber spoon works well for this). Stir in the capers.

Make deep (but don't cut all the way through) 1½- to 2-inch (3.8- to 5-cm) slits in the sides of each salmon fillet. Stuff the slits with equal portions of the Neufchâtel mixture. Lay the fillets out evenly in the prepared baking dish and drizzle olive oil over each of them.

Sprinkle the fillets lightly with salt and pepper, and lay 2 lemon slices on top of each one, overlapping slightly, if necessary. Bake for 18 to 20 minutes, or until just done—do not overbake or the salmon will dry out. Squeeze the lemon half over all, just before serving.

Yield: 4 servings
Per Serving: 284.4 calories; 18.8 g fat (59% calories from fat); 25.5 g protein; 6.6 g carbohydrate; 2.1 g dietary fiber; 83.8 mg cholesterol; 206.2 mg sodium

From Chef Jeannette

Depending on the size and how much juice you use, you will need two to three lemons for the completed dish.

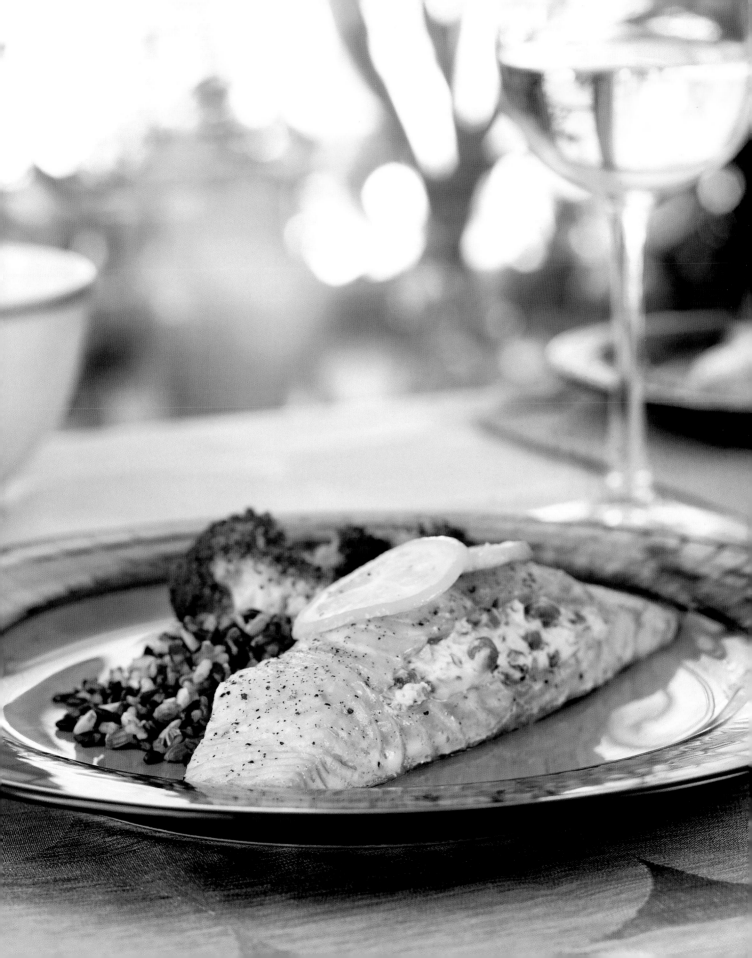

Ingredients

12 ounces (340 g) whole-wheat egg noodles

1 tablespoon (15 ml) olive oil

1 tablespoon (14 g) butter

1 sweet onion, diced

8 ounces (225 g) sliced mushrooms (cremini or baby bella work well)

¼ cup (60 ml) dry white wine

1 cup (225 g) silken tofu

⅔ cup (160 ml) milk (low-fat cow's or plain, unsweetened soy or almond)

¾ teaspoon salt, or to taste

½ teaspoon fresh-ground black pepper, or to taste

2 cups (240 g) grated sharp Cheddar cheese

2 cans (each 6 ounces, or 170 g) high-quality tuna (chunk light or skipjack) in water, drained

2 cups (260 g) frozen baby peas

¼ cup (12 g) diced chives, optional

3 tablespoons (20 g) ground flaxseed

½ cup (25 g) whole-wheat panko bread crumbs, optional

Tempting Tuned-Up Tuna Casserole

From Dr. Jonny: Ah, tuna casserole. The best way in the world to get kids to eat fish. But the old standby, with white pasta and cream of mushroom soup from the can, is a bad way to do it. Our version has the same creamy "mouthfeel," but it's made with whole-grain egg noodles. Even better, there's flax for more fiber (not to mention cancer-fighting substances called lignans) and silken tofu for extra protein. Mushrooms are one of the most healing foods on Earth, and—surprisingly, given all the buzz about the exotic mushrooms such as reishi—the plain old cremini "button" mushrooms turn out to be quite a nutritional bargain. (One cup, or 70 g, of mushrooms contains more than 200 mg of potassium and a decent dose of niacin, all for about 15 calories!) Note: When it comes to tuna, the least-expensive cuts such as chunk light and skipjack are the lowest in mercury (or you could do as we do and order the best tuna ever directly from Vital Choice in Alaska, available through a link on my website, www.jonnybowden.com, under "healthy food"). We also recommend organic white Cheddar—no pesky yellow dyes but the same soothing, satisfying taste.

Preheat the oven to 400°F (200°C, or gas mark 6).

Bring a large pot of water to a boil. Cook the pasta until al dente according to package directions. Drain in a colander and set aside.

While the pasta is cooking, heat the oil and butter in a large Dutch oven over medium-high heat. Add the onion and sauté for 2 minutes. Add the mushrooms and cook for 4 minutes. Add the wine and cook until evaporated and the mushrooms are tender, 4 to 5 minutes.

Meanwhile, combine the tofu and milk in food processor or blender and process for 20 seconds, or until smooth and creamy.

Reduce the heat to medium and pour the tofu-milk mixture over the vegetables in the pan. Stir in the salt, pepper, and cheese until well combined. Stir in the tuna and peas, and gently fold in the pasta and chives. Remove from the burner, sprinkle the flaxseed over the top, sprinkle the panko over the flaxseed, and bake, uncovered, for 16 to 18 minutes, until lightly browned.

Yield: 8 servings

Per Serving: 353.5 calories; 17.3 g fat (43% calories from fat); 26 g protein; 23.4 g carbohydrate; 4.7 g dietary fiber; 54.8 mg cholesterol; 657.1 mg sodium

Ingredients

One 12- to 15-inch x 6-inch (30- to 38-cm
    x 15-cm) natural cedar grilling plank

3¼ cups (770 ml) apple cider, divided

¼ cup (60 ml) apple cider vinegar

¼ cup (85 g) honey

1 tablespoon (13 g) Sucanat or sugar

½ teaspoon dry mustard

1 wild Alaskan salmon fillet (20 ounces,
    or 565 g)

Salt and fresh-ground black pepper, to taste

From Chef Jeannette

If the plank catches fire while cooking,
put it out with a spritz of water and move
the plank to a cooler part of the grill.

Protein-Packed, Apple-Glazed Wild-Caught Alaskan Salmon

From Dr. Jonny: That pure-sugar goo they put on "glazed salmon" in restaurants probably gets more people to eat fish and makes salmon more appetizing to many people who otherwise wouldn't touch it— that's good news. The bad news is that pure-sugar goo is pure-sugar goo. Plus, it's invariably slapped on farm-raised fish, which is not nearly as good for you as the wild variety. (Example: Farm-raised salmon gets its color from dyes; wild salmon comes by it naturally via its enormously healthy diet of crustaceans.) Looking for a way to get the delicious, sugary gooey taste of the restaurant glaze while minimizing the negatives, Chef Jeannette came up with the idea of using fresh apple cider as the glaze base. Good choice! We also enhance the flavor by grilling on a soaked cedar plank, and strongly recommend you use wild Alaskan salmon from Vital Choice, available through the shopping/ healthy foods menu item on my website, www.jonnybowden.com. (You can also get wild Alaskan salmon at better grocery stores and fish markets.) Smoky and sweet, this recipe is nothing short of freaky good!

Soak the plank for at least 1 hour in 2 cups (475 ml) of the cider plus enough water to cover completely.

While the plank is soaking, prepare the glaze. In a small saucepan, whisk together the remaining 1¼ cups (295 ml) cider, vinegar, honey, Sucanat, and dry mustard over medium-high heat. Bring the mixture to a boil, stirring often to dissolve the honey. When the mixture reaches a boil, reduce the heat to a simmer and cook until it reaches the desired glaze consistency, about 15 to 20 minutes. Set aside.

Preheat the grill to 350°F (180°C) and sprinkle the salmon lightly with salt and pepper. Drain the plank and place on the grill, cover, and heat for 3 minutes. Flip the plank and place the fish, skin-side down, on the plank. Cover the grill and cook for 15 to 20 minutes (more or less time depending on the thickness of the fillet) or until the fish is nearly cooked to desired doneness. Do not flip the fish while cooking.

When the fish is nearly done, brush the top surface heavily with the glaze and cook for 3 to 4 minutes, or until caramelized and cooked to your liking (about 135°F or 57°C on a meat thermometer). Drizzle a little extra glaze over the fish before serving, if desired.

Yield: 4 servings

Per Serving: 370.7 calories; 9.2 g fat (22% calories from fat); 28.3 g protein; 43 g carbohydrate; 0.2 g dietary fiber; 77.7 mg cholesterol; 69.8 mg sodium

Ingredients

Juice of 2 large limes (at least 4 tablespoons, or 60 ml)

1½ tablespoons (30 g) Thai sweet chili sauce

1 tablespoon (15 ml) plus 1 teaspoon peanut oil or more, if necessary, divided

Pinch of salt

1 pound (455 g) raw medium shrimp

1 package (12 ounces, or 340 g) fettuccini-style Thai rice noodles or rice sticks

⅓ cup (80 ml) Thai fish sauce

3 tablespoons (40 g) Sucanat or sugar

2 tablespoons (28 ml) unseasoned rice wine vinegar (or white wine vinegar)

1 tablespoon (15 ml) low-sodium tamari (or low-sodium soy sauce)

¾ teaspoon tamarind concentrate, optional

½ teaspoon red pepper flakes, or more for more heat

3 cloves garlic, minced

4 eggs, lightly beaten

¾ cup (75 g) chopped scallion

2 cups (100 g) mung bean sprouts

½ cup (73 g) chopped roasted unsalted peanuts

½ cup (8 g) chopped fresh cilantro

1 lime, quartered, for garnish

From Chef Jeannette

Time-Saver Tip: To save a little time, you can skip the marinating step and use thawed frozen cooked shrimp instead. Just add it when you add the noodles to briefly heat.

Tempting Four-Flavors Shrimp Pad Thai

From Dr. Jonny: Pad Thai is one of Thailand's national dishes and a huge favorite everywhere else. Chef Jeannette lowered the sugar in our version but designed it to hit several flavor receptors on the tongue so that it remains a deeply comforting dish. Tamari makes it just salty enough to be delicious, red pepper flakes and chili sauce give it some heat, and lime and vinegar make it piquant. Peanuts contain a wide range of nutrients and are especially high in fiber (3 grams per ounce) and protein (7 grams per ounce). In a 2004 study published in the *Journal of the American College of Nutrition*, peanut consumers had higher intakes of a number of key nutrients, including vitamin A, vitamin E, folate, magnesium, iron, and zinc. Fun fact: Ounce for ounce, peanuts contain about half the amount of resveratrol as red wine. (Resveratrol is a plant compound found to extend life in every species studied, hence its reputation as an anti-aging nutrient.)

Set aside 2 tablespoons (28 ml) of the lime juice and add the rest to a glass storage container. Whisk in the chili sauce, 1 teaspoon of the peanut oil, and the salt into the lime juice in the glass container. Add the shrimp and toss to coat. Marinate, covered, in the refrigerator for 15 to 30 minutes. Drain well.

While the shrimp are marinating, prepare the rice noodles according to the package directions and set aside.

In a small bowl, whisk together the fish sauce, Sucanat, reserved 2 tablespoons (28 ml) lime juice, vinegar, tamari, tamarind concentrate, and red pepper flakes, to taste. It's okay if the tamarind paste stays a little clumpy; it will incorporate when it is heated. Set aside.

Heat the remaining 1 tablespoon (15 ml) peanut oil in a wok or large skillet over high heat and swirl to coat the surface. Add the marinated shrimp and stir-fry for 1 to 2 minutes, or until just pink. Remove from the pan and set aside. Add another drizzle of peanut oil if necessary to recoat the wok. Add the garlic and cook for 30 seconds. Add the eggs and whisk them around the wok for about a minute, or until they are almost set. Add the sauce and stir for a minute or two until the sugar and tamarind concentrate dissolve. Add the scallions and bean sprouts and toss to combine. Add the cooked noodles and peanuts and toss to coat and heat through. Remove from the heat, sprinkle with the cilantro, and serve each plate with a wedge of lime.

Yield: 4 to 6 servings

Per Serving: 480.7 calories; 13.9 g fat (25% calories from fat); 25.6 g protein; 67 g carbohydrate; 2.7 g dietary fiber; 256.3 mg cholesterol; 1,438.7 mg sodium

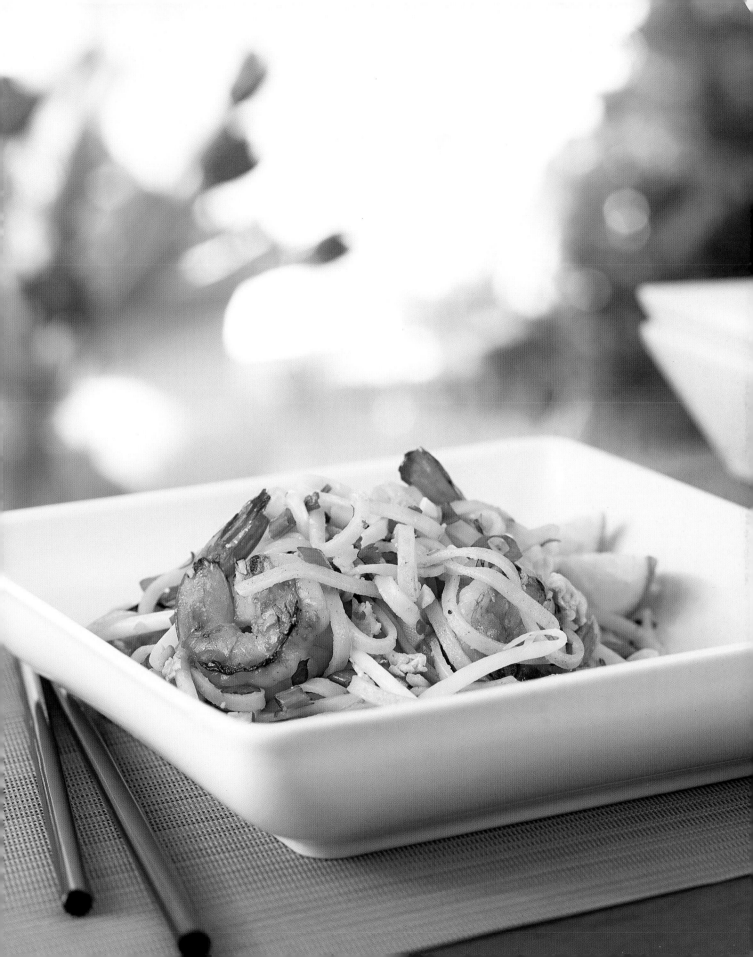

Backyard New England Clambake: Bounty of the Sea

From Dr. Jonny: Without going into the whole history of how I met my dear friend and writing partner, Chef Jeannette Bessinger, let me just say that we grew up in very different circumstances with very different traditions. I grew up in New York City and the only place I ever saw an actual clam was in the Oyster Bar at Grand Central Station. Jeannette grew up in Newport, Rhode Island, and went to clambakes. Which I didn't even know existed. But just because many of us can't do clambakes in the traditional way that Jeannette grew up with, it doesn't mean we can't replicate that same delicious and comforting blend of seaside ingredients in a regular home kitchen. Or outside on an ordinary backyard grill, which works perfectly well for this version of the old fave. Clams and lobsters are a fine source of protein and low in calories to boot. And although corn gets a bad rap for being high in carbs (and by association, for being the source of the dreaded high-fructose corn syrup), fresh corn on the cob is actually pretty good for you. For a measly 59 calories per ear of corn, it's got a fair amount of potassium and folate, and even a gram or two of fiber. And corn also contains a carotenoid known as beta-cryptoxanthin (a relative of the better-known beta-carotene), which has been found to significantly lower the risk for lung cancer. (To keep calories reasonable, just don't overdo the butter and portion size.) Leeks, by the way, are a member of the Brassica family of vegetable royalty. They're loaded with nutrients, including iron, magnesium, potassium, folate, and calcium. This is a tasty, healthy, high-protein dish that really satisfies!

From Chef Jeannette

Even Healthier: As Jonny mentioned, I grew up in New England, and clambakes were a regular part of my childhood. We did them on the beach, in the traditional way, not too differently from how they've been done for the past 300 years in this area. Early in the morning you dig a pit in the sand (about 3 feet [0.9 m] deep and as far across as you need to fit all the food—up to 10 feet [3 m] if you're having a huge party) and line it with skull-size, granite rocks. It's important to select them from above the tide line so you know they're dry. Then build a big, blazing hardwood fire (maple or oak work really well) on the rocks and let it burn down all morning. When the fire is out, scoop out the ashes and pile about 1 foot (30.5 cm) of rockweed (the dark, flat seaweed that clings to rock faces on the shoreline) on top of the hot rocks. Quickly lay out your shellfish (lobsters, oysters, clams, mussels, etc.), then pile on a few more inches of seaweed and lay out your veggies (scrubbed potatoes, ears of corn in their husks, etc.). We added large links of sausage, too, just folded them up into brown paper bags to absorb some of the oils. Top with just enough seaweed to cover, pull a big canvas tarp over the whole thing, and "seal" it closed by piling sand all around the outer edges. Then we played games all afternoon on the beach while everything steamed to perfection in its moist, briny sand pit. Nothing else like it in the world!

Ingredients

4 ears fresh corn, husks intact, preferably organic to avoid GMO

20 littleneck clams

4 large fresh lobster tails in their shells

2 cups (208 g) chopped leeks, tender sections only, well rinsed

2 cups (120 g) chopped fresh parsley

2 lemons, halved

2 tablespoons (28 g) ghee, melted (or organic butter)

Trim the corn silk and tips of the husks and soak the whole ears of corn in lots of fresh water for 1 hour. Drain.

Preheat the grill to medium.

Scrub the littlenecks clean. Using sharp kitchen shears, snip the soft inner shell in the middle of each lobster tail from the base to the fan and drain any liquids.

To make the grilling packets, lay out 4 sets of 2 sheets of heavy-duty aluminum foil, each 24 inches (61 cm) in length. For each packet, lay out 1 length of foil, then lay the other one across it on top like a + sign. Place ½ cup (52 g) leeks and ½ cup (30 g) parsley into the middle of each foil "cross." Lay 1 lobster tail and 5 littlenecks over the veggies in each foil cross. Squeeze half a lemon over each set of seafood and veggies, then drizzle 2 teaspoons (10 ml) melted ghee over all. Fold the ends of the foil neatly over the top of each packet of food to make a tight seal.

Place the soaked ears of corn and 4 packets (seam-side up) onto the preheated grill. Grill for 20 to 25 minutes, until the littlenecks are open and the lobster shells have turned bright red.

Yield: 4 servings

Per Serving: 590 calories; 10.3 g fat (15% calories from fat); 67.2 g protein; 48.4 g carbohydrate; 4.5 g dietary fiber; 163.6 mg cholesterol; 884.6 mg sodium

Ingredients

1 to 1¼ pounds (455 to 565 g) skinless flounder fillets

1 tablespoon (15 ml) olive oil

1½ cups (355 ml) tomato juice (we like Knudsen organic Very Veggie)

1 small yellow onion, chopped

1 cup (125 g) whole-wheat pastry flour

¼ cup (26 g) ground flaxseed

2 eggs

1½ cups (110 g) crushed cereal flakes (bran, corn, or heirloom whole-grain cereal)

1½ tablespoons (25 ml) olive oil or 1½ tablespoons (21 g) butter

From Chef Jeannette

Variation: I generally don't cook with grain flours, so I tried this dish using blanched almond flour in place of the whole-wheat flour to omit the wheat, decrease the carbs, and increase the fiber and healthy fats. (Honeyville makes an excellent blanched almond flour that is light enough to use in place of whole-wheat flour in many types of dishes.) I had to drag the fillets through the almond flour, though, because it clumped up in the bag, and cooked it for a minute or two longer because it made the crust a little heavier. But it crisped up beautifully and tasted divine.

Thanks to my Real Food Moms partner, Tracee Yablon Brenner, for this concept.

Fresh and Fiber-Full Fish Fingers

From Dr. Jonny: Nothing says "bland and uninteresting" like fast-food or frozen fishcakes. Not so this flavorful alternative, which, by the way, is a terrific way to get more fish into your diet. Remember, fish is a low-calorie source of the highest quality protein. The whole-grain flour and whole-grain cereal add a lot of fiber to this high-protein dish, and the flaxseed adds a nice nutty touch, not to mention cancer-fighting lignans and some omega-3s. (Best brand for our money: Barlean's Forti-Flax!) Flounder is a low-mercury fish, but do try to get the Pacific kind because Atlantic flounder is way overfished!

Slice the fillets in half lengthwise to make 10 to 12 strips.

Gently whisk the oil and tomato juice together in a shallow baking dish.

Stir in the onion, add the fish fillets, cover, and marinate in the refrigerator for at least 30 minutes.

Combine the flour and flaxseed in a 1-gallon (3.8-L) resealable plastic bag. In a shallow bowl, beat the eggs. Pour the crushed cereal onto a plate.

Remove the fillet strips from the marinade and gently place into the bag. Shake gently to coat the fish. Heat the olive oil (or melt the butter) in a Dutch oven or large skillet over medium heat. Remove and dip the fish strips into the egg, then roll in the crushed cereal flakes to coat evenly. Add the fish strips to the hot pan and cook for about 2 to 3 minutes on each side, until the crust is lightly browned and the fish is flaky.

Yield: about 4 servings

Per Serving: 500.4 calories; 17.9 g fat (31% calories from fat); 33.6 g protein; 51.3 g carbohydrate; 6.3 g dietary fiber; 160.4 mg cholesterol; 141.9 mg sodium

Ingredients

2 tablespoons (28 g) high-quality
    mayonnaise

2 teaspoons (10 ml) fresh-squeezed lemon
    juice

¾ teaspoon lemon zest

Pinches of salt, white pepper, and cayenne
    pepper

1 stalk celery, finely chopped

¼ cup (25 g) finely chopped scallion greens

2 tablespoons (8 g) chopped fresh parsley
    (or cilantro)

1¼ pounds (565 g) cooked lobster meat, cut
    into bite-size pieces

Four 10-inch (25-cm) whole-grain wraps (try
    it in a warmed sprouted corn wrap with
    cilantro for a Mexi-twist)

1 cup (70 g) shredded lettuce

½ Hass avocado, thinly sliced

Luscious Low-Carb Lobster Rolls

From Dr. Jonny: The first time I tasted a lobster roll was up in Chef Jeannette's neck of the woods—Newport, Rhode Island, in the heart of New England, where lobster rolls are high on the list of comfort foods. I remember the rich boiled lobster with gobs of mayo on white hot dog rolls. (Oh, to be young and foolish again. Or even just young.) But listen, you can have your lobster roll cake and eat it, too, by simply upgrading the concept to a wrap-style sandwich on whole grains. Bingo, you've reduced the starchy carb load. For your second trick, cut way back on the mayo (or even better, just serve it on top of a generous bed of crisp lettuce greens, chopped tomatoes, and cukes, in which case you've got a really healthy, high-protein, low-carb comfort food on your hands). Finally, for the nutritional trifecta, introduce some high-nutrient veggies for better nutrition and flavor. Presto bingo, you've got a winner! The avocado more than makes up for the reduced mayo, except that avocado is surprisingly high in fiber and absolutely teeming with potassium—one small avocado has twice the potassium of a banana, and that's really, really good for your heart!

In a large bowl, combine the mayonnaise, lemon juice, zest, salt, and peppers and mix well to combine. Stir in the celery, scallions, and parsley.

Gently fold in the lobster meat to coat.

Lay out the wraps and place one-fourth of the lettuce and one-fourth of the avocado into the center of each one. Divide the lobster salad evenly among the wraps and roll up to serve.

Yield: 4 servings

Per Serving: 305.2 calories; 7.2 g fat (20% calories from fat); 33.3 g protein; 28.7 g carbohydrate; 5.9 g dietary fiber; 101.5 mg cholesterol; 600 mg sodium

Creamy, Lower-Fat New England Clam Chowder

Ingredients

24 to 30 littleneck clams

1/4 cup (60 ml) dry white wine

1 cup (235 ml) water

4 strips smoked turkey bacon

1/4 cup (30 g) finely chopped celery

1 1/2 cups (155 g) clean chopped leeks (or 1 cup, or 160 g, chopped sweet onion)

2 medium Yukon gold potatoes, unpeeled and diced into small cubes

2 teaspoons (9 g) butter

1 1/2 tablespoons (12 g) flour

2 teaspoons (10 g) organic chicken Better Than Bouillon

3 or 4 drops liquid smoke, or to taste

1/2 teaspoon fresh-ground black or white pepper, or to taste

2 cans (each 12 ounces, or 355 ml) evaporated skim milk

1/4 cup (25 g) sliced scallion greens, optional, for garnish

From Chef Jeannette

Time-Saver Tip: Use two 6-ounce (170-g) cans of minced clams in place of the fresh. Drain them, reserving the juice. Add enough water to make 1 cup (235 ml).

From Dr. Jonny: Chef Jeannette asked me one day which clam chowder was the most "authentic": New England or Manhattan. So I did a little digging. The cream-based New England version—traditionally made with clams, broth, diced potato, bacon or salt pork, and flour—wins the historical battle. It's been around since the mid-eighteenth century, while there doesn't appear to be any mention whatsoever of Manhattan clam chowder before about 1930. In terms of preference, it's a no-brainer for my partner Jeannette, who grew up in Rhode Island. And truth be told, that's my fave, too, even though I grew up in Manhattan. But I rarely order it because it's just too darn high in calories. We lightened the caloric burden by swapping heavy cream for evaporated skim milk. And instead of pork or bacon fat, we used just the oils from some nice turkey bacon. (Which makes my dogs, Emily and Lucy, very happy because they are the beneficiaries of the actual turkey bacon.) This dish is rich in calcium and protein, not to mention flavor.

Scrub the littlenecks clean. Add the wine and water and cleaned clams to a large stockpot over high heat. Once boiling, steam them for 2 to 3 minutes, or until they just open (discard the ones that don't open). Cool, shuck, clean the clams, and chop them roughly.

Reserve 1 cup (235 ml) of the liquid in the pan, but it will be sandy, so strain it before using (a double-mesh sieve lined with a damp paper towel works well for this).

In a large, heavy-bottomed saucepan, cook the bacon over medium heat until crisp. Remove the bacon and reserve for another use or discard. Drizzle a little olive oil into the pan if the bacon didn't release enough fat. Add the celery and leeks and sweat them for 4 minutes. Stir them and add the potatoes. Cook for about 4 minutes more, stirring occasionally. Remove the veggies from the pan and set aside.

Add the butter to the pan to melt, and stir in the flour to make a roux. Stir constantly until the roux turns a light brown, and then add the reserved clam juice, whisking constantly to blend. Add the cooked vegetables, Better Than Bouillon, liquid smoke, and pepper, to taste, mixing well. Bring to a boil, reduce the heat, cover, and simmer until all the vegetables are tender, about 12 minutes. Slowly stir in the evaporated milk and bring just to a boil. Add the clams, return to a simmer, reduce the heat, and cook for about 1 minute, or until the clams are hot. Adjust the seasonings, if necessary. Sprinkle with the scallions and serve.

Yield: 4 servings

Per Serving: 523.9 calories; 5.2 g fat (9% calories from fat); 56.5 g protein; 44.9 g carbohydrate; 2.7 g dietary fiber; 83.9 mg cholesterol; 739.9 mg sodium

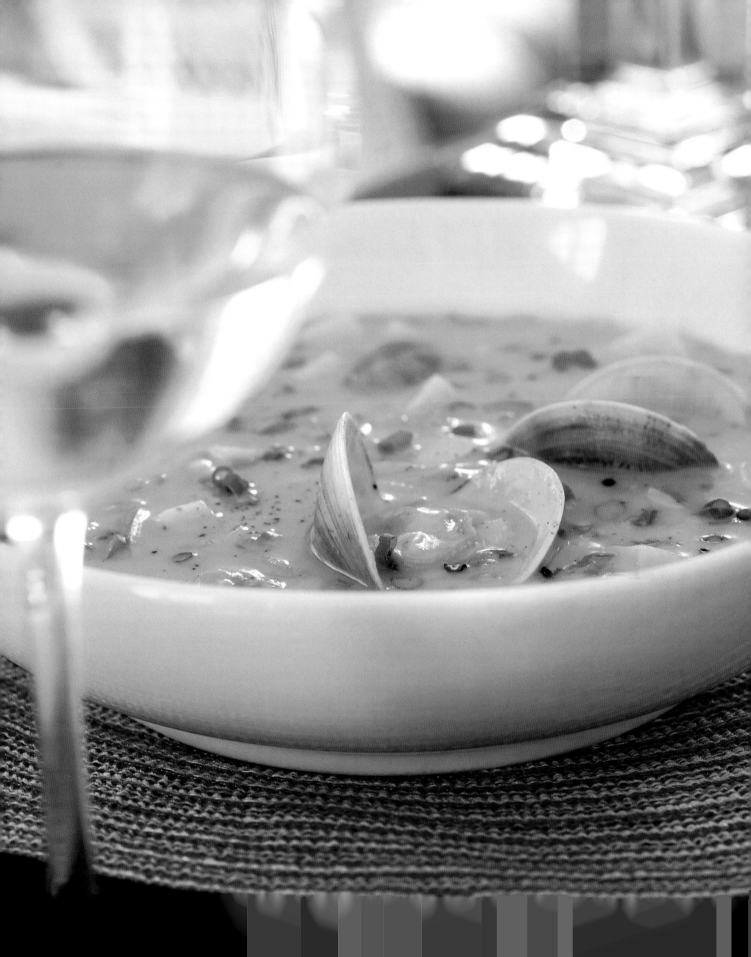

All-in-One Spicy Shrimp and Brown Rice Jambalaya

Ingredients

1 tablespoon (15 ml) olive oil

3 links (each 4 ounces, or 115 g) hot Italian turkey sausage, sliced into ¼-inch-thick (6-mm-thick) rounds

1 yellow onion, chopped

4 large cloves garlic, minced

2 stalks celery, thinly sliced

1 small red bell pepper, seeded and chopped

1 small green bell pepper, seeded and chopped

1 can (15 ounces, or 425 g) whole tomatoes, undrained

1 can (14 ounces, or 400 g) diced tomatoes in sauce, undrained

Pinch of Sucanat or sugar

2 cups (475 ml) chicken broth, plus more as needed

2 bay leaves

1 teaspoon sweet paprika

¾ teaspoon thyme

½ teaspoon oregano

½ teaspoon basil

½ teaspoon onion powder

½ teaspoon salt

½ teaspoon fresh-ground black pepper

½ to 1 teaspoon cayenne pepper, to taste (or more for more heat)

½ teaspoon red pepper flakes, or to taste

1 cup (190 g) parboiled brown rice

½ lemon, optional

1 pound (455 g) medium fresh shrimp, shelled and deveined

⅔ cup (67 g) sliced scallion

From Dr. Jonny: "Jambalaya and a crawfish pie and fillet gumbo." That phrase comes from a song by Hank Williams celebrating the famous creole dishes that originated in the French Quarter of New Orleans—truly a traditional American comfort food if there ever was one! But jambalaya is usually made with heavy sausage and instant white rice, about which the less said the better. Our version substitutes a small amount of turkey sausage and parboiled brown rice. The parboiling makes cooking quicker, but you still get more fiber and nutrients than you ever would with the white rice version. We also loaded this baby up with richly colored bell peppers, a terrific source of vitamins (like vitamin C and vitamin A) as well as fiber and the eye-friendly carotenoids, lutein, and zeaxanthin, and of course, seafood for extra protein ("crawfish pie"). Flavorful and spicy—this very satisfying dish will make you sweat a bit. But isn't that the whole point?

In a large Dutch oven, heat the oil over medium heat. Add the sausage and cook for about 10 minutes. Add the onion and cook for 2 minutes. Add the garlic, celery, and peppers, stirring to combine, and cook for about 5 minutes or until the veggies just start to soften and the sausage is browned. Pour in the whole tomatoes and break them up into smaller pieces with a spatula or spoon. Add the diced tomatoes, Sucanat, and broth, stirring to combine. Add the bay leaves, paprika, thyme, oregano, basil, onion powder, salt, peppers, and pepper flakes, and stir to combine. Increase the heat and bring just to a boil. Decrease the heat, stir in the rice, cover, and cook, keeping it just under a simmer, for 30 to 45 minutes, or until the rice and veggies are soft and most of the liquid is absorbed. Lower the heat or add more broth if the jambalaya starts to boil. If the mixture gets too dry, add more broth (or use tomato juice) to keep it moist. Squeeze the lemon into the jambalaya and gently fold in the shrimp and scallions. Cook for 1 to 3 minutes, or until the shrimp are just cooked through. Adjust the seasonings, if necessary.

Yield: about 8 servings

Per Serving: 398.7 calories; 13.4 g fat (29% calories from fat); 24.3 g protein; 50.2 g carbohydrate; 5.4 g dietary fiber; 120.3 mg cholesterol; 914.7 mg sodium

From Chef Jeannette

Time-Saver Tip: To save time preparing fresh shrimp, buy shelled and cleaned frozen shrimp. No need to thaw before adding—just add an extra minute or so to the shrimp cooking time.

Savory, Protein-Rich Chicken and Shrimp Paella

Ingredients

1 cup (190 g) short-grain brown rice

2½ cups (570 ml) chicken broth

¼ teaspoon saffron threads

¼ teaspoon turmeric, optional

2 tablespoons (28 ml) olive oil, divided

1 link (4 ounces, or 115 g) spicy chicken sausage

¾ pound (340 g) boneless, skinless chicken thighs, chopped into bite-size pieces

¾ pound (340 g) medium shrimp, peeled and deveined

1 large yellow onion, chopped

2 cloves garlic, crushed and chopped

½ pound (225 g) mushrooms, stemmed and chopped (cremini or portobello work well)

¼ cup (60 ml) dry sherry

1 red bell pepper, seeded and chopped

3 large, ripe heirloom tomatoes, chopped

1 teaspoon smoked Spanish paprika (sweet or hot, to taste)

½ teaspoon each salt and fresh-ground black pepper

¼ to ½ teaspoon cayenne pepper, to taste

1 cup (130 g) frozen baby peas

From Dr. Jonny: Paella is a basic dish in traditional Spanish cuisine. Usually, you sauté the vegetables and meat till they're cooked through, then you add water, followed by rice. Assuming you use the right ingredients, it can be one of the healthiest one-pot dishes on Earth. Problem is, most paella is filled with pork sausage (about which the less said the better) or chourico, and made with white rice. Here, we substituted lean chicken sausage and chicken thighs for the low-quality meat. We used brown rice instead of the more typical arborio, which changes the texture somewhat, but adds more fiber and vitamins. We kept added fats to a minimum as well, and spiced the whole thing up with vitamin C–rich peppers and antioxidant-rich mushrooms. Yes, it takes some time. Yes, it's a labor of love. Yes, it's worth it.

Note: Traditional paella is usually seasoned with saffron, which adds flavor, scent, and a beautiful color to the final dish.

Combine the rice, broth, saffron, and turmeric in a large saucepan and bring to a boil over high heat. Stir once, reduce the heat, cover, and simmer for about 45 minutes, or until the rice is tender but some liquid remains in the pot.

While the rice is cooking, preheat the oven to 400°F (200°C, or gas mark 6).

In a large Dutch oven, add 1 tablespoon (15 ml) of the olive oil and heat over medium-high heat.

Remove the sausage from the casing and crumble into the pan. Cook for about 2 minutes. Add the chicken pieces and cook for 1 to 2 minutes, turning occasionally, until browned on all sides and just cooked through. Remove from the pan and set aside.

Add the shrimp to the Dutch oven and cook for about 1 minute, or until they just turn pink. Remove from the pan and set aside with the chicken.

Add the remaining 1 tablespoon (15 ml) olive oil and onion and cook for 3 to 4 minutes, or until the onion has softened. Add the garlic and mushrooms and cook about 3 to 4 minutes, or until the mushrooms have released their juices. Add the sherry and cook until it is mostly evaporated. Reduce the heat, add the bell pepper, and cook for 3 minutes. Add the tomatoes, paprika, salt, and peppers, and cook, stirring frequently, until the tomatoes have started to break down and all the veggies are relatively soft. Fold in the rice and extra liquid until well combined. Adjust the seasonings, if necessary. Pour the peas over the top and bake in the oven for about 10 minutes.

Yield: about 6 generous servings

Per Serving: 355.6 calories; 10.1 g fat (25% calories from fat); 30 g protein; 36.1 g carbohydrate; 4.2 g dietary fiber; 136.4 mg cholesterol; 685.1 mg sodium

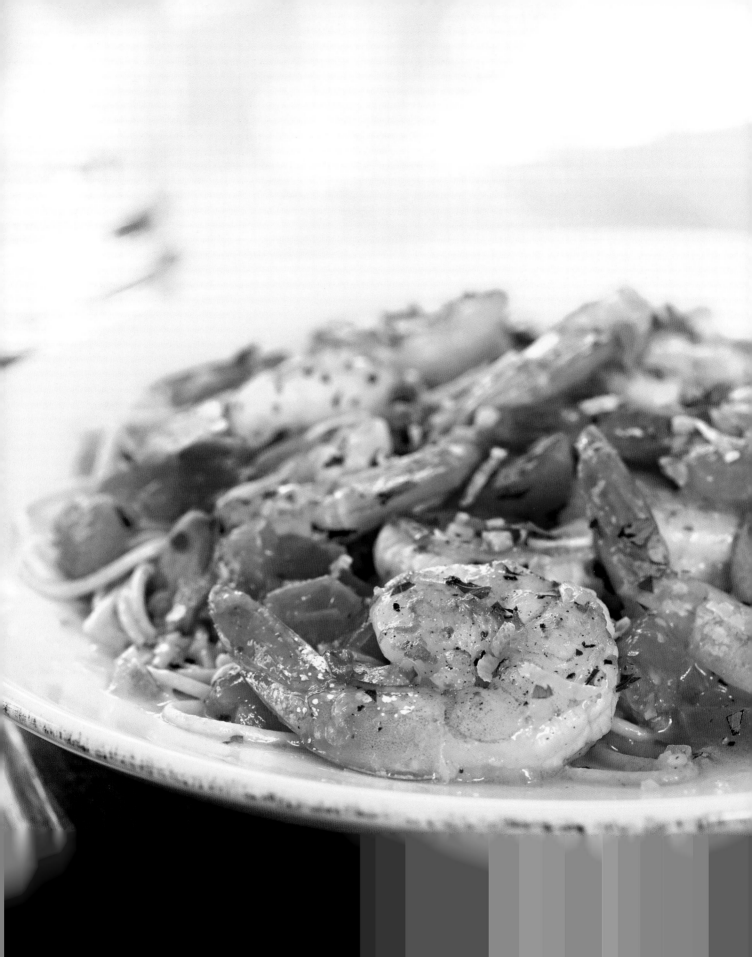

Superfresh and Lemony Olive Oil–Rich Shrimp Scampi

Ingredients

3 tablespoons (45 ml) olive oil, divided

Juice of 1 lemon, divided, optional

3 large cloves garlic, minced, divided

1/4 teaspoon red pepper flakes, optional

1 pound (455 g) large fresh shrimp, shelled and deveined

12 ounces (340 g) fresh whole-wheat fettuccini

Salt and fresh-ground black pepper, to taste

2 large shallots, finely chopped

1 large ripe heirloom tomato, diced

1 teaspoon lemon zest

1/3 cup (80 ml) dry white wine

2 tablespoons (8 g) chopped fresh parsley

From Dr. Jonny: According to the excellent website FoodTimeLine .org, the term *scampi* actually has two meanings—the name of a shrimp and the name of the dish. Shrimp scampi actually became popular right after World War II, when many Italian dishes went mainstream. Though there are lots of ways to make scampi, most recipes call for jumbo shrimp, olive oil, garlic, and parsley. Every scampi dish I've tasted in American restaurants pretty much swims in butter or olive oil or both, and that much fat really ups the calories in the dish. So we dropped the butter completely and marinated the shrimp for a bit to boost the over-all flavor. Fresh ripe tomatoes plus the always-delightful fresh parsley keeps this dish feeling light and summery. We used fresh whole-wheat pasta—higher in fiber and nutrients than the typical flabby white kind. The seafood sauce is light and refreshing and the dish won't break the calorie bank. Fun fact: According to *The Encyclopedia of American Food and Drink* (New York: Lebhar-Friedman, 1999), the true scampo (scampi is the plural) of Italy is a small lobster or prawn, of the family Nephropidae, which in America is called a *lobsterette*.

Optional marinating step: In a glass storage dish, whisk together 1 table-spoon (15 ml) of the olive oil, juice from 1/2 lemon, 1 clove of the minced garlic, and the red pepper flakes. Add the shrimp, toss to coat well, and mar-inate in the refrigerator for 30 minutes to 1 hour. Drain and use as directed.

Bring a large pot of lightly salted water to a boil. Fresh whole-grain pasta will only take about 2 minutes to cook, so put it into the water just before the shrimp is ready so you can drain it and immediately add the pre-pared scampi.

Heat the remaining 2 tablespoons (28 ml) olive oil in a medium sauté pan over medium heat. Add the marinated shrimp, season lightly with salt and pepper, and sauté for 1 to 2 minutes, until they begin to turn pink, flipping them occasionally. Add the remaining 2 cloves garlic and sauté for 30 seconds. Remove the shrimp from the pan and set aside. Add the shal-lots and cook for 2 to 3 minutes, until starting to soften. Add the tomato and cook for 1 minute. Add the remaining lemon juice, zest, and white wine, bring to a light simmer, and cook for a couple of minutes, or until the wine is greatly reduced. Return the shrimp to the pan and simmer until they are cooked through but still tender, just a minute or two. Season lightly with salt and pepper and toss with the parsley. Serve over the hot pasta.

Yield: 4 servings

Per Serving: 680.1 calories; 13.7 g fat (18% calories from fat); 41.3 g protein; 103.8 g carbohydrate; 1.8 g dietary fiber; 172.4 mg cholesterol; 203.6 mg sodium

Higher-Protein, Lower-Cal Creamy Fettuccini Alfredo

Ingredients

8 ounces (225 g) whole-grain fettuccini (our favorite for nutrition and mouthfeel is Barilla Plus)

12 ounces (340 g) broccoli florets

2 tablespoons (28 g) butter

1 onion, finely chopped

3 cloves garlic, minced

12 ounces (340 g) soft silken tofu (or evaporated low-fat milk plus 2 tablespoons, or 16 g, flour)

1 cup (235 ml) chicken broth

1½ teaspoons (8 g) organic chicken Better Than Bouillon

⅓ cup (33 g) freshly grated Parmesan cheese, divided

½ teaspoon fresh-ground black pepper, or to taste

¼ cup (28 g) sundried tomato strips (if in oil, well drained; if dry, plumped for 10 minutes in warm water and well drained)

¼ cup (10 g) slivered fresh basil, optional (or 1 teaspoon dried)

From Chef Jeannette

Even Healthier: To boost the protein content of this dish even more, add 1 to 2 cups (225 to 450 g) cooked shredded chicken or small cooked or frozen shrimp during the last 2 minutes of cooking.

From Dr. Jonny: Creamy, delicious fettuccini Alfredo tops many a list of favorite comfort foods, including my own. But calories? Fuggedaboudit. Restaurant versions are particularly scary—a lunch-size portion at most restaurants tips the scale at approximately 900 calories, and the average dinner size is more than twice that amount! (And that's without adding bread, Parmesan cheese, an appetizer, dessert, or wine. Get my drift?) But who wants to give up fettuccini Alfredo? Not me. So we improved the overall nutritional impact by substituting Barilla Plus pasta for the fat white noodles. And with one simple substitution—silken tofu for the cream base—we upped the protein and reduced the calories. For that rich flavor we're all looking for we used chicken broth, Parmesan cheese, and a hint of butter. Voilà. Add onion for sulfur and antioxidants, a bunch of lightly steamed broccoli for fiber and cancer-fighting plant chemicals known as indoles, sundried tomatoes to make the flavor pop (and add still more antioxidants in the bargain), and you're in business! Enjoy!

Cook the pasta until al dente according to package directions. Reserve ½ cup (120 ml) of the cooking liquid.

Steam the broccoli over boiling water for 2 to 3 minutes until tender-crisp, drain, and set aside.

In a large skillet, melt the butter over medium heat. Add the onion and sauté for about 5 minutes or until soft. Add the garlic and sauté for 1 minute.

While the onion is cooking, add the tofu to a food processor and blend until creamy and smooth. Add the chicken broth and Better Than Bouillon and process until well mixed. Stir in ¼ cup (25 g) of the Parmesan cheese. Pour the tofu cream into the skillet with the onions and garlic. Sprinkle in the pepper, add the sundried tomatoes, and simmer until hot and the flavors are well combined, 2 to 4 minutes. Stir in the broccoli and basil and remove from the heat. Add the sauce to the pasta, to taste, and toss to combine, thinning with a small amount of the pasta water, if necessary, to coat well. Sprinkle with the remaining Parmesan and serve immediately.

Yield: 4 servings

Per Serving: 399.6 calories; 12 g fat (27% calories from fat); 22.6 g protein; 56.1 g carbohydrate; 1.2 g dietary fiber; 22.6 mg cholesterol; 752.1 mg sodium

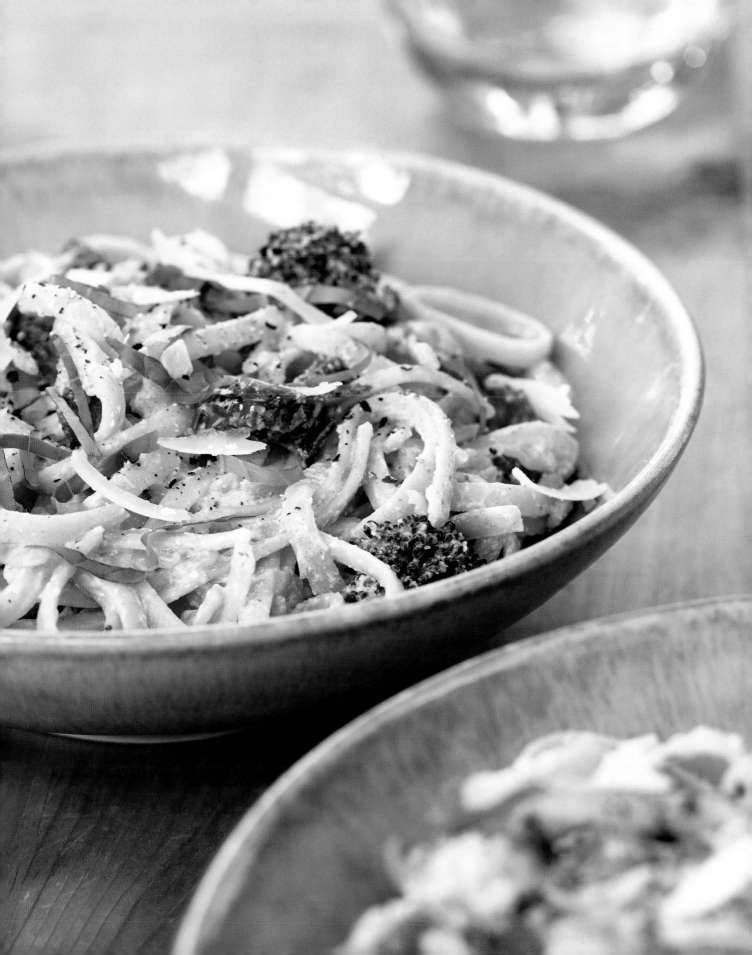

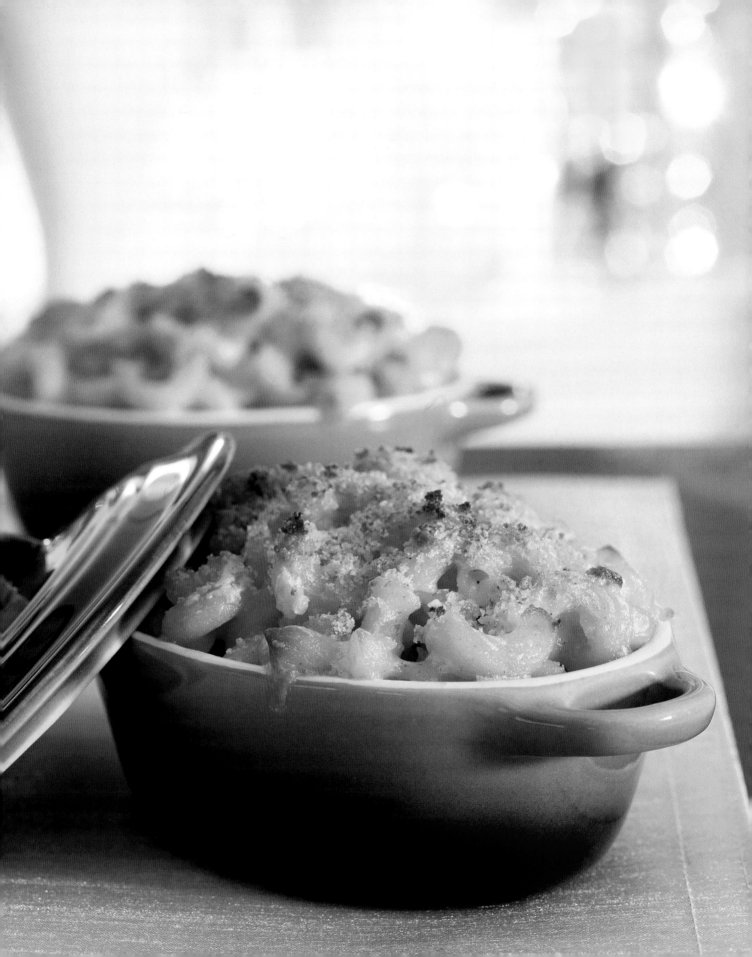

Madeover Mac and Cheese—a Calcium and Vitamin D Bonanza

From Dr. Jonny: Anja Christy, our top weight loss coach on www .jonnybowden.com, is fond of telling audiences that when she met me eight years ago, she thought mac and cheese out of a box was a fine healthy meal. At the very least, the familiar box is a popular American family favorite, but healthy? Not so much. High in sodium and calories, most popular versions also include a ton of artificial ingredients (you didn't think that scary orange color was natural, did you?), and the macaroni is almost always the most processed of white pastas, high in glycemic impact and low in nutrition. Our makeover version uses a whole-grain pasta so smooth your family will never notice the difference. It's high in both fiber and protein, two elements sorely lacking in the boxed version. Chef Jeannette also uses reasonable amounts of fresh whole cheese (not powdered "cheese food") that is high in both calcium and vitamin D. And if you really want to reduce the total calorie count even further, choose the low-fat versions with little loss of taste or satisfaction.

Ingredients

10 ounces (280 g) whole-grain Barilla elbow noodles
Cooking spray
2 tablespoons (28 g) butter
2 cups (475 ml) milk (low-fat cow's or plain, unsweetened soy or almond)
2 tablespoons (16 g) whole-wheat pastry flour
1/2 teaspoon salt
1/4 teaspoon nutmeg
1 1/2 teaspoons (4.5 g) dry mustard
1/2 teaspoon white pepper
1 cup (115 g) grated sharp Cheddar cheese (choose low-fat to reduce calories)
1 cup (115 g) grated Monterey Jack cheese (choose low-fat to reduce calories)
3/4 cup (90 g) whole-wheat bread crumbs
3 tablespoons (20 g) ground flaxseed
1/4 cup (25 g) fresh-grated Parmesan cheese

In a large pot, cook the pasta until al dente according to package directions, reserving 1/4 cup (60 ml) of the cooking liquid. Drain, rinse, and set aside in the empty cooking pot with 1/4 cup (60 ml) reserved liquid to prevent sticking.

While the pasta is cooking, preheat the oven to 400°F (200°C, or gas mark 6). Lightly oil a medium casserole dish with cooking spray.

Melt the butter in a medium saucepan over low heat. Add the milk and warm for 2 minutes. Whisk in the flour, salt, nutmeg, mustard, and pepper. Stir in the cheese until well mixed. Remove from the heat and spoon the cheese mixture over the pasta (in the cooking pot), folding gently to combine well. Transfer the pasta mixture to the prepared casserole dish and sprinkle with the bread crumbs, flaxseed, and Parmesan. Bake for 30 to 35 minutes, or until bubbly and lightly browned on top.

Yield: about 6 servings
Per Serving: 483.5 calories; 23.7 g fat (43% calories from fat); 22.8 g protein; 51.6 g carbohydrate; 7.6 g dietary fiber; 56.9 mg cholesterol; 636.8 mg sodium

From Chef Jeannette

To make this gluten-free, substitute rice pasta for the Barilla noodles (we like Tinkyada brand), and just undercook them by about 3 minutes so they will hold their shape when baked.

Even Healthier: To improve the nutritional impact of this tasty, satisfying dish even more, add 1 pound (455 g) lean ground turkey. This will both increase the protein content and lower the total glycemic load of your meal. Cook the turkey in a large nonstick skillet over medium-high heat for 8 to 10 minutes, or until cooked through and all the pink is gone. Drain well and fold into the cheese mixture just before combining it with the pasta.

Chuck's Healthy Eggplant Parm

From Dr. Jonny: Eggplant Parmesan is a treat, but that breading, deep-frying, and excess cheese tends to dominate any discussion of the health benefits of this terrific vegetable. You can do better. We lightened up on the heavy breading by substituting a small amount of whole-wheat pastry flour, and cut back on the cheese, leaving just enough to make it taste great but not so much that you forget there's eggplant under there! Our version uses a roasted, fresh tomato sauce and plenty of the main attraction: eggplant, a vegetable that's reasonably high in fiber and ridiculously low in calories (how does 35 calories per cup sound to you? Are you surprised? I thought so!). In this version, a couple of slices of good-old turkey bacon replaces the pancetta, enriching the flavor substantially without adding many calories. Remember to take the time to drain the eggplant 3 to 12 hours ahead of time—this is "slow food" at its best! Fun fact: Eggplants are a member of the nightshade family of vegetables, along with tomatoes and potatoes. Besides the usual vitamins and minerals, they're also rich in a powerful antioxidant known as nasunin, which functions by scavenging excess iron in the body, basically stopping the formation of certain kinds of free radicals that can damage your cells and DNA. The nasunin is found in the skin of the eggplant, so don't peel it!

From Chef Jeannette

The sauce can be prepared ahead of time, if desired.

This recipe is a makeover of a spectacular comfort-food version by Chuck Hripak, partner of my longtime client and friend Diane Welsch. I worked to preserve the rich complexity of flavor in the roasted sauce, while lightening up significantly on the calories by reducing the cheeses, swapping turkey bacon for pancetta (and removing it!), and sautéing the eggplant instead of deep-frying it.

Ingredients

1 large eggplant, sliced into ³/₈-inch (1-cm) slices

Salt and fresh-ground black pepper, to taste

1 pound (455 g) ripe, red heirloom tomatoes, coarsely chopped

1 yellow onion, diced

¼ cup (10 g) fresh basil, finely chopped

¼ cup (60 ml) olive oil, divided

2 tablespoons (32 g) tomato paste

½ teaspoon Sucanat or sugar

2 slices turkey bacon, optional, for richer flavor

½ cup (120 ml) red wine

1 tablespoon (15 ml) Marsala wine

1 egg

½ cup (120 ml) milk (low-fat cow's or plain, unsweetened soy or almond)

½ cup (63 g) whole-wheat pastry flour

2 cups (300 g) grated part-skim mozzarella

¼ cup (25 g) fresh-grated Parmigiano-Reggiano

¼ cup (25 g) fresh-grated Pecorino Romano

Lightly salt the sliced eggplant and lay the slices in a dish between clean dish towels to remove some of the eggplant's natural liquids. Allow the eggplant to release liquid and drain at room temperature for up to 3 hours, or in the refrigerator for up to 12 hours.

To prepare the sauce, preheat the oven to 450°F (230°C, or gas mark 8).

Place the tomatoes and onion in a 9 x 12-inch (23 x 30-cm) roasting pan. Add the basil, 2½ tablespoons (35 ml) of the olive oil, and salt and pepper to taste, and gently toss to coat. Roast for 20 minutes, turning twice while cooking. After 20 minutes, increase the heat to broil and cook just until the tomatoes begin to brown. Remove from the oven and transfer the mixture to a medium saucepan over medium heat. Add the tomato paste, Sucanat, bacon, and wines. Cook until most of the liquid has evaporated or been absorbed, and the sauce is medium thick. Remove the bacon and discard. Remove the pan from the heat and set aside.

Whisk the egg and milk together in a pie plate (or shallow bowl).

Whisk the flour and salt and pepper, to taste, together in a second pie plate.

Heat the remaining 1½ tablespoons (25 ml) olive oil in a large nonstick sauté pan over medium heat.

Dredge the sliced eggplant in the egg-and-milk mixture, then lightly coat the tops and bottoms with the flour mixture. Sauté the eggplant on both sides until lightly browned. Remove the eggplant from the pan and place on paper towels to remove excess oil.

To bake, preheat the oven to 375°F (190°C, or gas mark 5).

Coat the bottom of a 9 x 12-inch (23 x 30-cm) baking dish with a thin layer of sauce. Make layers of eggplant and mozzarella with 1 tablespoon (5 g) each of Parmigiano-Reggiano and Romano, and sauce to cover. Top with the remaining cheeses. Bake for 30 minutes, or until the top layer of cheese is melted and lightly browned.

Yield: 12 servings

Per Serving: 188.1 calories; 11.2 g fat (52% calories from fat); 10.3 g protein; 10.8 g carbohydrate; 2.8 g dietary fiber; 39.9 mg cholesterol; 304 mg sodium

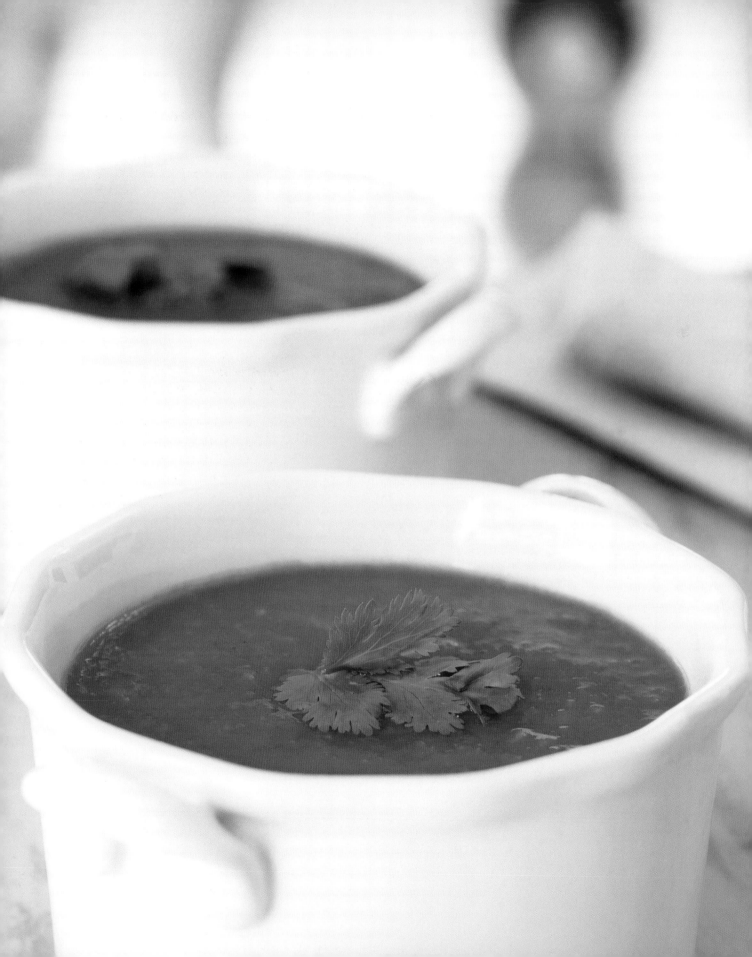

Ingredients

1 tablespoon (15 ml) olive oil

1 yellow onion, chopped

²/₃ cup (75 g) prepared shredded carrots (or grated fresh)

1 stalk celery, sliced into 3 pieces

2 cups (475 ml) low-sodium chicken or vegetable broth

1 can (28 ounces, or 795 g) crushed tomatoes

1 tablespoon (15 ml) red wine vinegar

1 teaspoon Sucanat, sugar, or xylitol, or to taste

½ teaspoon each salt and fresh-ground black pepper

¾ cup (175 ml) plain unsweetened soy or rice milk (or low-fat cow's)

3 tablespoons (3 g) chopped cilantro, optional

From Chef Jeannette

Even Healthier: For more protein and a creamier consistency, substitute ½ cup (115 g) blended silken tofu for the ¾ cup (175 ml) milk.

Tangy, No-Cream of Tomato Soup

From Dr. Jonny: Chef Jeannette reminded me of how creamy tomato soup brings back memories of being home from school with a winter bug—deeply soothing and satisfying, and associated with love. But the regular kind is full of calories from all that cream, not to mention that if you get it from a can it's a sodium nightmare. Make it better by dumping the cream and choose vegan milks for the lowest calorie count. You'd be surprised at how little richness gets lost with this substitution. Fun fact: Tomatoes are filled with a powerful antioxidant known as lycopene. According to the American Cancer Society, "People who have diets rich in tomatoes, which contain lycopene, appear in some studies to have a lower risk of certain types of cancer, especially cancers of the prostate, lung, and stomach."

Heat the oil in a large soup pot over medium heat. Add the onion, carrots, and celery and cook for 6 to 7 minutes, or until the vegetables have started to soften, but before the onion browns. Add the broth, tomatoes, vinegar, Sucanat, salt, and pepper, increase the heat, and bring to a low, steady boil for 15 minutes, or until all the vegetables are very tender. Remove the celery and discard. Using an immersion blender (or regular blender or food processor), purée the soup until mostly smooth. Stir in the milk and simmer for 1 to 2 minutes until the soup is hot. Stir in the cilantro and adjust the seasonings, if necessary.

Yield: 4 servings

Per Serving: 163 calories; 5.6 g fat (31% calories from fat); 7.9 g protein; 23.4 g carbohydrate; 5.2 g dietary fiber; 3.7 mg cholesterol; 978.3 mg sodium

Frozen, Fresh, or Canned?

Fresh fruits and vegetables are usually your best choice, but not always.

Sound confusing? It really isn't.

See, when a vegetable's just been pulled out of the ground that morning and finds its way to your table by the afternoon, you've hit the nutritional bull's-eye. All those fabulous vitamins and minerals are intact, and—assuming you've harvested the vegetable at the height of its readiness—you've got all the wonderful protective plant chemicals (also known as phytonutrients) available to do their work in your body. Same thing, of course, with fruit. Pluck an apple from a tree and bite right in—that's the way nature intended it.

But—yes, there's a but—fresh isn't always really as fresh as it seems.

When you go to the supermarket to buy produce, that stuff has probably been sitting around for a fair amount of time. Even if it just came in that day, it's probably spent a few days on a truck being transported from the farm where it was grown to the supermarket where you buy it. Every day that passes between harvesting and eating diminishes the nutritional value of the fruit or vegetable—not a ton, mind you, but still it adds up. Cutting up the veggies or fruits also reduces the amount of certain vitamins (like vitamin C, for example), so those little bags of precut carrots and apples are a little less potent than when they're eaten as soon as they're cut.

Does this mean you shouldn't buy fresh? Of course it doesn't. Fresh is the way to go, but just be aware that "fresh" may have been sitting around for a week or more. If you can get locally grown stuff, like at a farmers' market, you reduce the odds that it's been traveling for a week from Florida or California, or wherever it was grown, and then sitting on your grocer's shelf for a few days after that.

This is why frozen fruits and vegetables are such a good nutritional deal. Picked or plucked at the height of their ripeness, they're usually flash frozen right when you'd want to be eating them—and the freezing locks in all the nutritional goodies so they're ready for you just when you want them.

You should feel perfectly safe choosing either fresh (again, be sure it's really fresh) or frozen. What you should not do is choose canned. (There are exceptions and I'll get to them in a minute.)

Most canned vegetables are soggy and overcooked, and what's inside the can rarely resembles what a real vegetable looks like or tastes like. (Want proof? Try canned string beans. Ugh.) Canned vegetables are almost invariably loaded with sodium (read the label—it'll scare you.) And canned fruits, like "fruit salad," are chock-full of added syrups and sugar.

The exceptions to the no-canned rule are pumpkin, beans, and pineapple. Pumpkin is just a terrific vegetable and it's hard to get except at holidays, plus it's a bear to prepare. And there are a number of canned beans (chickpeas, black beans, kidney, and navy beans) that are awfully good, including organic and low-sodium versions (though if you'd prefer to cook them on your own that's fine with me!). And while pineapple is always best fresh, the canned (or frozen) kind is a very decent second. Note: Watch out for added sugar in some brands of baked beans, and always buy any fruits canned in water or 100 percent juice only, never in syrup.

Ingredients

1 tablespoon (15 ml) olive oil

⅓ leek, tender whites and greens, carefully cleaned and thinly sliced (about ¾ cup, or 75 g)

3 cups (710 ml) low-sodium vegetable broth

¼ cup (60 g) plain low-fat Greek yogurt

1 small clove garlic, minced

2 teaspoons (10 ml) fresh-squeezed lemon juice

2 tablespoons (6 g) minced fresh chives

1 pound (455 g) fresh sweet peas (or frozen baby peas)

Salt and fresh-ground black pepper, to taste

¼ cup (60 ml) low-fat evaporated skim milk

Pork-Free Fresh Pea Soup

From Dr. Jonny: I know I'm going to get in trouble with some readers for saying this, but I won't eat pork. While the factory farming of animals like chickens and cows is barbaric and horrible, the treatment of pigs, whose intelligence and sociability is on a par with dogs, is possibly the worst of all, and too cruel to contemplate. So call me a tree-hugger if you like, but I can't bring myself to eat pork, at least until someone finds a way to raise pigs in a truly humane fashion. All of which is a long-winded way of explaining why we ditched the big old hambone in this comfort food favorite, but I can assure you that you won't miss it. Made with fresh peas, this light and lovely soup is a nutrient-loaded, superfresh counterpart to traditional split peas. Peas, by the way, are a nutritional heavyweight. They contain a generous amount of protein and fiber, quite a bit of vitamin A, plus calcium, potassium, choline, and a nice helping of lutein and zeaxanthin, two nutrients that are essential for the health of the eyes. We replaced the high-calorie cream that usually forms the base of this soup with low-fat evaporated skim milk so you can eat more of it for the same number of calories! Luscious, low-cal, and high in fiber, this is the poster child for healthy comfort food.

Heat the oil in a large saucepan over medium heat. Add the leeks and cook for 3 to 4 minutes, or until beginning to soften. Add the broth, increase the heat to high, and bring to a boil. Reduce the heat and simmer for about 15 minutes, or until the leeks are very tender.

While the leeks are cooking, in a small bowl, mix together the yogurt, garlic, lemon juice, and chives until well combined. Set aside.

Add the peas, salt, and pepper, return to a boil, reduce the heat, and simmer until the peas are tender, about 3 minutes. Purée the soup until very smooth using an immersion blender, regular blender, or food processor. Return to low heat and mix in the evaporated milk. Adjust the seasonings, if necessary, and serve each bowl with a dollop of the yogurt garnish.

Yield: 4 servings

Per Serving: 167.3 calories; 5.3 g fat (30% calories from fat); 8 g protein; 19.8 g carbohydrate; 5 g dietary fiber; 5.5 mg cholesterol; 257.5 mg sodium

Smoky Bean Baked Nachos

From Dr. Jonny: Whenever I go out to eat at Mexican restaurants with friends, I'm always amazed at how many nachos they can consume without coming up for air. Personally, I think restaurant nachos can be . . . well, frankly, gross—piles of low-quality ground beef, sour cream, fried chips, and humongous portions. And movie nachos? Please. Weird fake nacho cheese (or should I say "cheese food," which is to cheese what Spam is to meat). We use baked chips, a delicious and flavorful base of pinto beans with smoky chipotle pepper, lots of fresh salsa, and just a smattering of high-quality cheese (not, let me point out, "cheese food"). The result is scrumptious. You still can't eat an entire bowl of them, but you won't go wrong with a decent-size nosh.

Ingredients

2 cans (each 15 ounces, or 425 g) pinto beans, rinsed and drained
⅓ cup (80 ml) chicken or vegetable stock (or water)
¼ cup (65 g) tomato paste
1 to 2 teaspoons chipotle adobo purée, to taste
2 cloves garlic, minced
1¼ teaspoons (3 g) ground cumin
1½ teaspoons (4 g) chili powder
¼ teaspoon salt
12 ounces (340 g) hearty baked corn chips
1 cup (115 g) shredded jack or Cheddar cheese
2 pickled jalapeño peppers, thinly sliced (or more, to taste)
1 cup (260 g) high-quality jarred salsa
⅓ cup (50 g) finely diced avocado
3 tablespoons (45 g) plain low-fat Greek yogurt
¼ cup (4 g) chopped cilantro

Preheat the oven to 350°F (180°C, or gas mark 4).

Combine the beans, stock, tomato paste, adobo, garlic, cumin, chili powder, and salt in a medium saucepan over medium heat and bring to a low simmer. Reduce the heat to low and cook, gently stirring occasionally, for about 10 minutes. Remove from the heat, cool slightly, and partially purée the beans using an immersion wand (or mash with a potato masher). Set aside.

Lay the chips out thickly in a large Dutch oven or casserole dish. Gently spread the beans over the chips, taking care not to crush them. Sprinkle the cheese evenly over the beans. Place the jalapeño slices evenly around the cheese and bake for 8 to 10 minutes, until the cheese is melted. Top with the salsa, avocado, yogurt, and cilantro.

Yield: 4 to 6 servings
Per Serving: 527.5 calories; 22 g fat (37% calories from fat); 18.2 g protein; 66.2 g carbohydrate; 11.6 g dietary fiber; 17.5 mg cholesterol; 1,098.1 mg sodium

From Chef Jeannette

Most large grocery stores carry chipotles in adobo sauce in 6- or 8-ounce (170- or 225-g) cans in the Mexican food section. They are very spicy; a little goes a long way, so start with less and add more if desired. To make the purée, blend the entire contents of the can in a blender or food processor to make a smoky, hot sauce that will keep for several weeks in your refrigerator. Use it to spice up beans, as in this recipe, as well as meats, veggies, or salad dressings.

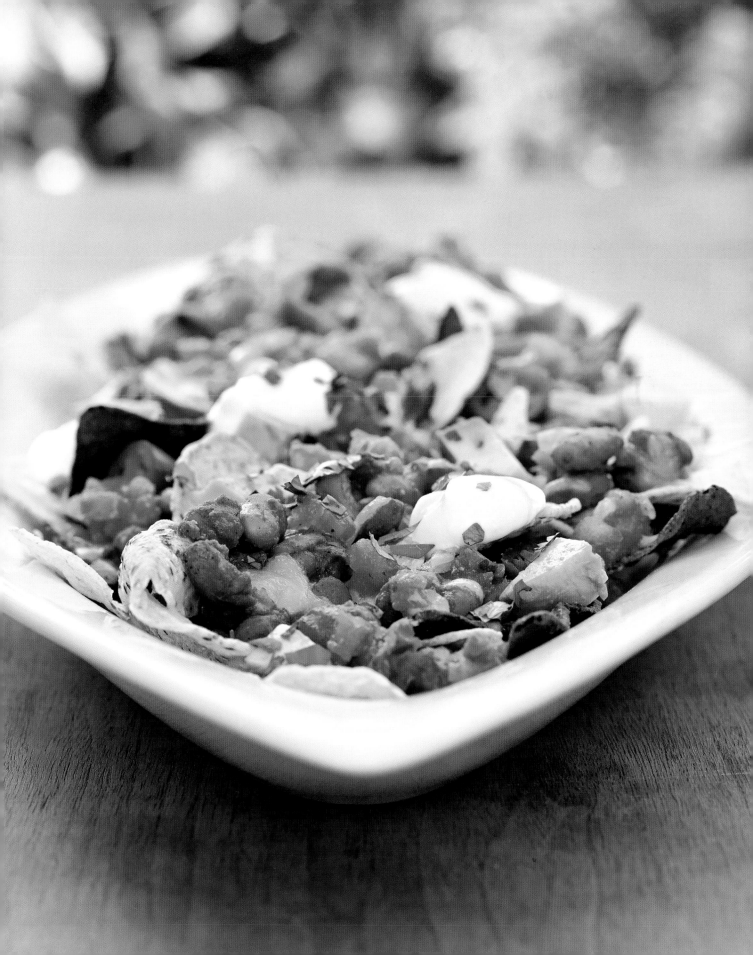

Ingredients

12 ounces (340 g) soba noodles (or other hearty whole-grain pasta)

1/2 cup (130 g) natural peanut butter (without salt, sweetener, or other additives, or use almond butter)

1/4 cup (60 g) tahini

3 cloves garlic, minced

2 to 3 tablespoons (12 to 18 g) minced ginger, to taste

1/4 cup (60 ml) warm water

1 tablespoon (15 ml) peanut oil

1 tablespoon (15 ml) sesame oil (light, toasted, or a combination)

1 to 2 tablespoons (15 to 28 ml) chili oil, to taste

1/4 cup (60 m) low-sodium tamari (or low-sodium soy sauce)

1 tablespoon (13 g) Sucanat, xylitol, or sugar, or more to taste

2 tablespoons (28 ml) apple cider vinegar

2 tablespoons (28 ml) fresh-squeezed lime juice (or omit and add 2 more tablespoons, or 28 ml, cider vinegar)

1 cup (100 g) chopped scallion

1 cup (110 g) shredded or julienned carrot

1 large cucumber, peeled, seeded, and julienned

1/4 cup (35 g) roasted peanuts or toasted sesame seeds

Lower-Oil Spicy Sesame Peanut Noodles

From Dr. Jonny: I am so crazy about peanut noodles it's ridiculous. Unfortunately, they make me fat because they're loaded with sugar and fat (not that the fat is a bad thing, but it sure does add calories). What to do, what to do? How about cutting sugar and fat by a third? That's exactly what Chef Jeannette did without sacrificing any of the sweet, peanut-y flavor and "mouthfeel" of the original. We replaced 1/4 cup (65 g) of the peanut butter with tahini, which gives a better blend of nutrients than just peanut butter alone (it's rich in iron, as well as phosphorus and potassium). Tahini, by the way, is made from sesame seeds, which contain valuable compounds (including sesamin and sesaminol) that enhance vitamin E absorption, improve lipid profiles, and help normalize blood pressure! Then we added extra vegetables for even more nutrients and fiber. Beef up the protein by adding a couple of cups of cooked or chilled shrimp or chicken breast!

Cook the soba noodles until al dente according to package directions. When draining, reserve one-fourth of the cooking liquid and pour it back into the empty cooking pot with the drained noodles to help prevent sticking.

In a food processor, add the peanut butter, tahini, garlic, ginger, water, peanut oil, sesame oil, chili oil, tamari, sweetener, vinegar, and lime juice, and process until smooth, scraping down the sides as necessary.

Toss the prepared noodles with 1 cup (235 ml) of the sauce or to taste, and fold in the scallions, carrots, and cucumber, topping with peanuts or sesame seeds. Serve warm, at room temperature, or cold.

Yield: 4 to 6 servings plus 3/4 cup (175 ml) extra sauce

Per Serving: 765.7 calories; 39.1 g fat (43% calories from fat); 28.6 g protein; 87.5 g carbohydrate; 6 g dietary fiber; 0 mg cholesterol; 1,570 mg sodium

Ingredients

8 ounces (225 g) Barilla Plus thin spaghetti

¼ cup (35 g) pine nuts, plus extra for garnish

1 packed cup (30 g) chopped baby arugula

⅓ cup (13 g) fresh basil

2 tablespoons (10 g) Parmesan cheese (grated or shaved), plus optional extra to finish

¼ teaspoon each salt and fresh-ground black pepper

2 tablespoons (28 ml) balsamic vinegar

¼ cup (60 ml) olive oil, plus more if necessary

2 large, ripe heirloom tomatoes, seeded and chopped

Tender Greens Pesto with Protein-Packed Pasta

From Dr. Jonny: One of the many things that define a comfort food is the associations you have to it. And it's hard to think of pasta without associating it with big family dinners. (I mean, what bachelor or bachelorette whips up huge pots of pasta to eat in front of the television?) So by any definition pasta qualifies as a comfort food. Problem is, it's usually piles of white pasta made with all-purpose white flour. A simple tweak improves it: use Barilla Plus pasta. Barilla Plus is whole-grain, making it higher in fiber, and it's also a high-protein variety. You can cut calories considerably by using a bit less pasta and a bit less cheese, as Chef Jeannette has done here. Fresh basil is one of the great "go-to" spices; it perks everything up. And it's also a source of protective flavonoids, as well as antibacterial compounds from the unique volatile oil that gives basil its characteristic aroma. Add chopped tomatoes for the incredibly potent antioxidant lycopene and punch up the flavors even more with arugula. If you want to make this meal even healthier, add a piece of grilled chicken or fish for more protein. Fun fact: It's estimated that there are more than 350 different shapes and varieties of pasta in Italy, where the average person consumes about 60 pounds of pasta per year; Americans eat about 20 pounds!

Cook the pasta until al dente according to package directions.

While the pasta is cooking, add the pine nuts, arugula, basil, Parmesan, salt, pepper, and vinegar to a food processor and pulse five times or so to break down the greens. Process until well combined and at the desired consistency, scraping down the sides as necessary. Pulse or process briefly as you add the olive oil in a thin stream to incorporate. Pesto should be wet enough to easily disburse in the pasta, but not puddle.

Gently toss the pasta with the pesto, to taste. Add the extra Parmesan. Fold in the chopped tomatoes, sprinkle with the additional pine nuts, and serve.

Yield: 4 servings

Per Serving: 421 calories; 21.5 g fat (44% calories from fat); 10.4 g protein; 47.6 g carbohydrate; 3.1 g dietary fiber; 2.2 mg cholesterol; 194.7 mg sodium

From Chef Jeannette

To Store Extra Crust: Roll it into balls for individual crusts, lightly oil the surfaces, and wrap them tightly in plastic wrap for refrigerator storage. Most sources advise using refrigerated dough within 24 hours, but others say the yeast will hold for 2 or 3 days. To freeze, follow the same process, but double-wrap in freezer-safe plastic and store for up to one month. Thaw frozen dough in the refrigerator overnight, then allow refrigerated dough to rest on the counter at room temperature for 1 hour to lose its chill (it's much harder to roll out cold dough).

Variations: Try a red pizza sauce and light sprinkling of grated, part-skim mozzarella on your grilled pizza in place of the pesto and tomatoes. Use other sautéed or grilled veggies to top, such as spinach, mushrooms, onions, or bell peppers, but use sparingly so as not to overload the thin crust.

Whole-Grain Home-Grilled Pizza

From Dr. Jonny: If anybody's counting, pizza is right up there on Dr. Jonny's top ten comfort food indulgences, along with chocolate chip cookies, rice pudding, bread pudding, chocolate pudding, and ice cream. (There, I've said it! Now we have no secrets!) And the thing of it is, pizza isn't really inherently unhealthy. In fact, one highly publicized study from Harvard Medical School found that four foods were associated with a low risk of developing prostate cancer, and pizza with tomato sauce was one of them! (Although it was pizza as a food that was associated with the lower risk, researchers suspect that it was the cooked tomatoes that accounted for the results, particularly the lycopene found in tomatoes.) That said, you can make pizza a lot better than the usual fast-food takeout. Use a fresh, whole-wheat crust, swap out the cheese for delicious pesto, and ditch the processed meats for fresh heirloom tomatoes.

To make the crust: Combine the yeast and water in a small bowl and stir until it dissolves. Set aside.

Spread a thin layer of flour over a smooth surface for kneading: A clean countertop or large cutting board work well. Combine the flour and salt in a large mixing bowl and whisk to combine. Scoop out a well in the middle and gently pour the yeast water into the well, making a little pool. Add the olive oil and slowly work the flour into the liquid. Use a pastry cutter or a fork at first, switching to your hands if the mixture becomes too sticky. As the flour and liquid combine, it will become a dough. Once the dough is formed, turn out of the bowl and onto the floured surface. Knead the flour for 10 to 15 minutes, adding extra flour when it gets too sticky, until the dough becomes very smooth and elastic. It should no longer be sticky; this is important so you can move the crust easily.

Ingredients

Crust

1 package (2¼ teaspoons, or 9 g) active dry
yeast

1½ cups (355 ml) warm water

3½ cups (440 g) white whole-wheat flour,
or 2 cups (250 g) whole-wheat flour and
1½ cups (190 g) unbleached flour, plus
more as needed

1 teaspoon salt

2 tablespoons (28 ml) olive oil, plus extra
for bowl

High-heat oil (avocado or peanut oil work
well)

Topping

3 tablespoons (45 g) fresh pesto, or to taste
(see Tender Greens Pesto recipe on
page 103)

1 or 2 ripe heirloom tomatoes, thinly sliced

1½ tablespoons (7.5 g) fresh-grated
Parmigiano-Reggiano

Coat the surface of a medium bowl with olive oil. When the dough is ready, roll it into a ball and place it in the bowl, rolling it around to coat the whole surface with oil. Lay a dish towel over the top and place the bowl in a warm area to rise for about an hour, or until it doubles in size.

Preheat the grill to high.

Once the dough has risen, flour your surface again, and roll it out. Punch down the dough to deflate it. Knead it for a couple more minutes and then divide it into 4 parts to make 4 medium thin-crust pizzas.

To make one pizza, gently stretch and pull one ball of dough with your hands. Before it begins to tear, lay it on the floured surface and roll it out into a flat oval or a circle (depending on the pan you're using) with a floured rolling pin. Keep rolling it out, coming from different directions, until you have a nice thin crust, ⅛ to ¼ inch (3 to 6 mm) thick. Try to keep the dough from breaking apart or sprouting holes. Store any dough you won't use right away in the refrigerator or the freezer.

Oil a flat baking sheet (no edges) with a high-heat oil and gently lay the crust on the pan. Lift or slide the pizza crust gently from the pan and lay it directly on your preheated grill. Grill the crust for only 1 to 2 minutes, watching carefully to prevent scorching. Remove the crust using a large spatula and flip it over back onto the oiled baking sheet so the grill marks are visible on top.

To make the topping: Spread the pesto on the grilled side in a thin, even layer, arrange the tomato slices on the pesto, top with the grated cheese, and return the pizza to the grill. Cover and cook for another 1 to 2 minutes or so, until the toppings are warmed and the crust is lightly browned and crisp.

After cooking, allow the pizza to cool to desired temperature and then cut it into quarters or eighths.

Yield: 4 servings
Per Serving: 481.4 calories; 7.4 g fat (13% calories from fat); 15.2 g protein; 87.1 g carbohydrate; 4 g dietary fiber; 5.1 mg cholesterol; 699.3 mg sodium

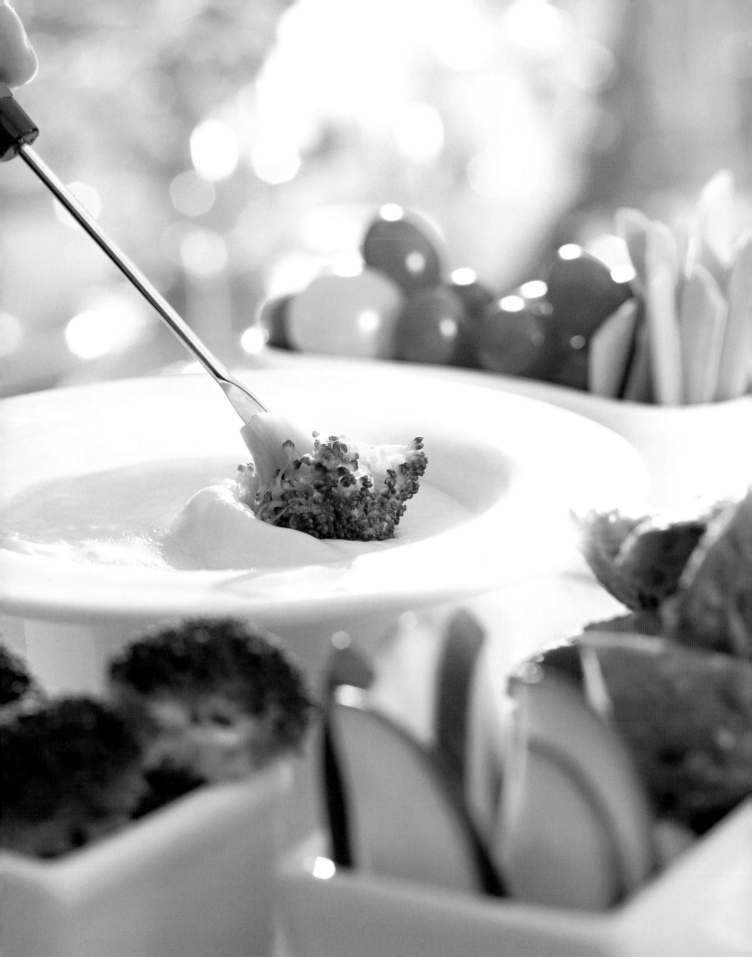

Ingredients

2 cups (240 g) grated Gruyère cheese

2 cups (240 g) grated Cheddar cheese

8 ounces (235 ml) dark beer, plus more
if necessary

1 tablespoon (15 ml) Worcestershire sauce
(organic to avoid high-fructose corn
syrup)

6 dashes hot sauce, or to taste

1½ teaspoons (4.5 g) dry mustard

1 cup (150 g) each sliced carrot sticks,
celery sticks, zucchini sticks, and red,
yellow, or orange bell pepper sticks
(6 inches, or 15 cm, in length)

1 pint (340 g) cherry tomatoes

2 cups (142 g) blanched broccoli florets

2 cups (100 g) cubed sprouted-grain
peasant bread, optional

From Chef Jeannette

If you don't have a fondue pot, you can
warm ingredients on the stove in a large,
nonstick pan and then transfer to a slow
cooker set to high to serve.

Rich Cheesy Crudités Fondue

From Dr. Jonny: Fondue brings me back to my bachelor days as a struggling musician. Back when I was living in New York City and going to Juilliard, fondue was a dish that signaled to all the girls that you were sophisticated. It was easy to make, easy to serve, tasted great, and impressed the ladies. What more could a bachelor ask for? Of course in those days we made it with piles of low-grade cheese and as much white bread as we could stuff down our throats. (Remember, folks, I wasn't thinking about nutrition, I was thinking about looking cool!) Anyway. This twenty-first-century version uses rich cheese and replaces the wads of high-glycemic white Italian bread with loads of fresh raw veggies for dipping. (Believe me, you won't miss the bread when the cheese is this high in quality.) Dark beer adds some extra antioxidants, the red peppers are loaded with vitamin C, and the carrots are stuffed with vitamin A, beta-carotene, and other nutrients. Use a little bit of chewy, fiber-rich sprouted-grain bread if you want a healthy update on the old-fashioned (and unhealthy) version.

Place a heavy ceramic fondue pot on the stovetop over medium heat and add the Gruyère, Cheddar, beer, Worcestershire, hot sauce, and dry mustard, and gently mix. Cook, stirring frequently, until the cheeses have melted and the ingredients have combined thoroughly, about 15 to 20 minutes. If the cheese becomes too thick or begins to separate, add another splash of beer. Transfer the fondue pot to a tabletop warmer and serve with the prepared veggies and bread for dipping.

Yield: 5 to 6 servings
Per Serving: 416.8 calories; 27 g fat (57% calories from fat); 26 g protein; 15.7 g carbohydrate; 2.9 g dietary fiber; 86 mg cholesterol; 851.2 mg sodium

Smoky Hot Whole Grains and Beans Chili

From Dr. Jonny: Chili has been a favorite of mine since the days when I was a musician, traveling the country with various road companies, and stuck in efficiency apartments that weren't exactly ideal for cooking. But you could always open a can of the stuff, or go to the local greasy diner and order it up. Problem was, typical chili has a lot of poor-quality, greasy meat, and the canned stuff is loaded with sodium. Chef Jeannette's version has all the stuff that makes chili healthy and none of the stuff that doesn't. This is a meatless version that still has plenty of protein and fiber courtesy of the quinoa combined with a nice mix of kidney and pinto beans. Onion provides sulfur, so good for the skin, and the red pepper has capsaicin, which is a potent anti-inflammatory that may also help with energy. If that weren't enough, we replaced the sour cream and cheese with something even better—Greek yogurt. It's high in protein and lower in calories and you'll hardly notice the difference. Tip: Garnish the yogurt with the bright flavor of cilantro and citrus to cut down on the naturally smoky heat of this delicious dish.

Ingredients

1 tablespoon (15 ml) olive oil
1 tablespoon (7.5 g) chili powder
1 teaspoon cumin
½ teaspoon coriander
1 small yellow onion, chopped
1 red bell pepper, seeded and chopped
2 cans (each 14.5 ounces, or 410 g) fire-roasted diced tomatoes, undrained
2 cups (475 ml) low-sodium vegetable broth, water, or dark beer
1 can (6 ounces, or 170 g) tomato paste
½ cup (88 g) quinoa, rinsed
1 teaspoon oregano
½ teaspoon salt, or to taste
1 tablespoon (15 g) chipotle adobo purée, or more to taste
1 can (15 ounces, or 425 g) kidney beans, drained and rinsed
1 can (15 ounces, or 425 g) pinto beans, drained and rinsed

Optional Garnish

⅓ cup (77 g) plain low-fat Greek yogurt
⅓ cup (5 g) chopped fresh cilantro
1 tablespoon (15 ml) fresh-squeezed lime juice

In a large Dutch oven, heat the oil over medium heat. Add the chili powder, cumin, and coriander and cook, stirring frequently, for about 1 minute. Add the onion and bell pepper, stir to combine, cover, and cook the vegetables for 5 to 6 minutes, until slightly softened, stirring occasionally. Add the tomatoes, broth, and tomato paste and stir well to combine. Add the quinoa, oregano, salt, and chipotle purée, increase the heat, and bring to a boil. Stir in the beans, reduce the heat, partially cover, and cook for 25 to 30 minutes, or until the grains and vegetables are soft and the chili has thickened slightly.

To make the optional garnish, in a small bowl whisk together the yogurt, cilantro, and lime juice and place a dollop on top of each bowl of chili.

Yield: about 7 servings
Per Serving: 315.5 calories; 4 g fat (13% calories from fat); 10.8 g protein; 49.1 g carbohydrate; 13.8 g dietary fiber; 0 mg cholesterol; 1,047.2 mg sodium

From Chef Jeannette

To make the purée, look for canned chipotle peppers in adobo sauce. They are widely available in the ethnic sections of major supermarkets or Hispanic grocers. Purée the entire contents of the can in the blender until smooth. The remaining purée will keep in your refrigerator for a few weeks or in the freezer for a couple of months. It makes a wonderful smoky and pungent seasoning, and a little goes a long way. Have caution when working with the purée: Don't touch it with bare skin and keep it away from your eyes. The capsaicin in the peppers can really burn.

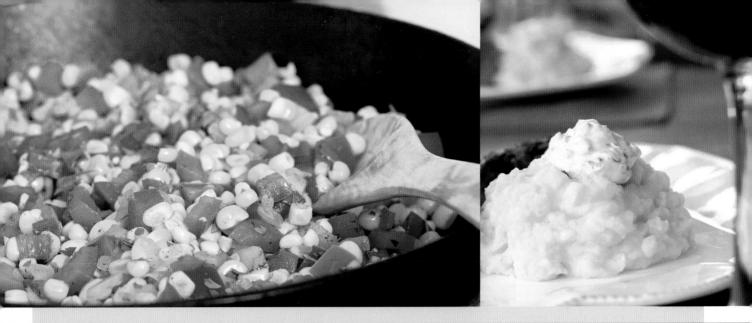

Side Dishes

This section is what I call the "accessory" counter of the cookbook. It's where you'll find a rich array of vegetables, soups, and other goodies that can complement your main dish and make your meal a real expression of your taste and style. Express your creativity by putting them together in unique and unusual ways. (Hint: Mix colors and textures. Remember, presentation counts!) A personal favorite: the Aromatic, Antioxidant-Rich Orange-Sweet Potato Casserole. But that's just me! You're sure to find your own personal favorites.

Two-Corn Cheesie Grits with Roasted Veggies

Nutted Shiitake Brown Rice Pilaf

Sweet-Tart Omega-Rich 3-Bean Salad

Zingy Whole-Grain Broccoli Corn Bread

Nutty, Iron-Rich Creamed Spinach

Not-Your-Grandmother's Green Bean Casserole

Creamy Creamless Skillet Corn

Healthier, Whole-Grain Lemon Veggie Rice

Aromatic, Antioxidant-Rich Orange-Sweet Potato Casserole

Lower-Cal Cheesy Scalloped Potatoes

Creamy Low-Fat Mashed Potatoes

Fluffy Twice-Baked Potatoes with Chèvre and Roasted Shallots

A Lighter Touch: Tangy German Potato Salad

Tender Lower-Fat French Fries

Sweet and Tangy No-Bake, High-Fiber Beans

Whole-Grain Veggie-Rich Macaroni Salad

Light and Bright Waldorf Salad

Tangy Raw Caesar Salad with Whole-Grain Croutons

Lean and Clean Dirty Rice

Lighter Cider Coleslaw

Ingredients

1 teaspoon unrefined corn oil (or olive oil)

3/4 cup (75 g) sliced scallion, whites and greens separated

2 cloves garlic, minced

1 cup (130 g) frozen roasted corn (such as Trader Joe's, or use regular), thawed

1 1/4 cups (295 ml) milk (low-fat cow's or plain, unsweetened soy or almond)

1 1/4 cups (295 ml) water

2/3 cup (85 g) stone-ground corn grits

2 tablespoons (8 g) diced green chiles, drained, optional

1 large roasted red pepper, chopped

1 1/2 teaspoons (7 g) butter

1/2 teaspoon each salt and fresh-ground black pepper

1/3 cup (38 g) grated pepper jack cheese

2 to 4 dashes hot pepper sauce, optional

From Chef Jeannette

You can use jarred prepared roasted peppers, but for best flavor roast your own fresh. See our directions in the Two-Cheese Fit and Flavorful Frittata recipe, page 186.

Two-Corn Cheesie Grits with Roasted Veggies

From Dr. Jonny: I grew up with a deep love of gospel music, jazz, and rhythm and blues. (I am still proud to say that I was actually there when the Temptations, the Miracles, Marvin Gaye, Mary Wells, Martha and the Vandellas, and "Little" Stevie Wonder performed together as the now-legendary Motown Review at the Apollo Theatre in 1962.) And my African-American friends used to talk fondly about "home cooking," which inevitably featured such (to me) esoteric menu items as "grits." Which I came to love (still do). But like a lot of comfort foods, the traditional recipe for this Southern favorite has an awful lot of calories. We do a calorie correction by reducing the amount of butter and cheese. The flavorful addition of scallion and roasted red pepper adds not only color but also an array of nutrients (albeit in small quantities): peppers are rich in vitamin C and onions are a good source of thiamine, riboflavin, magnesium, phosphorus, and copper, and a good source of dietary fiber, vitamin A, vitamin C, vitamin K, folate, calcium, iron, potassium, and manganese. Note: You don't want to use instant grits any more than you want to use instant oatmeal—both have been overly processed and have less fiber than the regular kind (and often added sugar). This slow-cooked version takes a little longer, sure, but believe me, it's worth it.

Heat the oil over medium heat in a medium, heavy-bottomed saucepan. Add the white slices of scallion and sauté for about 2 minutes. Add the garlic and sauté for 1 minute. Stir in the corn and cook for about a minute. Add the milk, water, grits, and chiles, and stir to combine. Bring to a boil over high heat, stir, reduce the heat to low, partially cover, and cook until the mixture has thickened and the grits reach the desired tenderness, 30 to 40 minutes.

Stir in the red pepper during the last few minutes of cooking time. Stir in the butter, salt, pepper, cheese, and hot pepper sauce. Adjust the seasonings. Fold in the green slices of scallion and serve hot.

Yield: 4 to 6 servings

Per Serving: 144.1 calories; 4.5 g fat (28% calories from fat); 5.9 g protein; 20.7 g carbohydrate; 1.7 g dietary fiber; 10.7 mg cholesterol; 444.5 mg sodium

Nutted Shiitake Brown Rice Pilaf

From Dr. Jonny: One thing I learned over the years was that food that comes in a box is rarely good for you. (I know, there are exceptions, but you can count them on the fingers of a three-fingered man!) White rice pilaf isn't one of those exceptions. The box mixes almost always have a ton of sodium and artificial ingredients, which range from the innocuous to the not-so-innocuous (e.g., MSG, or monosodium gluta-mate). Do yourself and your family a favor and make this comfort food from scratch. The texture and crunch come from delicious wild rice plus walnuts. We use a brown rice base for more fiber and added flavor and nutrient-rich shiitake mushrooms with a bit of basil to finish. Fun fact: In a recent study from Penn State researchers, a diet rich in walnuts and walnut oil was found to help the body deal better with stress. The walnuts (and walnut oil) lowered resting blood pressure as well as blood pressure response to stress in the laboratory. Researchers believe this may be due in part to walnuts' high concentration of an omega-3 fatty acid called ALA, or alpha-linolenic acid.

Ingredients

³/₄ cup (140 g) long-grain brown rice

¹/₄ cup (40 g) wild rice

2 cups (475 ml) low-sodium chicken broth

2 teaspoons (10 ml) olive oil

¹/₂ small white onion, finely chopped

¹/₄ cup (30 g) finely chopped celery

4 ounces (115 g) shiitake mushroom caps, julienned

1 teaspoon low-sodium tamari (or low-sodium soy sauce, or ¹/₂ teaspoon salt)

¹/₄ teaspoon fresh-ground black pepper

¹/₄ cup (30 g) chopped roasted unsalted walnuts

2 tablespoons (5 g) slivered basil, optional

Bring the rices and broth to a boil in a medium saucepan over high heat. Stir, reduce the heat, and simmer for 45 to 50 minutes, or until the liquid is absorbed and the rice is tender. Stir, remove from the heat, and fluff with a fork.

At the end of the rice cooking time, heat the oil in a large sauté pan over medium heat. Add the onion and celery and cook for 4 minutes. Push the onion and celery to the outer edges of the pan and add the shiitakes in a single layer in the middle and let them cook, undisturbed, for about 3 minutes. Flip the shiitakes and cook until lightly browned. Stir to mix the veggies and remove from the heat.

In a large bowl combine the rice, vegetable mixture, tamari, and pepper, and gently toss to combine. Fold in the walnuts and basil just before serving.

Yield: about 6 servings

Per Serving: 171.7 calories; 5.8 g fat (29% calories from fat); 6.1 g protein; 27.7 g carbohydrate; 3.7 g dietary fiber; 0 mg cholesterol; 71.7 mg sodium

Ingredients

1 pound (455 g) fresh green beans, halved and ends trimmed

1 can (15 ounces, or 425 g) dark red kidney beans, drained and rinsed

1 can (15 ounces, or 425 g) white kidney beans, drained and rinsed

½ green or red bell pepper, finely chopped

¼ large Vidalia onion, finely chopped

½ cup (120 ml) raw apple cider vinegar

¼ cup (50 g) Sucanat, sugar, or xylitol

⅓ cup (80 ml) flaxseed oil (or olive oil)

¾ teaspoon salt

¼ teaspoon fresh-ground black pepper

From Chef Jeannette

Time-Saver Tip: To save on prep time without a heavy nutrient sacrifice, use 12 to 16 ounces (340 to 455 g) frozen green beans in place of the fresh. Steam them until tender-crisp according to package directions.

Sweet-Tart Omega-Rich 3-Bean Salad

From Dr. Jonny: Back in the '80s when I was a professional musician touring the country with productions including *Joseph and the Amazing Technicolor Dreamcoat*, one thing we'd try to do whenever we were in town for any length of time was see whether we could find a cookout or a picnic (like a fundraiser for the local fire department or something like that). You could always get amazing homemade food, lovingly prepared, and it was always a good way to meet local people. One of the dishes I found consistently at these events, especially all over the Midwest, was three-bean salads. At the time I didn't know any better, but these days I think this great dish could be made so much better without the canned green beans and unneeded sugar. So we went to work! First we used fresh, lightly steamed green beans. Next we used two high-powered legumes, red and white kidney beans, both of which are among the highest fiber-containing foods. Raw bell pepper adds vitamin C and minerals, and onions—well, substantial research has shown that onions are chock-full of anticancer chemicals. Onions contain many members of the flavonoid and phenol family (chemicals that help protect plants against bacteria, fungi, and viruses. They're powerful antioxidants that help prevent cancer by sweeping up cell-damaging rogue molecules called free radicals. And they make your three-bean salad taste even better!). Note: Don't panic about the reduced sugar—we left enough in to get that signature sweet-but-tart tang that makes this dish such a classic comfort food.

Steam the green beans in a large pot for 5 to 10 minutes or until tender-crisp. In a large bowl, combine the green beans, both kinds of kidney beans, bell pepper, and onion.

In a small bowl, whisk together the vinegar, sweetener, flaxseed oil, salt, and pepper.

Dress the beans, to taste, and toss to coat. Let the beans marinate for 3 hours to overnight in the refrigerator, stirring occasionally to recoat. Drain off the excess marinade and serve cold or at room temperature.

Yield: about 6 servings

Per Serving: 287.7 calories; 12.7 g fat (26% calories from fat); 8.8 g protein; 34.9 g carbohydrate; 10.2 g dietary fiber; 0 mg cholesterol; 669 mg sodium

Ingredients

Drizzle of unrefined corn oil

3/4 cup (105 g) stone-ground cornmeal, fine grind

1/4 cup (42 g) whole-wheat pastry flour

1 teaspoon Sucanat, sugar, or xylitol

1 tablespoon (14 g) baking powder

1/2 teaspoon salt

1/3 cup (80 ml) milk (low-fat cow's, or unsweetened vanilla almond or soy milk)

1 egg

2 tablespoons (28 ml) melted butter or unrefined corn oil

1 to 2 tablespoons (9 to 18 g) pickled jalapeño peppers, drained and minced, to taste

1 package (9 ounces, or 255 g) chopped frozen broccoli, thawed and drained well

From Chef Jeannette

Extra helpings freeze like a dream: Cool completely, chill in the refrigerator for at least 2 hours, wrap individual pieces in waxed paper, place them in an airtight resealable freezer bag, and store in the freezer. Thaw overnight and toast lightly to serve.

Zingy Whole-Grain Broccoli Corn Bread

From Dr. Jonny: There are dozens of ways to prepare delicious corn bread: sweet, savory, cakey, or spiced, and there are probably more than a few regional varieties that I've never heard of but are equally great-tasting. Chef Jeannette has opted for a more traditionally Southern-style choice, but in the name of great health, she's made a few tweaks. Number one: Maximize cornmeal while minimizing flour. Number two: Keep the sweetener at a minimum and use just enough to mimic the taste of fresh corn. Number three: Add an egg for extra protein and density. Number four: Add broccoli for a boost of anticancer phytochemicals called isothiocyanates. The jalapeños add a piquant heat—kicky and tasty. Tip: Choose organic corn oil and cornmeal to avoid rampant GMO.

Preheat the oven to 425°F (220°C, or gas mark 7). Lightly coat an 8 x 8-inch (20 x 20-cm) metal baking pan (glass can shatter at this temperature) with corn oil and set aside.

In a large bowl, add the cornmeal, flour, sweetener, baking powder, and salt and whisk to combine well.

In a medium bowl, add the milk, egg, and butter and whisk to combine. Stir in the jalapeños. Pour the wet mixture into the dry and mix gently until just combined. Fold in the broccoli and bake for 18 to 20 minutes, or until a toothpick inserted into the center comes out clean.

Yield: 9 servings

Per Serving: 103.9 calories; 3.7 g fat (31% calories from fat); 3.3 g protein; 15.4 g carbohydrate; 1 g dietary fiber; 30.7 mg cholesterol; 317.8 mg sodium

Ingredients

1 pound (455 g) spinach, stemmed and
    chopped into bite-size pieces

½ cup (115 g) soft silken tofu

2 tablespoons (30 g) tahini

1 tablespoon (15 ml) low-sodium tamari (or
    low-sodium soy sauce)

2 teaspoons (10 ml) fresh-squeezed lemon
    juice

⅛ teaspoon cayenne pepper, optional

2 teaspoons (10 ml) olive oil

2 cloves garlic, minced

From Chef Jeannette

Time-Saver Tip: You can skip cleaning,
chopping, and blanching the spinach if
you use two 10-ounce (280-g) boxes of
thawed, frozen chopped spinach. Just
squeeze against a double-mesh sieve to
remove as much moisture as possible and
follow directions from heating the oil.

Variation: This sauce is great on all
different types of greens. Try it with
collards or kale. Just add a couple more
minutes of blanching time for tougher
leaves.

Nutty, Iron-Rich Creamed Spinach

From Dr. Jonny: There's good news and bad news about creamed
spinach. The good news is it's spinach. The bad news is it's really heavy
on the calories. And let's face it—is it really fair to take this flavorful
veggie superstar and bury it beneath scads of high-calorie dairy? Of
course not. Our version takes a nutty twist on things. We use a bit of
silken tofu to give the dish a shot of low-cal protein and then flavor
it up with a luscious mix of tahini, tamari, and garlic—sounds like
a vaudeville act, doesn't it? Tahini is a thick paste that's made from
ground-up sesame seeds and is rich in B vitamins, protein, and minerals. Okay, it's a different taste than you may be used to for creamed
spinach, but wait until you try it! It's creamy as can be, delicious,
satisfying, and a real nutritional powerhouse.

Blanch the spinach in a large pot of boiling water until wilted, 1 to 2 minutes. Drain and run under very cold water to stop the cooking process.
Drain well and set aside.

In a small bowl whisk the tofu until smooth and creamy. Add the tahini,
tamari, lemon juice, and cayenne and whisk again until well combined
and creamy.

Heat the oil in a large skillet or sauté pan over medium heat. Add the
garlic and cook for about 1 minute. Add the drained greens and toss to
combine. Add the sauce and heat for about 2 minutes, or until well coated
and very hot.

Yield: 4 servings

Per Serving: 113.8 calories; 7.1 g fat (54% calories from fat); 7.2 g protein;
7.8 g carbohydrate; 3.3 g dietary fiber; 0 mg cholesterol; 283.7 mg sodium

Ingredients

Olive oil cooking spray

1 pound (455 g) fresh green beans (French beans or haricots verts are great, if in season), trimmed and cut into 2-inch (5-cm) pieces

2 teaspoons (9 g) butter

2 teaspoons (10 ml) olive oil

4 shallots, chopped

8 ounces (225 g) sliced white mushrooms

2 teaspoons (1.6 g) chopped fresh thyme (or ³/₄ teaspoon dried)

Salt and fresh-ground black pepper, to taste

¹/₂ cup (115 g) soft silken tofu

1 cup (235 ml) chicken broth

2 teaspoons (10 ml) low-sodium tamari

¹/₄ cup (25 g) fresh-grated Parmesan cheese, divided

3 tablespoons (9 g) whole-wheat panko bread crumbs

Not-Your-Grandmother's Green Bean Casserole

From Dr. Jonny: There's a reason Andy Warhol chose Campbell's soup as a model for one of his most iconic works—he grew up with it, as did I, and probably you, too. But ye olde cream of mushroom soup from a can—any can—is hardly a health food, whether eaten by itself or used as a base for your grandmother's green bean casserole. So this version, in my case anyway, is aptly named because the recipe is most certainly not my grandmother's green bean casserole—but it's probably not your grandmother's, either. We upgraded the typical grandma version with a nice dose of fresh mushrooms, which are much higher in nutrients than most people know. We used a light hand with the butter and added a drop of olive oil, but the comforting cream base remains—it just comes from high-protein tofu and chicken broth (rather than canned cream with a sodium chaser!). A tiny bit of fresh-grated Parmesan pops the flavors really nicely. The result? A remarkably light and tasty upgrade of an old comfort favorite!

Preheat the oven to 400°F (200°C, or gas mark 6). Spray a 9 x 13-inch (23 x 33-cm) ceramic baking dish with olive oil and set aside.

Bring a large pot of water to a boil and add the prepared beans. (Use no-sodium chicken broth in place of the water for richer flavor.) Boil for 2 to 5 minutes, depending on the type and freshness of the beans, until just tender. Drain and run under cold water for a couple of minutes to quickly cool and set aside.

In a large sauté pan, heat the butter and olive oil over medium heat. Add the shallots and sauté for about a minute. Add the mushrooms and thyme and cook until the mushrooms are soft and the released juices have mostly evaporated, 8 to 10 minutes. Season lightly with salt and pepper.

While the mushrooms are cooking, in a small bowl whisk the tofu until creamy and smooth. Add the broth and tamari and whisk until smooth and well incorporated. Pour the broth mixture over the mushrooms and stir to combine.

In a large bowl, combine the cooked beans and mushroom mixture and fold together. Pour half the mixture into the prepared baking pan. Sprinkle evenly with 2 tablespoons (10 g) of the Parmesan. Add the other half of the beans and top with the panko crumbs and remaining 2 tablespoons (10 g) Parmesan. Bake for 10 to 15 minutes, until hot throughout and the beans are very tender.

Yield: 4 to 6 servings
Per Serving: 281.8 calories; 5.2 g fat (16% calories from fat); 12.8 g protein; 51 g carbohydrate; 1.9 g dietary fiber; 6.9 mg cholesterol; 322.2 mg sodium

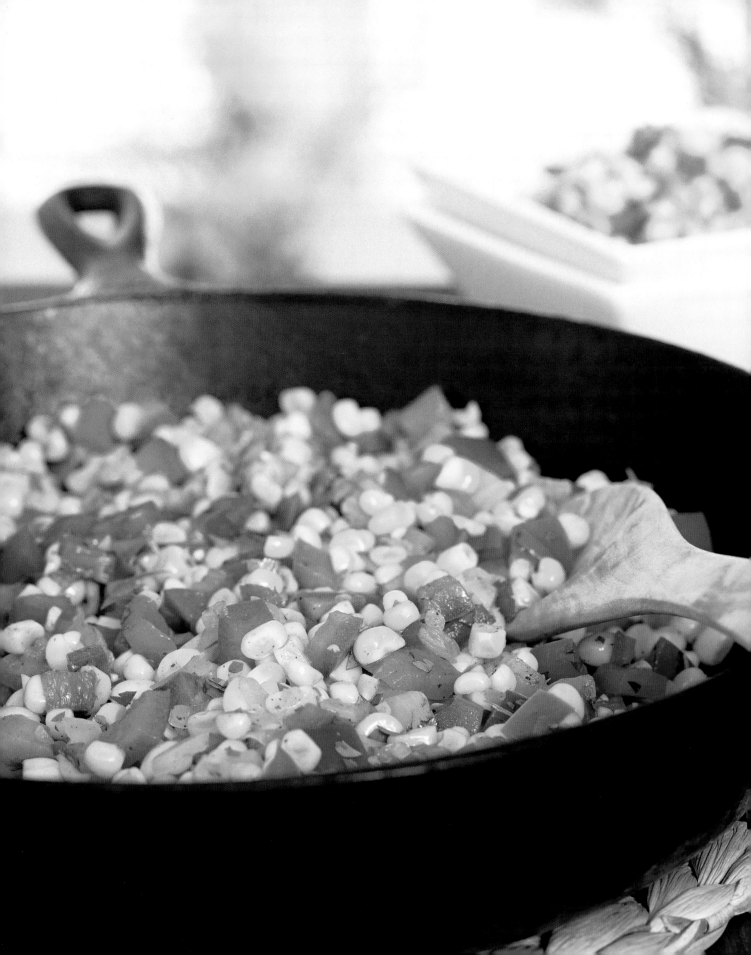

Ingredients

6 to 10 ears fresh sweet corn, shucked
(or 4 cups, or 520 g, frozen kernels)

1 tablespoon (14 g) butter

1½ tablespoons (25 ml) olive oil

1 small yellow onion, finely diced

1 teaspoon cumin

1 green bell pepper, seeded and diced small
(about ½-inch, or 1.3-cm, square or
smaller)

1 red bell pepper, seeded and diced small
(about ½-inch, or 1.3-cm, square or
smaller)

½ cup (120 ml) vegetable broth or water,
plus more as needed

½ teaspoon each salt and fresh-ground
black pepper

2 or 3 dashes hot pepper sauce, or to taste,
optional

¼ cup (4 g) chopped fresh cilantro

From Chef Jeannette

This recipe is best made with superfresh
corn, but it also works with slightly older
corn, and I have even used it as a way to
finish up cold cooked ears left over from
a big barbecue.

Creamy Creamless Skillet Corn

From Dr. Jonny: I love corn as much as the next person, but I love it on the cob, freshly made. What I don't love is canned "creamed" corn—it's loaded with sugar, sodium, and artificial ingredients and tastes like yellow chalk (not that I know what chalk tastes like, but I bet I'm right). And if you make creamed corn from scratch you're still likely to have a high-calorie dish, because real fresh cream (delicious and wholesome as it is) is not exactly a diet food. Try our version. It's a nutrient-rich dish that's way lower in calories than either of the two above-mentioned options, and you don't sacrifice a drop of taste. Corn gets a bad rap from us "low-carb" enthusiasts, but even though it's high in carbs it also has a fair amount of nutrition—about 4 grams of fiber per cup, a couple mg of niacin and other B vitamins, some beta-carotene, vitamin A, and a nice helping of the superstar eye nutrients, lutein and zeaxanthin (more than 1,100 mcg). Red peppers and onions are also loaded with antioxidants and healthy plant compounds. Enjoy!

If using fresh corn, place the thick side of each ear of corn firmly on a plate or shallow bowl and run a sharp chef's knife down four sides, shearing the kernels away from the cob.

Heat the butter and olive oil in a large cast-iron skillet over medium heat until the butter is melted. Add the onion and sauté for about 4 minutes. Add the cumin and sauté for 1 minute. Add the bell peppers, broth, salt, and pepper, and stir gently to combine. Increase the heat to high and bring the liquid to a boil, stirring frequently. Reduce the heat to low, cover, and simmer for about 20 minutes, until the vegetables are tender and fragrant. Stir and check the liquid level about every 5 minutes, adding a few additional tablespoons of broth if the mixture gets too dry. Add the hot sauce to taste during the last 2 to 3 minutes of cooking time, remove from the heat, and stir in the cilantro just before serving.

Yield: about 6 servings

Per Serving: 148.6 calories; 6.7 g fat (39% calories from fat); 3.3 g protein; 22.2 g carbohydrate; 3.6 g dietary fiber; 5.1 mg cholesterol; 616.1 mg sodium

Ingredients

1 cup (190 g) brown basmati rice

2¹⁄₂ cups (570 ml) no-sodium vegetable broth

Juice from ¹⁄₂ small lemon

Zest from small lemon

2 teaspoons (10 ml) low-sodium tamari (or ³⁄₄ teaspoon salt)

¹⁄₄ teaspoon fresh-ground black pepper

1 clove garlic, minced

¹⁄₂ cup (65 g) peeled and finely diced carrot

¹⁄₂ cup (50 g) finely diced celery

¹⁄₂ cup (80 g) finely diced onion

¹⁄₄ cup (15 g) chopped fresh parsley, optional

From Chef Jeannette

Time-Saver Tip: Omit the soaking step and cook everything in a rice cooker equipped for brown rice. I love my Zojirushi Neuro Fuzzy rice cooker. Expensive, but it cooks everything with no fuss, even other grains and combinations!

Healthier, Whole-Grain Lemon Veggie Rice

From Dr. Jonny: One of the biggest misconceptions about rice is that it's a health food. I love it when people debate me on this, pointing out that no one in China, where they eat a ton of rice, is fat. (Unfortunately, that's just not true—almost 18 percent of Chinese are overweight or obese.) Regardless, white rice is completely useless when it comes to providing real nutrition. What's more, it's a high-glycemic food, meaning it sends your blood sugar (and fat-storing hormones) through the roof, particularly when you eat typical American-size portions. But no reason to pass on the rice—just make it healthier by using brown basmati, which has the additional advantage of being easy to digest. Basmati is infinitely more flavorful, and we made it even more so with the light piquancy of fresh lemon juice. The celery, carrots, and onions add fiber plus a nice amount of nutrition (including vitamin A, vitamin K, and potassium). This dish is nourishing and satisfying and makes a great side dish for many protein main dishes—try it with grilled bass!

Rinse the basmati well and drain. Cover the rice with water in a bowl, cover the bowl, and let soak for 15 minutes. Drain well. In a large, heavy-bottomed saucepan with a tight-fitting lid, mix together the soaked rice, broth, lemon juice, zest, tamari, pepper, garlic, carrot, celery, and onion, and bring to a boil, stirring occasionally. Reduce the heat to keep a low simmer, cover, and cook for about 35 to 40 minutes, or until the rice and veggies are tender. Remove from the heat, adjust the seasonings, fold in the parsley, and serve.

Yield: about 6 servings

Per Serving: 117.5 calories; 1.1 g fat (8% calories from fat); 2.8 g protein; 24.9 g carbohydrate; 2.7 g dietary fiber; 0 mg cholesterol; 151.8 mg sodium

Ingredients

4 medium sweet potatoes, peeled and coarsely chopped (or garnet yams, if you can find them)

Cooking oil spray

1 egg

1 teaspoon vanilla extract

1 tablespoon (15 ml) 100 percent maple syrup (grade B for more nutrients and flavor)

2 to 4 tablespoons (28 to 60 ml) fresh-squeezed orange juice

1½ teaspoons (3 g) orange zest

4 drops orange extract, optional

3 tablespoons (42 g) butter, softened

3 tablespoons (40 g) Sucanat, brown sugar, or xylitol

¾ cup (83 g) chopped toasted pecans

Aromatic, Antioxidant-Rich Orange–Sweet Potato Casserole

From Dr. Jonny: As someone who tries to keep his carbohydrate intake moderate, I'm very careful about what carbs I eat. Rarely do I eat white rice, potatoes, pasta, or most cereals (notice I said "rarely," not "never"!). More important, when I do eat starchy carbs I try to choose carefully—and sweet potatoes make the cut. They're far richer in nutrients than white potatoes—1 cup (225 g) of sweet potatoes contains 950 mg of potassium (more than twice that in a banana), some calcium, iron, vitamin C, and about 6½ grams of fiber! Not exactly a shabby resume! You can make a pretty darn delicious sweet potato casserole using just a little less butter and sugar and kicking up the nutritional value with a generous helping of chopped pecans (extra fiber, magnesium, and potassium, not to mention heart-healthy monounsaturated fat). The orange boosts not only the vitamin C content but also the flavor so you don't miss (or need!) the excess sweetener (or other mystery ingredients in the marshmallow topping sweet potato casseroles everywhere). The egg adds protein and also gives the casserole a lighter feel. Fragrant, sweet, and satisfying.

Place the sweet potatoes in a large pot of boiling water. Cook for 15 to 20 minutes, or until soft, and drain well.

While the potatoes are boiling, preheat the oven to 350°F (180°C, or gas mark 4). Spray a 7 x 11-inch (18 x 28-cm) baking pan with a neutral cooking oil and set aside.

In a mixer beat together the cooked sweet potatoes, egg, vanilla, syrup, 2 tablespoons (28 ml) of the orange juice, zest, and extract until smooth and creamy. If the potatoes are a little dry, add more orange juice, 1 tablespoon (15 ml) at a time, until you reach the desired consistency. Spread the mixture into the prepared baking pan. In a medium bowl, mix together the butter, Sucanat, and pecans. Crumble the mixture evenly over the top of the potatoes and bake for 25 to 30 minutes, or until hot and fragrant.

Yield: about 6 servings

Per Serving: 259.5 calories; 16.5 g fat (54% calories from fat); 3.8 g protein; 26.1 g carbohydrate; 4 g dietary fiber; 50.3 mg cholesterol; 100.1 mg sodium

From Chef Jeannette

Even Healthier: Turn this dish from an indulgence into something truly healthy by swapping the white potatoes for peeled sweet potatoes and omitting the cheese entirely. This is also a time-saver. Preheat the oven to broil. Simmer the sweet potatoes in enough skim milk to cover by ½ inch (1.3 cm) in a large saucepan until they are tender, 8 to 10 minutes. Drain well, reserving ¼ cup (60 ml) of the milk. In a small bowl, whisk together the reserved milk, ½ cup (115 g) of sour cream (low-fat to reduce calories further), ½ teaspoon thyme, ½ teaspoon onion powder, ½ teaspoon salt, and ½ teaspoon fresh-ground black pepper until well combined. Layer the drained potatoes in an oiled, broiler-safe baking dish and pour the sour cream mixture evenly over the potatoes. You can also sprinkle on a few crushed walnuts, if desired. Broil for about 3 minutes to heat the topping through.

Lower-Cal Cheesy Scalloped Potatoes

From Dr. Jonny: You can easily "health up" your scalloped potatoes by giving all that extra cream and butter an "attitude adjustment." (Let me repeat, for those who might have missed one of the other times I've said this, that I don't think there's a thing wrong with cream and butter as whole foods—but they are wildly high in calories when combined and used freely, and are definitely not the best things to OD on, especially if you're eating a conventional American diet!) So we cut the butter down to almost nothing, reduced the cheese, and swapped the cream for low-cal evaporated milk. (Who invented that stuff, anyway? It's way better than you might think, and does an admirable job of standing in for the richer stuff.) Leaving the skins on the potatoes gives this old favorite another instant upgrade because so many of the nutrients in potatoes (such as fiber, vitamin C, vitamin B$_6$, iron, manganese, and copper) are found in the skins as well as the flesh. Note: For a truly lightened-up and higher-fiber version, check out the sweet potato option under "Even Healthier." Fun fact: Though potatoes are high in starchy carbohydrates, which some people need to limit, they are also high in phenolic compounds, plant chemicals that have a wide range of health-promoting properties, including antioxidant activity. Agricultural Research Service scientists have turned up sixty different phytochemicals and vitamins in potatoes, including compounds called kukoamines, which have been found to have blood pressure–lowering properties!

Ingredients

1 clove garlic, lightly crushed

Olive oil cooking spray

1 pound (455 g) Yukon gold potatoes, unpeeled and thinly sliced (about 3 potatoes, about $\frac{1}{8}$ inch, or 3 mm, thick—a mandolin works beautifully for this)

1 small yellow onion, thinly sliced

Salt and fresh-ground black pepper, to taste

$\frac{3}{4}$ teaspoon thyme

1 teaspoon granulated garlic

1 cup (120 g) grated Gruyère cheese

3 tablespoons (15 g) fresh-grated Pecorino Romano or Parmesan cheese

1 egg

1 can (12 ounces, or 355 ml) evaporated skim milk

1 tablespoon (14 g) butter, quartered

Preheat the oven to 350°F (180°C, or gas mark 4).

Using a heavy hand, rub the crushed garlic all over the inside of a shallow casserole dish or 7 x 11-inch (18 x 28-cm) baking dish.

Spray the dish with olive oil and lay down one-third of the sliced potatoes in a neat layer covering the bottom. Spread half the sliced onion on top in an even layer, season lightly with salt and pepper, half the thyme, and half the garlic. Sprinkle $\frac{1}{2}$ cup (60 g) of the Gruyère and 1 tablespoon (5 g) of the Pecorino evenly over the onions, and top with another one-third of the potatoes in an even layer. Cover with the remaining onion slices, and season lightly with salt, pepper, and the remaining halves of the thyme and garlic.

Top with $\frac{1}{4}$ cup (30 g) of the Gruyère, and 1 tablespoon (5 g) of the Pecorino. Cover with the remaining potatoes.

In a small bowl, whisk the egg into the evaporated milk until well incorporated and gently pour the mixture over the potatoes. Top with an even layer of the remaining $\frac{1}{4}$ cup (30 g) Gruyère and 1 tablespoon (5 g) Pecorino. Add the 4 small pieces of butter, seal with aluminum foil (be careful not to touch the potatoes with the foil or the cheese will stick), and cook for about 40 minutes.

Remove the foil and continue to bake for 15 to 20 minutes, until the potatoes are tender and the cheese on top is lightly browned. Let rest for 10 to 15 minutes before serving; the sauce will thicken slightly as it cools.

Yield: 6 servings

Per Serving: 233 calories; 10 g fat (38% calories from fat); 15.1 g protein; 23.3 g carbohydrate; 2 g dietary fiber; 67.4 mg cholesterol; 183.9 mg sodium

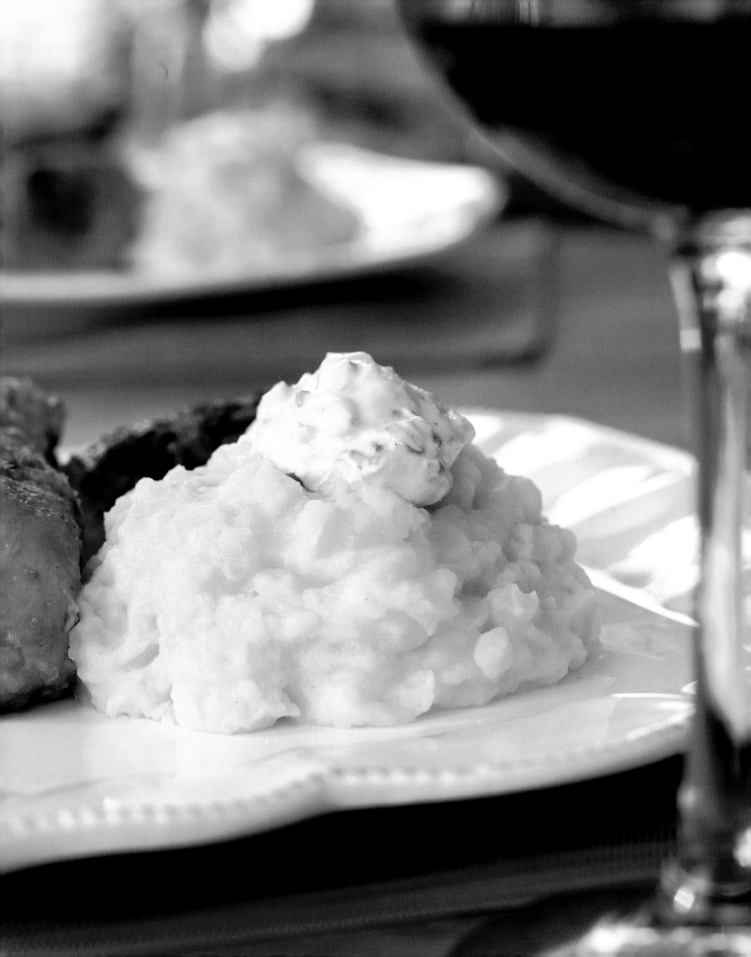

Creamy Low-Fat Mashed Potatoes

From Dr. Jonny: It's no secret that I've been an advocate of lower-carb eating for many years, and I'm as guilty as the next guy of making white potatoes the poster food for bad carbs. But what isn't common knowledge is that I grew up on mashed potatoes, and to this day they remain one of my all-time favorite foods even though I rarely eat them. Until now. The pure creamy delight of a steaming bowl of mashed potatoes has to be the ultimate comfort food. I used to drown mine in butter, salt them to death, and—don't tell anyone—cover them with ketchup. But I digress. Our madeover version uses the sweet pungent flavor of roasted garlic with just a dab of creamy butter and a low-sodium broth. P.S. There are those who argue that white potatoes deserve a reputation makeover. Roy Navarre, a plant geneticist with the Agricultural Research Service of the U.S. Department of Agriculture, states that "potatoes can actually be packed with phenolic compounds, which have a wide range of health-promoting properties, including antioxidant activity." Even someone raised on the traditional style will love this healthier version of the old favorite.

Ingredients

1 small head garlic

Drizzle of olive oil

1½ pounds (680 g) Yukon gold potatoes, peeled and quartered

Salt and fresh-ground black pepper, to taste

⅓ cup (77 g) plain low-fat yogurt, optional

⅓ cup (33 g) sliced scallion, optional

1 tablespoon (14 g) butter

⅓ cup (80 ml) low-sodium chicken or vegetable broth or low-fat milk (cow's milk or plain, unsweetened soy)

Preheat the oven to 400°F (200°C, or gas mark 6).

Peel away the papery outer skins of the garlic head, leaving all the cloves intact. Using scissors or a sharp paring knife, cut away the upper portions of each clove (about ⅓ inch, or 8 mm) to expose the flesh of the cloves. Place the garlic head upright in a small, high-heat baking dish, and drizzle olive oil lightly over each clove (about 1 teaspoon). Cover the garlic in aluminum foil and bake for 25 to 35 minutes, or until tender to the squeeze. Remove from the oven. When cool enough to handle, squeeze out the individual cloves and set aside. Snipping the tough skins can help with this.

While the garlic is cooking, prepare the potatoes. Place the potatoes in a large pot. Add water to cover and a sprinkle of salt and bring to a boil over high heat. Cook, partially covered, for 15 to 20 minutes, or until tender. Remove from the heat and drain well.

While the potatoes are cooking, prepare the dressing, if using. Select 3 or 4 (peeled) cloves of the roasted garlic (to taste) and smash them with a fork in a small bowl. Add the yogurt and a sprinkle of salt and pepper, and mix until well incorporated. Gently stir in the scallions and set aside.

(continued on page 124)

From Chef Jeannette

Because you are already taking the time to roast the garlic, roast several heads at once to use for other dishes. Roasted garlic makes a delicious, low-cal, nutrient-packed replacement for butter on grilled whole-grain bread. It will also give a flavor and nutrient boost to soups, salads, and stews. The immune-strengthening power of garlic is so strong that eating extra garlic in the cold months can help stave off those pesky winter ailments.

One of the great secrets to making fantastic, fluffy mashed potatoes that are actually good for you is to choose Yukon gold potatoes over standard russets or Idaho potatoes. They contain a little less starch and tend to hold their moisture well. Plus, the skins are not as heavy or gritty, so it's easy to leave them in for the added nutrients and fiber: See tip below.

Even Healthier: To retain more of the natural fiber and nutrients of the potatoes in the dish, scrub them well but leave them unpeeled. To decrease the carb content and add a cruciferous punch, replace 1/2 pound (225 g) of the potatoes with 1 1/2 cups (150 g) bite-size cauliflower florets. Add them to the cooking potatoes once the water is boiling and follow the same directions (they will need 15 to 20 minutes of cooking time to get tender, depending on the size of the florets).

Select 5 to 7 additional (peeled) cloves of the roasted garlic (to taste) and smash them with a fork in a large bowl. Add the potatoes and butter and mash them with the garlic using a potato masher. Add the broth a little at a time until your potatoes reach the consistency you like. Do not overmix them or they will get gummy. Season to taste with salt and pepper. Serve with a dollop of the garlic yogurt "sour cream," if desired.

Yield: 4 servings
Per Serving: 169.2 calories; 3.3 g fat (17% calories from fat); 6.7 g protein; 34.4 g carbohydrate; 3.8 g dietary fiber; 8.7 mg cholesterol; 100.8 mg sodium

Fluffy Twice-Baked Potatoes with Chèvre and Roasted Shallots

Ingredients

4 large russet potatoes

Drizzle of olive oil

6 shallots

⅓ cup (77 g) plain low-fat Greek yogurt

½ cup (120 ml) evaporated skim milk

½ teaspoon salt

½ teaspoon white pepper

½ cup (75 g) chèvre (fresh goat cheese)

¼ cup (12 g) chopped fresh chives

2 tablespoons (10 g) fresh-grated Parmesan cheese

From Dr. Jonny: There's good news and bad news about our old comfort food favorite, twice-baked potatoes. First the good news—they're delicious. The bad news is that they have all the butter, cream, and sour cream of baked and mashed potatoes, plus—if that weren't enough—a nice extra helping of cheese and salt. So we mimicked the creamy delicious texture, but we ditched the butter, sour cream, and heavy cream. How did we keep the flavor? Simple. Protein-rich Greek yogurt and evaporated skim milk. We also boosted the flavor with crispy roasted shallots and fresh, tangy chèvre, topping it all off with just a touch of fresh-grated Parmesan for a nice cheesy, crusty top. It's beyond delicious. Fun fact: Research from the Department of Physiology of the University of Granada shows that goat's milk has more beneficial properties to health than cow's milk, such as helping prevent iron deficiency and softening of the bones.

Preheat the oven to 400°F (200°C, or gas mark 6). Scrub and dry the potatoes well. Poke a few times with a fork. Rub with a light coating of olive oil, place them on a baking sheet or in a roasting pan, and bake for about 1 hour and 15 minutes, or until they are tender to the squeeze.

Peel the shallots but leave them whole. Rub with a light coating of olive oil and place them in the roasting pan with the potatoes about 20 minutes before the end of the potato cooking time. Turn them a couple of times and remove when they are crispy and lightly browned (should be about the same time as the potatoes). Allow the potatoes to cool enough to handle.

Reduce the oven to 350°F (180°C, or gas mark 4).

Cut off a thin slice lengthwise across the top of each potato. Carefully scoop out the insides, leaving a thin shell of potato and skin (about ¼ inch, or 6 mm), and place the potato fillings in a large mixing bowl. Add the yogurt, evaporated milk, salt, and pepper and beat just to desired consistency. Do not overbeat potatoes or they can become gluey.

Coarsely chop the roasted shallots and fold into the potatoes with the chèvre and chives, gently mixing by hand until evenly distributed. Adjust the seasonings as necessary.

Refill the potato skins with equal amounts of the potato mixture and top each with ½ tablespoon (2.5 g) of the Parmesan cheese. Place the potatoes back into the roasting pan and bake for 15 to 20 minutes, or until heated through.

Yield: 6 servings

Per Serving: 460.2 calories; 5.5 g fat (11% calories from fat); 17.5 g protein; 91.7 g carbohydrate; 2.8 g dietary fiber; 15.1 mg cholesterol; 341.6 mg sodium

A Lighter Touch:
Tangy German Potato Salad

Ingredients

1¼ pounds (565 g) small baby Yukon gold potatoes, unpeeled and quartered

3 slices nitrate-free turkey bacon

⅓ cup (55 g) chopped Vidalia onion

1 tablespoon (13 g) Sucanat, sugar, or xylitol

½ teaspoon salt

¼ teaspoon fresh-ground black pepper

½ cup (120 ml) plus 1 tablespoon (15 ml) low-sodium vegetable broth (or water), divided

¼ cup (60 ml) apple cider vinegar

1 teaspoon kudzu

1 teaspoon mustard seed

3 hard-boiled eggs, peeled and chopped

⅓ cup (33 g) sliced scallion, optional

From Dr. Jonny: What's a picnic without comfort food like potato salad? Our sweet-tart German version replaces the heavy canned mayo of classic potato salad with a tangy shot of apple cider vinegar. As I wrote in *The 150 Healthiest Foods on Earth*, apple cider vinegar has a long tradition of being used as an all-purpose medicinal food. If you use the organic, less-processed version, you'll be getting a hefty dose of the antioxidants and vitamins found in apples, and the vinegar will help regulate your blood sugar and "alkalize" your system (trust us, that's a good thing). Many of the nutrients found in potatoes are concentrated in the skin, so you'll get some fiber, iron, vitamin C, B$_6$, potassium, copper, and manganese as well as many other antioxidants. Oh yes, one more thing. Dump the all-fat pork bacon traditional to German potato salad and try the leaner turkey version. The eggs, one of nature's greatest foods, add more protein.

In a large saucepan, add the potatoes and enough water to generously cover them. Bring to a boil over high heat, lower the heat, partially cover, and simmer for about 15 minutes, or until the potatoes are fork-tender. Drain.

While the potatoes are cooking, in a large Dutch oven, cook the turkey bacon over medium heat until crisp. Remove the bacon and set on paper towels to drain.

Add the onion to the hot pan and cook in the oil left by the bacon for 4 to 5 minutes, until softened but not browned. Stir in the Sucanat, salt, pepper, ½ cup (120 ml) of the broth, and vinegar until well combined. Increase the heat to medium-high and simmer for about 3 minutes.

While the vinegar mixture is simmering, in a small cup stir the kudzu into the remaining 1 tablespoon (15 ml) broth until dissolved. Pour the kudzu mixture into the vinegar mixture and simmer for 1 minute, or until slightly thickened. Reduce the heat to medium-low and crumble the bacon strips into the mixture. Fold in the potatoes and heat for 2 to 3 minutes, until warm throughout.

Gently fold in the mustard seed, eggs, and scallion. Adjust the seasonings if necessary and serve warm.

Yield: 4 servings

Per Serving: 215.4 calories; 6 g fat (28% calories from fat); 10.7 g protein; 29.5 g carbohydrate; 3.5 g dietary fiber; 168 mg cholesterol; 639.7 mg sodium

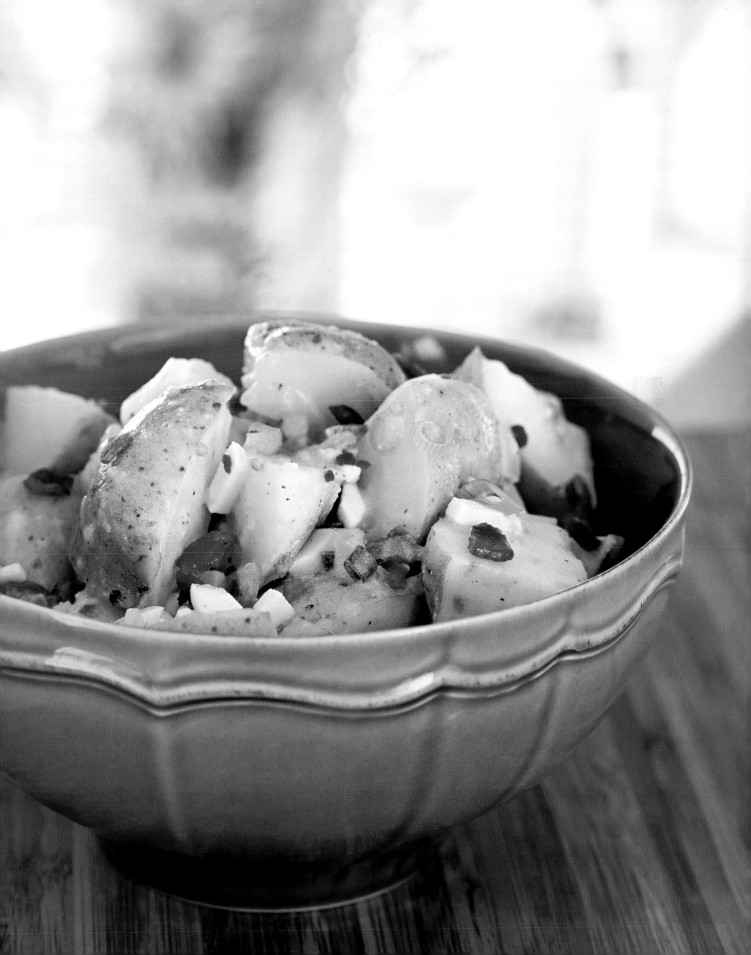

Ingredients

2 large Yukon gold potatoes, unpeeled and sliced lengthwise into ½ x ¼-inch-thick (1-cm x 6-mm-thick) strips

1 tablespoon (15 ml) olive oil

½ teaspoon each salt and fresh-ground black pepper

1 tablespoon (1.7 g) fresh chopped rosemary, optional

From Chef Jeannette

Even Healthier: For less starch, more fiber, and more vitamin A, substitute peeled sweet potatoes for the white potatoes. For the lowest-carb, lowest-starch option, use peeled rutabagas and add about 5 minutes (or more until tender) to the cooking time.

Tender Lower-Fat French Fries

From Dr. Jonny: It's hard to separate foods into "good" and "bad" categories because most foods have a combination of qualities, some of which are good, some of which are not so good. Except, of course, those on the extreme ends of the scales—broccoli, for example, which has nothing really bad about it, and French fries, which have absolutely nothing that's good. (In fact, French fries and sodas are two of my candidates for the all-time hall of fame of really, really unhealthy foods with nothing to recommend them except that kids like 'em.) These "substitute" fries taste just as good as the original. Just bake them instead of frying, leave them unpeeled, choose lower-starch Yukon gold potatoes, and spice 'em up with fresh herbs like rosemary. (Note: This recipe is officially "kid-tested" on my friend Michelle's twin seven-year-olds, and it passes!) Fun fact: In European herbalism, sprigs of rosemary were considered a love charm, a sign of remembrance, and a way to ward off the plague. Rosemary is also used to this day to help with indigestion and digestive disorders.

Preheat the oven to 400°F (200°C, or gas mark 6).

In a medium bowl, add the potato strips and drizzle the oil over all. Sprinkle with the salt, pepper, and rosemary and toss gently to coat. Spread the strips out evenly in a single layer on a baking sheet and bake, turning occasionally, for about 15 minutes, or until tender and lightly browned.

Yield: 4 servings

Per Serving: 81.5 calories; 3.5 g fat (37% calories from fat); 2 g protein; 13.3 g carbohydrate; 1.6 g dietary fiber; 0 mg cholesterol; 291 mg sodium

Ingredients

2 teaspoons (10 ml) olive oil

1 yellow onion, finely chopped

½ green bell pepper, seeded and finely chopped

½ cup (120 ml) no-salt chicken or vegetable broth, plus more as needed

⅓ cup (80 g) low-sugar ketchup

⅓ cup (80 ml) apple cider vinegar

¼ cup (85 g) blackstrap molasses

1 tablespoon (15 g) Dijon mustard

½ teaspoon chipotle pepper, or to taste (or cayenne)

¼ teaspoon each salt and fresh-ground black pepper, or to taste

1 can (15 ounces, or 425 g) red kidney beans, drained and rinsed

1 can (15 ounces, or 425 g) white kidney beans, drained and rinsed

2 slices nitrate-free turkey bacon

Sweet and Tangy No-Bake, High-Fiber Beans

From Dr. Jonny: Beans are one of the few foods I know of where it's perfectly acceptable to use the canned version (look for low- or no-sodium versions), and in this case, that also cuts the cooking time by a whopping 90 minutes. To avoid that sweet, syrupy goo that unfortunately goes with a lot of canned Boston baked beans, we dumped the brown sugar, so it won't be quite as sweet as the canned version, but it will be a whole lot better for you. We also used turkey bacon instead of lumps of pork fat or even a ham hock. And don't think that because there's no syrup or sugar these won't taste sweet—we used blackstrap molasses, which is as good a sweetener as sweeteners can be. It's loaded with iron, calcium, magnesium, and potassium, a claim no other sweetener I know of can make! Onions, with their high concentration of anti-inflammatory anticancer flavonoid quercetin, and bell peppers, with their high concentration of vitamin C and potassium, round out the picture for this delicious, high-fiber version of an old favorite.

Heat the oil over medium heat in a large, heavy-bottomed saucepan. Add the onion and bell pepper and cook for about 6 minutes. Stir in the broth, ketchup, vinegar, molasses, mustard, chipotle pepper, salt, and pepper until well mixed. Gently stir in the beans and raw bacon, increase the heat, and bring the mixture just to a simmer. Reduce the heat to low, cover, and cook for about 20 to 30 minutes, stirring occasionally and adding a little more broth, if necessary. Adjust the seasonings, if necessary. Remove the bacon strips and discard before serving the beans.

Yield: 4 to 6 servings

Per Serving: 210.8 calories; 3 g fat (8% calories from fat); 8.8 g protein; 36.2 g carbohydrate; 8 g dietary fiber; 4.2 mg cholesterol; 816.1 mg sodium

Ingredients

8 ounces (225 g) dry whole-grain elbow or
    macaroni pasta (we like Barilla Plus)
1/4 cup (60 g) plain low-fat Greek yogurt
3 tablespoons (42 g) high-quality natural
    mayonnaise
1 tablespoon (15 g) Dijon mustard
1 teaspoon apple cider vinegar
1/2 teaspoon Sucanat, sugar, or xylitol,
    optional
1/4 teaspoon each salt and fresh-ground
    black pepper, or to taste
1 large roasted red pepper, chopped
1/3 cup (40 g) finely chopped celery
1/2 cup (55 g) freshly grated carrot
1/3 cup (33 g) sliced scallion greens
3 hard-boiled eggs, peeled and chopped

From Chef Jeannette

Use prepared roasted red peppers in
jars or roast your own fresh. See our
directions in the Two-Cheese Fit and
Flavorful Frittata recipes, page 186.

Even Healthier: Swap out the creamy
base for a vinaigrette rich in good fats—
this is also a time-saver. Omit the yogurt
and mayo dressing and use 3 tablespoons
to 1/4 cup (45 to 60 ml) of a high-quality,
olive oil- or flaxseed oil-based Italian or
balsamic vinaigrette in its place.

Whole-Grain Veggie-Rich Macaroni Salad

From Dr. Jonny: You know how I know that macaroni salad is a comfort food? Because when I'm stressed it looks really attractive to me! Now all the reasons why it's so easy and natural to reach for high-carb foods when we're feeling stressed is beyond the scope of this book, but trust me, it's true. Which wouldn't be so bad in the case of macaroni salad except that it's usually a study in white pasta and mayo—not exactly a health bonanza. So upgrade it a bit by adding nutrient-rich veggies such as bell pepper (high in vitamin C), celery (good source of vitamin K), onions (great source of the anti-inflammatory compound quercetin), and a few other goodies. Because protein makes you feel satisfied (and also significantly lowers the blood sugar impact of a high-carb dish like macaroni), we upped the protein quotient in several ways. One, we used high-protein Barilla Plus pasta. Two, we swapped half the mayo for an equal amount of low-cal, high-protein Greek yogurt. And three, we included three eggs—a food that's been called one of the most perfect protein sources in the world (which it is, by the way). Hint: Choose a high-quality, all-natural mayo. Or . . . if you've got the time and inclination—make your own!

Cook the pasta until al dente according to package directions, rinse under cold water, and drain.

In a large bowl, combine the yogurt, mayo, mustard, vinegar, Sucanat, salt, and pepper, and whisk to mix well. Add the red pepper, celery, carrot, scallion, chopped egg, and pasta and mix gently to coat. Adjust the seasonings to taste. Chill for at least 1 hour in the refrigerator before serving.

Yield: 4 servings
Per Serving: 360.3 calories; 13.3 g fat (33% calories from fat); 14.6 g protein; 48.8 g carbohydrate; 6.3 g dietary fiber; 163.3 mg cholesterol; 336.5 mg sodium

Ingredients

2 tablespoons (30 g) plain low-fat yogurt

2 tablespoons (28 g) mayonnaise

1 tablespoon (15 ml) fresh-squeezed
    lemon juice

2 teaspoons (13 g) honey, or to taste

3/4 teaspoon lemon zest

1 green apple, unpeeled and chopped

1 cup (150 g) green grapes, halved

1 stalk celery, sliced thinly

1/4 cup (33 g) chopped unsulphured dried
    apricots, optional

1/3 cup (40 g) toasted chopped walnuts or
    sliced almonds

6 cups (540 g) chopped hearts of romaine
    lettuce

Light and Bright Waldorf Salad

From Dr. Jonny: To this day I think of Waldorf salad as more of a dessert than a salad, but the conventional version really does a disservice to the term "salad" by glopping it up with too much heavy mayonnaise. Lighten it up a bit by swapping out half that mayo for yogurt; you'll get all those friendly bacteria known as probiotics, which help your digestion and immune system. You'll also have a lower-calorie dish (which means you can eat more of it!). Add fresh fruit and nuts for minerals, antioxidants, and fiber. It's light, bright, and delicious! And still tastes like dessert. Note: Dried apricots are an incredibly nutritious fruit—1 cup (130 g) contains more than 1,000 mg of potassium (2½ times that in a banana), not to mention more than 3,100 IUs of vitamin A and a whopping 6½ grams of fiber!

In a small bowl, whisk together the yogurt, mayonnaise, lemon juice, honey, and zest and set aside.

In a large bowl combine the apple, grapes, celery, apricots, walnuts, and lettuce, dress lightly to taste with the yogurt mix, and scoop into a salad bowl.

Yield: 4 to 6 servings

Per Serving: 122.2 calories; 6.3 g fat (44% calories from fat); 2.7 g protein; 16.5 g carbohydrate; 3.7 g dietary fiber; 1.5 mg cholesterol; 51 mg sodium

Tangy Raw Caesar Salad with Whole-Grain Croutons

Ingredients

3 cloves garlic, minced

⅓ cup (80 ml) olive oil

½ loaf whole-grain peasant bread

1 egg (free-range organic raw, pasteurized, or poached in boiling water for 1 minute)

2 teaspoons (10 g) anchovy paste, or to taste

2½ tablespoons (38 ml) lemon juice

½ teaspoon Dijon mustard

¼ teaspoon each salt and fresh-ground black pepper

3 dashes Worcestershire sauce (organic, to avoid high-fructose corn syrup)

¼ cup (20 g) shaved Parmesan cheese, divided, or more to taste

1 large head romaine lettuce, torn into bite-size pieces

From Dr. Jonny: Go into any restaurant in America and you're sure to hear someone order "chicken Caesar, no croutons." (Well, if you wait around and listen to enough people order, that is.) The point is that in a world where carbs have been demonized (not entirely unfairly, I might add), croutons are the devil in the punchbowl, at least when it comes to Caesar salads. They're the unnecessary white bread carb devil in an otherwise Atkins-friendly salad, rich in protein, greens, and good fats. Well the crouton-banishers are only partly right. Certainly the stale white bread cubes are of no nutritional value and add a bunch of high-glycemic carbs that you don't need, but even without them Caesar salads can pack a big caloric punch. To counter this, we used smaller amounts of everything. We swapped out those ridiculous white bread cubes for dense crusts of whole-grain peasant bread, giving a nice bite to the salad without the big carb dump. Oh, and something you should know about that raw egg: Free-range, organic eggs are significantly less likely to contain salmonella than eggs from factory farms. The chickens are healthier and so are the eggs. A European Food Safety Authority study found that there was significantly higher salmonella risk from eggs that come from confined hens; in organic egg production the odds of salmonella contamination were 95 percent lower and in free-range production they were 98 percent lower.

Preheat the broiler.

Whisk the garlic into the oil until well mixed. Set aside.

Carve the crusts off of the loaf and tear them into 4-inch (10-cm) sections (save the bread insides for another use; for example, see our recipe for fondue, page 107). Brush the crusts very lightly all over with the garlic oil and arrange on a broiling pan. Broil for about 1 minute, turn the pieces, and broil again until just golden. Watch closely to avoid burning. Trim off any edges that accidentally char. Set aside.

Whisk the egg, anchovy paste, lemon juice, mustard, salt, pepper, and Worcestershire sauce into the remaining garlic oil until pale yellow and slightly emulsified. Stir in half the Parmesan. Taste and adjust the seasonings, if necessary.

In a large bowl, add ¼ cup (60 ml) of the dressing (or to taste) and the lettuce, and sprinkle with the remaining Parmesan. Break up the prepared croutons, add to the salad, toss well, and serve. Refrigerate the remaining dressing.

Yield: 4 to 6 servings

Per Serving: 377.1 calories; 24 g fat (56% calories from fat); 12.9 g protein; 29.7 g carbohydrate; 7.3 g dietary fiber; 66.4 mg cholesterol; 635.6 mg sodium

Ingredients

1 cup (190 g) brown basmati rice

2 cups (475 ml) plus 2 tablespoons (28 ml) no-sodium chicken broth, divided

2 slices nitrate-free turkey bacon

2 links (each 3 ounces, or 85 g) spicy chicken or turkey sausage

2 teaspoons (10 ml) olive oil

½ yellow onion, finely chopped

1 stalk celery, finely chopped

½ green bell pepper, seeded and finely chopped

½ teaspoon each salt and fresh-ground black pepper, or to taste

½ teaspoon cayenne pepper

½ teaspoon paprika

½ teaspoon garlic granules

3 tablespoons (12 g) chopped fresh parsley, optional

From Chef Jeannette

Time-Saver Tip: Omit the spices (except salt) and replace with 1 to 1½ teaspoons of a prepared salt-free creole or Cajun spice mix.

Lean and Clean Dirty Rice

From Dr. Jonny: Dirty rice is a classic Cajun rice made with pork sausage and chicken livers, sometimes with bacon added to the mix just for good measure. Yikes! Not that those foods are always bad (although I'm not taking bets on the medicinal value of that mystery sausage), but you can do a lot better. First, use nitrate-free turkey bacon. Then add just the perfect amount of classic Cajun spices. Finally, upgrade from plain-old white rice to brown basmati, which has more nutrients, has more fiber, and is a breeze to digest. Onion contributes its usual array of compounds known to help fight inflammation and cancer, and green peppers give you a nice dollop of vitamin C. Use the Cajun spices Chef Jeannette recommends and you'll feel like you're right in the Treme district of New Orleans!

Bring the rice and 2 cups (475 ml) of the broth to a boil in a medium saucepan over high heat. Stir, reduce the heat, cover, and simmer for 45 to 50 minutes, or until the liquid is absorbed and the rice is tender. Stir, remove from the heat, and fluff with a fork.

At the end of the rice cooking time, add the bacon to a large skillet or Dutch oven over medium heat. Remove the sausage from the casing and crumble into the pan. Cook for about 5 minutes or until beginning to brown. Flip the bacon and remove it from the pan when it is crisp to drain on a paper towel. Add the olive oil, onion, celery, and bell pepper, and cook for about 4 minutes. Stir in the salt, pepper, cayenne, paprika, and garlic and continue to cook until the vegetables are tender and the sausage is cooked through, stirring frequently—reduce the heat if the veggies brown too fast. Add the remaining 2 tablespoons (28 ml) broth to the pan and stir to release any stuck veggies, meat, or spices. Fold in the hot rice and parsley. Crumble the bacon and fold in. Adjust the seasonings to taste and serve piping hot.

Yield: about 6 servings

Per Serving: 168.4 calories; 5 g fat (26% calories from fat); 6.8 g protein; 26.1 g carbohydrate; 2.3 g dietary fiber; 12.8 mg cholesterol; 546.6 mg sodium

Ingredients

½ head green cabbage

2 small carrots, grated

½ cup (50 g) sliced scallion

⅓ cup (5 g) chopped fresh cilantro

1½ tablespoons (25 ml) flaxseed oil (or olive oil)

1½ tablespoons (25 ml) raw apple cider vinegar

1½ teaspoons (10 g) honey

¼ teaspoon cumin

¼ teaspoon cayenne pepper

¼ teaspoon each salt and fresh-ground black pepper

From Chef Jeannette

Time-Saver Tip: Use a 12-ounce (340-g) bag of prepared veggie slaw mix in place of the cabbage and carrots.

Lighter Cider Coleslaw

From Dr. Jonny: It has always amazed me why coleslaw doesn't have more of a reputation as a health food. After all, its primary ingredient is cabbage, one of the great superstars of the vegetable kingdom with its rich array of indoles, cancer-fighting plant chemicals that have a positive effect on hormonal metabolism. But then I realized why no one thinks of coleslaw as a health food—the veggies are overshadowed by piles of low-quality industrial-grade mayonnaise. In our lightened version, we dump the mayo altogether in favor of a light, flavorful dressing with a Southwestern flair. It's made from flaxseed oil (we recommend Barlean's High Lignan Flax Oil because it's highest in cancer-fighting lignans), plus one of the great traditional healing foods, apple cider vinegar. The result is a truly healthy coleslaw, lower in calories and definitely higher in flavor. What's not to like? Answer: absolutely nothing. Enjoy!

Halve and core the cabbage half, then slice each quarter thinly, or feed through the slicing attachment on the food processor to save time. In a large bowl, combine the prepared cabbage, carrots, scallion, and cilantro.

In a small bowl whisk together the oil, vinegar, honey, cumin, cayenne, salt, and pepper. Dress the veggies to taste, toss to coat, and serve. (You can also chill this dish for a whole day in the refrigerator—the flavors will combine and deepen.)

Yield: 4 servings

Per Serving: 84.2 calories; 5.9 g fat (62% calories from fat); 0.8 g protein; 7.8 g carbohydrate; 1.9 g dietary fiber; 0 mg cholesterol; 178.8 mg sodium

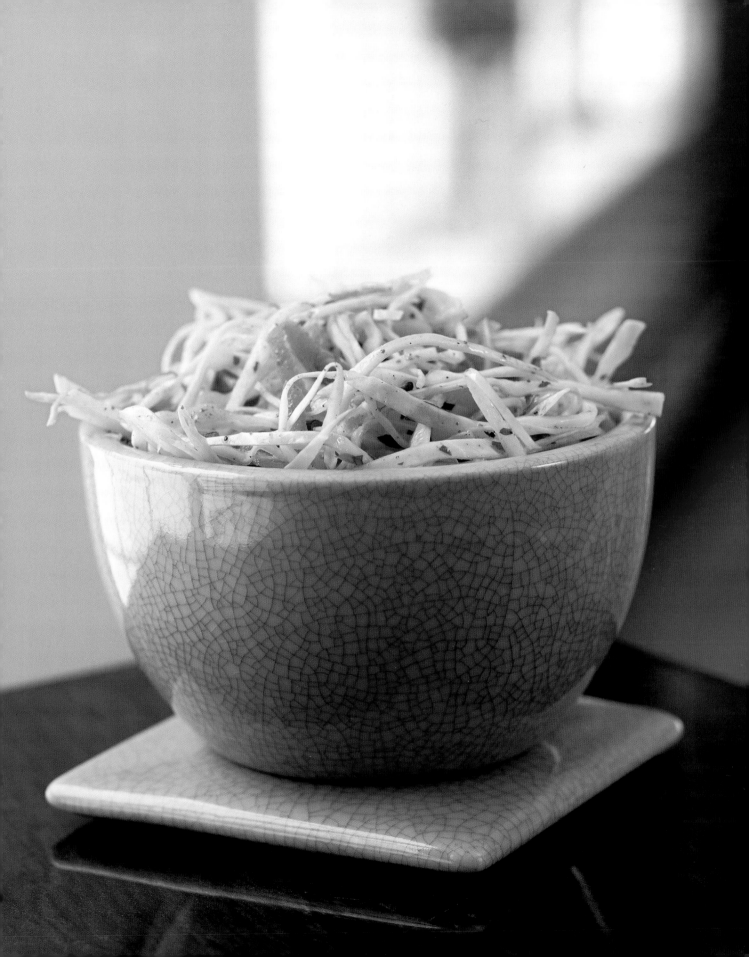

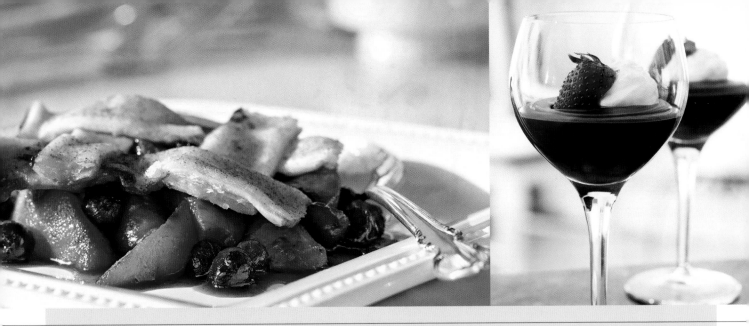

Desserts

In this section we did damage control on the usual dessert fare, creating scrumptious recipes but adding as little sweetener as possible and using only the best ingredients. You can have your nutritional "cake" and eat it too!

Satisfying Real-Food Piecrust

Organic Gingersnappy Piecrust

Giant Two-Crust Apple Dumpling Pie

Autumnal Fresh-Pumpkin Pie with Potassium

Memorable Freshest Blueberry Blast Pie

Dark and Mineral-Rich Coco-Fudgy Pie

Vitamin C-Rich Sweet-Tart Apple Rhubarb Crisp

Tender and Trans Fat-Free Peach and Blueberry Cobbler

Decadent Dark Chocolate Chip Multigrain Cookies

Simple Snappy Real Ginger Cookies

Dreamy, All-Natural Choco-Peanut Butter Cookies

Spiced, Lower-Sugar Cookies

Decadent Better-Fat Walnut Brownies

Jonny's Fudgy Chocolate Antioxidant Pudding

Creamy and Nutritious Coconutty Rice Pudding

Chocolate Peanut Butter Protein-Power Milkshakes

Light and Groovy Sorbet and Homemade Soda Floats

Lower-Cal, Moist Mock Sour Cream Chocolate Cake

Dense and Dreamy Fruit 'n Nut-Filled Carrot Cake

Rich and Creamy Lower-Cal Cream Cheese Frosting

Real Fresh, Real Fruit Strawberry Ice Cream

Magnificent Madeover Strawberry Shortcake

Iron-Strong Gingerbread Cake with Poire William

The Real Deal: Lightly Sweetened Fresh Whipped Cream

Tart Cherry Chocolate Whole-Grain Bread Pudding

Satisfying Real-Food Piecrust

From Dr. Jonny: In the olden days, cooks used real, honest-to-goodness ingredients like butter or lard as a shortening. (You may think I'm crazy, but lard is making a comeback—many health professionals now realize it was probably better for us than some of the things that replaced it, such as Crisco. But I digress.) These days, we make piecrusts with vegetable shortening, which is a huge source of trans fats—if you doubt me, go to the nutrition facts label and you will see "fully hydrogenated palm oil, partially hydrogenated palm and soybean oils," the precise definition of trans fats. So how do we make a really good, high-comfort, grandma-worthy piecrust without the trans fats? Simple. We use Chef Jeannette's recipe, which incorporates a real whole food (and one you needn't fear), butter! Butter, you may be surprised to know, is mostly monounsaturated fat, the same kind found in olive oil. You can make this crust with white flour if you want the most familiar taste and texture, but we recommend a nutritional upgrade: Try whole-grain pastry flour and you'll get some extra fiber and nutrients. (The whole-wheat kind works especially well for a savory dish like quiche.) As Chef Jeannette once told a reader, "If you encourage your palate gently, it will adjust over time and you—like us—will most likely grow to prefer the richer flavor and texture of whole-grain baked products over highly refined ones." I couldn't have said it better.

Ingredients

1¼ cups (155 g) whole-wheat pastry flour (or wheat flour), plus more for sprinkling

½ teaspoon salt

½ teaspoon sugar

½ cup (1 stick, or 112 g) well-chilled butter

2 to 4 tablespoons (28 to 60 ml) well-chilled milk (cow's milk works best)

In a large bowl, mix together the flour, salt, and sugar.

Add the cold butter to a food processor and pulse a few times to chop. Gently pour in the flour mixture and pulse until it forms moist crumbs, scraping down the sides, as necessary. Don't worry if you can still see bits of butter—they help with the flakiness. (You can also use a pastry cutter or two knives: Dice the chilled butter into pieces, or grate the butter using a cheese grater, and cut them into the flour until the mixture forms moist crumbs.)

Return the flour mixture to the large bowl. Pour the milk into the flour mixture a little at a time, mixing with a fork, until it begins to hold together. Knead the mixture with your hands just until it achieves a smooth, elastic consistency—do not overwork the dough or it will become tough.

Lay out a large piece of waxed paper and sprinkle it with flour. Place the dough in the center, flour a rolling pin (to help prevent sticking), and roll the dough into a circle to fit a 9-inch (23-cm) pie plate, about ¼ inch (6 mm) thick.

(continued on page 138)

From Chef Jeannette

Healthiest Version: You can also make a simple, delicious, high-fiber crust with no flour at all and substitute a small amount of nut oil for the butter. This increases the protein and fiber content. It is also much lower in gluten (gluten-free if you use certified gluten-free oats). This nutty crust comes together much more quickly than any traditional pastry crust and is completely "unfussy"–great for novice bakers.

Neutral cooking oil spray
½ cup (40 g) whole rolled oats
1 cup (125 g) blanched almond flour
    (we like Honeyville brand)
¼ teaspoon salt
¼ cup (60 ml) almond oil (or
    macadamia nut, avocado, or melted
    coconut oil)
1 tablespoon (15 ml) maple syrup

Preheat the oven to 350°F (180°C, or gas mark 4). Lightly spray a 9½-inch (24-cm) pie plate with cooking oil and set aside.

Process the oats in the food processor until they are coarse crumbs, about 5 seconds, twice. Add the almond flour, salt, almond oil, and maple syrup, and pulse until all ingredients are well combined, scraping down the sides as necessary. Using wet or lightly oiled fingers, press the mixture evenly into the pie pan. Prick two or three times with a fork and bake for 10 to 15 minutes until lightly browned. Cool and fill as desired.

Yield: One 9-inch (23-cm) piecrust, 9 servings

Per Serving: 147.4 calories; 12.6 g fat (72% calories from fat); 3.3 g protein; 35 g carbohydrate; 1.8 g dietary fiber; 0 mg cholesterol; 65.1 mg sodium

Invert the pie plate over the crust and gently lift the waxed paper with the crust, holding it close to the pie plate. Flip the pie plate upright again and gently peel the waxed paper away from the curst, fitting it into the plate. Press the dough lightly and evenly into the plate and flute the edges by pinching the crust between your thumb and two fingers all around the upper rim. If it tears, just seal the edges back together with your fingers.

Fill with the filling of your choice and bake according to recipe directions, or prebake the crust before filling: Preheat your oven to 450°F (230°C, or gas mark 8), poke a fork into the bottom of the crust three or four times to prevent air bubbles from forming, and bake for about 8 minutes, or until lightly browned.

Yield: One 9-inch (23-cm) piecrust, 9 servings
Per Serving: 154.4 calories; 10.3 g fat (59% calories from fat); 2 g protein; 13.5 carbohydrate; 0.5 g dietary fiber; 27 mg cholesterol; 132.2 mg sodium

Ingredients

Cooking oil spray

About 3 cups all-natural, high-quality gingersnaps (choose organic to avoid high-fructose corn syrup, such as MI-DEL organic Old-Fashioned Gingersnaps)

¼ cup (55 g) butter, melted

From Chef Jeannette

To make a 9-inch (23-cm) deep-dish crust, add ⅓ cup (38 g) more cookie crumbs plus 1½ tablespoons (25 ml) of almond oil (or melted butter).

You can also chill this crust to firm it rather than baking. This works well for cold fruity fillings, such as strawberry cream or our Memorable Freshest Blueberry Blast Pie on page 147.

Even Healthier: For more fiber and nutrients, substitute ¼ cup (30 g) almond meal or almond flour for ¼ cup (30 g) of the cookie crumbs, and substitute 2 tablespoons (28 ml) almond oil for half the butter.

Variation: Substitute high-quality, lower-sugar chocolate cookie crumbs (such as MI-DEL Swedish Style Chocolate Snaps) for the gingersnaps for a chocolate crust.

Organic Gingersnappy Piecrust

From Dr. Jonny: Making a standard cookie crust is easy: Start with a bunch of sugar-filled cookies and heap some more sugar into the mix. You and I both know you really don't need all that sugar. Seriously. We use flavorful, zingy gingersnaps as the cookie base (oh, they bring back childhood memories!) and choose high-quality, low-sugar organic cookies. Instead of any added sweetener (which it really doesn't need), we simply use a bit of butter to bind the whole mix together and—presto bingo—you've got a delicious, heart-and-belly-warming sweet crust that will brighten up just about any filling you decide to pour into it. Try it with our pumpkin pie filling (page 144)! Fun fact: Ginger is considered a tonic for the digestive tract. According to the great nutritional medicine guru Alan Gaby, M.D., it stimulates digestion and tones the intestinal muscles.

Preheat the oven to 325°F (170°C, or gas mark 3). Spray a 9-inch (23-cm) pie plate lightly with cooking oil and set aside.

Break the cookies up and add them to a food processor. Pulse and then process until the mixture forms crumbs. You'll need enough cookies to make about 1½ cups (175 g) crumbs. Drizzle in the butter and pulse until the mixture holds together. Press firmly into the pie plate to form a thin, even crust. Bake for 5 minutes, cool, and fill with desired filling.

Yield: One 9-inch (23-cm) piecrust, 9 servings

Per Serving: 277.1 calories; 11.6 g fat (39% calories from fat); 1.7 g protein; 36.7 g carbohydrate; 1.7 g dietary fiber; 13.1 mg cholesterol; 225.7 mg sodium

Good, Better, Best: What Cooking Oils Should I Use?

Choosing the right oil, like choosing the right tool, depends entirely on the job you want it to do.

Almost all cooking oils or cooking fats, such as butter, contain some mixture of three types of fatty acids: polyunsaturated, monounsaturated, and saturated. Each has certain advantages. (Even saturated fat has an advantage—it is much less subject to oxidative damage when heated!)

Polyunsaturated fats include both omega-3 and omega-6 fatty acids. Omega-3s, like flaxseed oil, are terrific for using on salads, but can't be used for cooking at high temperatures because of the delicate structure of the fats—any health benefit will be destroyed during the heating. On the other hand, omega-6s (found in corn oil, soybean oil, safflower oil, and the like) are "pro-inflammatory," and oils that have a high ratio of omega-6s should be used sparingly. We get far too many of these omega-6s in our diet (and far too few omega-3s). Plus, omega-6s are very susceptible to cell-damaging free radicals when heated. In addition, most vegetable oils are highly processed and refined, meaning many of the natural antioxidants have been destroyed.

Chef Jeannette and I recommend that you use only unrefined, cold-pressed oils whenever possible, regardless of the oil you choose.

Monounsaturated fats, also known as omega-9s, are found in olive oil and macadamia nut oil, two of the best oils to cook with. Macadamia nut oil stands up to heat quite well, and contains a ton of these heart-healthy monounsaturated fats. Extra-virgin olive oil is the least processed of the olive oils, and the one we most recommend. In addition, it has the added advantage of being a terrific salad dressing.

We're not big fans of canola oil, despite the hype. It's a highly refined oil that has to be chemically bleached, degummed, and deodorized at very high temperatures (much like many other refined vegetable oils). We think its so-called health benefits are oversold. For these very reasons our friend Fred Pescatore, M.D., author of *The Hamptons Diet*, says, "I would never use this oil."

When choosing an oil for cooking there's something else to consider: smoke point. Low smoke point oils such as flaxseed should, as mentioned, never be used for cooking, though you can certainly use them on salads or even cooked vegetables. Medium smoke point oils (such as corn oil, which has a smoke point of 350°F, or 180°C) can be used, but it's not our favorite because it's a very refined oil and extremely high in omega-6s. Instead, try peanut oil (smoke point 275°F to 300°F, or 140°C to 150°C, for unrefined peanut oil), which is much higher in monounsaturated fats and much lower in omega-6s. High smoke point oils we recommend include the aforementioned macadamia nut oil, coconut oil (our favorite), almond oil, and palm kernel oil (as long as it has not been hydrogenated it's perfectly fine!).

While we're at it, let's clear up some of the confusion about solid fats (like ghee, coconut oil, and butter). There's really no need to avoid them (even lard if you use the real, honest-to-goodness clean kind, not the hydrogenated trans fat-laden substitutes like Crisco). As noted above, saturated fat is very resistant to oxidative damage, so these fats can be used without creating carcinogenic compounds. (Vegetable oils, with their high concentration of omega-6s, are actually the oils most prone to oxidation!)

Coconut oil is an especially good choice (we love the organic Barlean's Extra-Virgin Coconut Oil). Butter and ghee, which is clarified butter, are also perfectly good choices. Remember, saturated fatty acids constitute at least 50 percent of your cell membranes, giving them their necessary stiffness and integrity. They play a vital role in the health of our bones and they lower certain substances in the blood, such as Lp(a), which indicates proneness to heart disease. They've been given a terrible rap, and while we don't advocate that you go out and eat containers of lard, we also don't think you need to obsessively avoid saturated fat at any cost.

Giant Two-Crust Apple Dumpling Pie

Ingredients

8 green apples, unpeeled, cored, and chopped

2 to 4 tablespoons (26 to 52 g) Sucanat, sugar, or xylitol, to taste

1 teaspoon cinnamon

1/2 teaspoon ginger

1/4 teaspoon cardamom, optional

Pinch of salt

2 tablespoons (16 g) flour

2 teaspoons (5.4 g) kudzu (or arrowroot or cornstarch)

1 1/2 tablespoons (25 ml) fresh-squeezed lemon juice or apple cider vinegar

2 unbaked 9 1/2-inch (24-cm) deep-dish piecrusts

1 egg, beaten

2 teaspoons (10 ml) cow's milk

From Dr. Jonny: The classic apple dumplings—pastry filled with apples, cinnamon, and sometimes raisins—involves a ton of shortening and enough sugar to choke a horse. The thing of it is that you don't need that much heavy syrup to create the warm, sweet, and satisfying flavor that defines comfort food desserts like this one. How do I know? 'Cause I tasted this version, which turns the individual dumplings into a pie, thus reducing the overall "crust factor" by a significant amount. So instead of eight individual dumpling wraps (normally made with shortening and sugar), we've got two simple piecrusts. That's an improvement right there. Chef Jeannette also used a light hand with the sweetener, always a good option, and chose green apples for their lower sugar content as well as their pleasant tang. (Don't forget to leave the skins on—many of the phytochemicals that make apples so good for you are found in the skin, not to mention the majority of the valuable fiber known as pectin.) We piled the apples up high to give the visual impression of one big fat dumpling! (Presentation is everything!) Lemon juice adds some antioxidants, or you can choose apple cider vinegar, which is loaded with nutrients and has an alkalizing effect on the body to boot. Added bonus: This pie is a snap to make!

Preheat the oven to 375°F (190°C, or gas mark 5).

In a large bowl, mix the apples and sweetener, to taste. Sprinkle with the cinnamon, ginger, cardamom, and salt, and toss to combine. In a small bowl, mix the flour and kudzu, crushing any kudzu clumps so everything is powder. Sprinkle evenly over the apples. Sprinkle the lemon juice over all and toss again to coat evenly.

Gently place one crust into a deep-dish pie plate. Carefully pour the apples into the crust—they will make a high pile. Gently lay the second crust over the top of the apples and pinch the edges together to make a seal. Slice four 1-inch (2.5-cm) slits at the top of the pie around the center for vents.

In a small bowl, whisk the egg and milk together until well beaten and brush all the crust you can reach liberally with the mixture. Bake for 50 to 55 minutes, until the crust is golden brown and the apples are soft.

Yield: 8 to 10 servings

Per Serving: 366 calories; 19.1 g fat (46% calories from fat); 4.4 g protein; 46.2 g carbohydrate; 5.1 g dietary fiber; 69.9 mg cholesterol; 245.5 mg sodium

Spicy, Multipurpose Cinnamon

Cinnamon is one of those spices that you don't have to convince anyone to eat. It adds terrific flavor and a sweet bite to everything from coffee to pumpkin pie. What you may not know is all the ways cinnamon can benefit your health.

Cinnamon has received a lot of attention because of studies showing that it can help lower blood sugar. One 2009 study found that in people with poorly controlled type 2 diabetes, cinnamon taken twice a day for 90 days improved hemoglobin A1c levels—a reflection of average blood sugar level for the past two to three months.

Though some of the research is conflicting, the majority of the studies on cinnamon show that it may lower postprandial (after eating) blood sugar even in nondiabetics. According to the Mayo Clinic (www.mayoclinic.com)," [C]innamon may be helpful as a supplement to regular diabetes treatment in people with type 2 diabetes."

But even if you don't have type 2 diabetes, cinnamon has a place in your diet. A 1999 study showed that 1 teaspoon of cinnamon killed almost 100 percent of *E. coli* bacteria present in apple juice samples, and it's also been found that cinnamon, along with cloves and garlic, are the most powerful spices when it comes to combating *E. coli* in raw ground beef and sausage. Bottom line: Cinnamon appears to have some nice antimicrobial activity.

Cinnamon—like many spices we use and recommend—is high in antioxidants and plant compounds known as polyphenols. And a little fun fact: Cinnamon trees grow in a number of tropical areas, notably parts of China, Madagascar, Brazil, the Caribbean, and parts of India.

Autumnal Fresh-Pumpkin Pie with Potassium

Ingredients

3 eggs

1 can (12 ounces, or 355 ml) evaporated skim milk

½ cup (100 g) Sucanat, sugar, or xylitol

¼ cup (60 ml) maple syrup

2 cups (490 g) fresh pumpkin purée (or one 15-ounce, or 425-g, can unsweetened pumpkin purée)

1½ teaspoons (3 g) orange zest, optional

2 teaspoons (4.6 g) cinnamon

1 teaspoon ginger

½ teaspoon nutmeg

¼ teaspoon ground cloves

½ teaspoon salt

One unbaked 9-inch (23-cm) deep-dish piecrust (page 137) or Organic Gingersnappy Piecrust, page 139

From Dr. Jonny: I'm frequently asked by magazine editors to come up with lists of foods we should all be eating, and I almost always include pumpkin. It always seems to surprise everyone to learn how good it is for you. One cup (245 g) of canned pumpkin has 7 grams of fiber, more potassium than a large banana, a fair amount of bone-building vitamin K, and a hefty dose of vitamin A and beta-carotene. All for—get this—a measly 83 calories. All things considered, pumpkin is one of the best possible fillings for a pie! (It also makes a great vegetable side dish.) So pumpkin, big thumbs-up. Pumpkin pie—not so much. Usually the crust is made with Crisco (don't even ask), and the pumpkin filling itself is mixed with cream and buckets of sugar. Our version lightens it up with one of our delicious crusts (flaky or gingersnap, your choice), and uses evaporated skim milk instead of cream (or condensed sweetened milk) for the pumpkin purée. We also pull back a bit on the sweetener and add cinnamon for its help with balancing blood sugar.

Preheat the oven to 425°F (220°C, or gas mark 7).

Beat the eggs lightly with a mixer. Add the milk, Sucanat, and syrup, and beat until well mixed. Add the pumpkin, zest, cinnamon, ginger, nutmeg, cloves, and salt, and beat on low until combined. Pour into the pie shell and wrap a thin ring of aluminum foil around the outer edges of the crust to prevent burning. Bake for 15 minutes. Then reduce the oven temperature to 350°F (180°C, or gas mark 4) and bake for 40 to 45 minutes, until the middle of the pie is set (a toothpick inserted into the center will come out mostly clean), removing the foil for the last 5 or 10 minutes of baking time. Allow the pie to cool for at least 1 hour before slicing.

Yield: 12 servings

Per Serving: 207.5 calories; 9.2 g fat (39% calories from fat); 5.9 g protein; 26.3 g carbohydrate; 1.6 g dietary fiber; 74.4 mg cholesterol; 253 mg sodium

From Chef Jeannette

To make fresh pumpkin purée, halve a good-size sugar pumpkin (about 4 pounds, or 1.8 kg) and scoop out the seeds with a heavy spoon. Cut away the peel (a heavy sharp chef's knife works best for this), cut it into large chunks, and cook it down for 5 to 7 hours on low in a slow cooker with a bit of apple cider or plain water. When it's soft, mash and cool it and it's ready for use. Extra purée freezes beautifully.

Even Healthier: This filling recipe is featured in another one of our books, *The Most Effective Ways to Live Longer Cookbook*. It boosts the health value even more with all the added protein from the silken tofu.

**1 package (12.3 ounces, or 350 g) extra-firm silken tofu
    (or 1¹/₂ cups)**
1 can (15 ounces, or 425 g) pumpkin purée
²/₃ cup (160 ml) maple syrup
1 teaspoon vanilla or orange extract
2 teaspoons (4.6 g) cinnamon
2 teaspoons (3.6 g) ginger
¹/₄ teaspoon ground cloves
¹/₄ teaspoon allspice

Preheat the oven to 350°F (180°C, or gas mark 4).

Drain the tofu and process in a food processor until it reaches the consistency of thick, smooth yogurt. Add the pumpkin purée, maple syrup, extract, and spices, and process, scraping down the sides periodically, until the mixture is smooth and creamy. Pour the mixture into the prepared piecrust and bake for 40 to 45 minutes, until the filling is set. The pie will continue to firm somewhat as it cools. Serve warm or chilled.

Yield: 12 servings

Per Serving: 195.8 calories; 8.7 g fat (39% calories from fat); 3.9 g protein; 26.4 g carbohydrate; 1.6 g dietary fiber; 20.3 mg cholesterol; 196.9 mg sodium

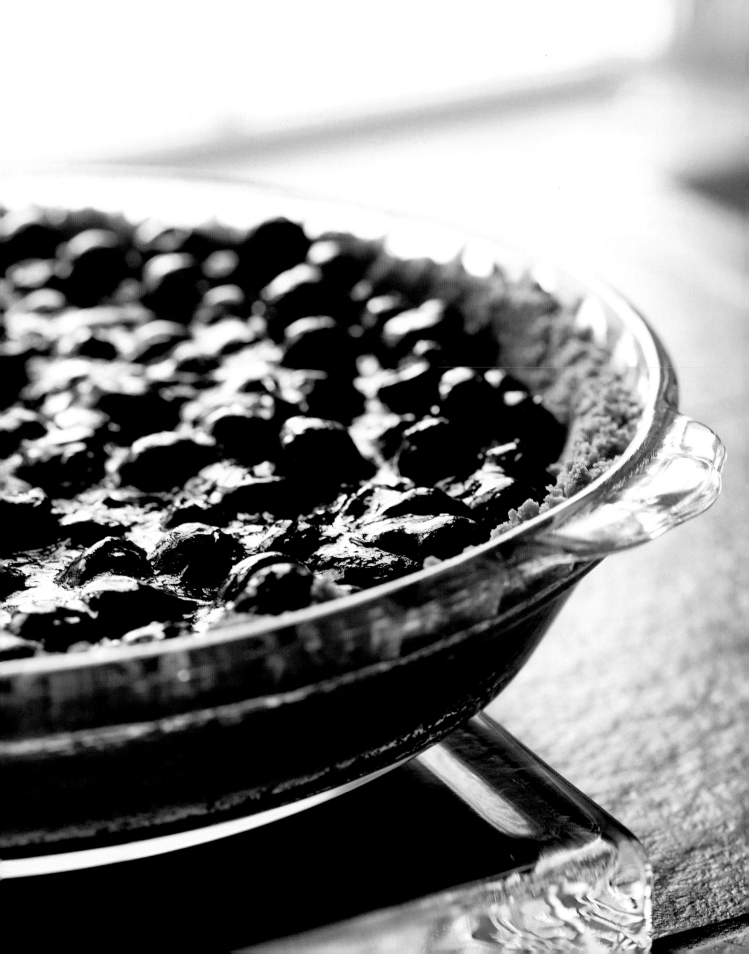

Ingredients

¾ cup (175 ml) cold water, divided

⅔ cup (135 g) sugar (or Sucanat)

Pinch of salt

2 pints (580 g) fresh blueberries, divided

2½ tablespoons (20 g) kudzu

1 cooked, premade crust (try our Organic
    Gingersnappy Piecrust, page 139, or
    Satisfying Real-Food Piecrust, page 137)

From Chef Jeannette

Even Healthier: To reduce the sugar
even further, use 100 percent pure apple
juice in place of the water and reduce the
sugar to ¼ cup (50 g).

Memorable Freshest Blueberry Blast Pie

From Dr. Jonny: So there's good news and bad news. The bad news first: This isn't exactly a low-cal treat. (But the news isn't really bad—just don't eat the whole pie, like some people I know. I'm not naming names, but his initials are Jonny. I'm just saying.) The good news, and it's really good news, is that you can feel great about eating this dessert because it's loaded with one of the healthiest foods on Earth, blueberries. Blueberries first got their reputation as a memory food from the published research of the late Jim Josephs, Ph.D., who found that old rats fed a blueberry concentrate acted like young rats, learning mazes faster, and generally just "dancing the Macarena," as Josephs put it. The whole fresh, nutrient-loaded berries will just burst in your mouth letting loose a taste that's light and sweet and about as far as you can get from that sticky, gluey, syrupy "gel" that fills most commercial blueberry pies. Best of all, ours is way lower in sugar and, as a special added attraction, you don't even have to bake it. Hint: Use our Satisfying Real-Food Piecrust and you'll be banishing trans fats to boot!

In a medium saucepan over medium heat, combine ½ cup (120 ml) of the water, sugar, and salt and whisk occasionally to help dissolve the sugar. When the sugar is completely dissolved, add 1 cup (145 g) of the blueberries and bring to a simmer. In a small bowl or cup, whisk the remaining ¼ cup (60 ml) cold water and kudzu until the kudzu is completely dissolved. Add the kudzu mixture to the blueberry mixture and simmer, stirring gently, for about 2 minutes, or until thickened. Fold in the remaining 3 cups (435 g) blueberries and pour the mixture into the prepared pie shell. Chill for at least 2 hours before serving.

Yield: 8 to 12 servings

Per Serving: 191.7 calories; 7.9 g fat (36% calories from fat); 17.2 g protein; 29.6 g carbohydrate; 1.7 g dietary fiber; 20.3 mg cholesterol; 99.7 mg sodium

Ingredients

2 ounces (55 g) high-quality unsweetened
chocolate (such as Scharffen Berger,
Dagoba, or Callebaut)

2 tablespoons (28 g) butter

1/4 cup (55 g) coconut oil

3/4 cup (150 g) sugar

2 tablespoons (16 g) whole-wheat pastry
flour

1/2 teaspoon cinnamon

2 eggs, lightly beaten

1 teaspoon vanilla extract

1 cup (100 g) chopped, toasted, unsalted
pecans (or slivered almonds)

1 unbaked 9-inch (23-cm) pie shell
(page 137)

From Chef Jeannette

Even Healthier: For less processed,
more natural sweetening, substitute
Sucanat for the sugar in an equal
amount. The pie will set in 25 to 30
minutes of cooking time and will be
a little drier in consistency.

Dark and Mineral-Rich Coco-Fudgy Pie

From Dr. Jonny: Here's a riddle: What do you get when you cross-
breed three of your favorite comfort foods—chocolate fudge, chocolate
pie, and a brownie? Give up? Well here's the answer: Chef Jeannette's
Dark and Mineral-Rich Coco-Fudgy Pie. Now, to get this kind of
gooey richness you usually have to be drowning in sugar and butter.
Personally, I don't mind butter as an ingredient, but replacing some of
it with coconut oil adds a lot of healthy fats called MCTs, as well as
certain fatty acids (such as lauric acid), which are well known to be antimicrobial and thus a boon to the immune system. Sugar, on the other
hand, is a different story. So we reduced the sugar (you'll never notice)
and added rich dark chocolate and a full cup of pecans, one of the
most mineral-rich nuts on the planet. The eggs add protein to the mix
and cinnamon helps modulate blood sugar (as well as adding a really
nice taste note). Healthwise, this isn't exactly a plate of steamed veggies—it's definitely an indulgence—but our version is a heck of a lot
healthier than, say, a chunk of fudge!

Do not preheat the oven. In a medium saucepan over medium heat, melt
the chocolate, butter, and coconut oil together, whisking occasionally, until
smooth. Remove from the heat, whisk in the sugar, and let cool. Whisk in
the flour, cinnamon, eggs, and vanilla. Stir in the pecans and spoon the
batter into the pie shell. Place the pie in a cold oven, set to 350°F (180°C,
or gas mark 4), and bake for 30 to 35 minutes, until mostly set. Cool for
30 minutes to 1 hour; the pie will be gooey and will set more with more
cooling time. Serve warm or chilled.

Yield: 12 servings

Per Serving: 246.3 calories; 17.6 g fat (62% calories from fat); 3.4 g
protein; 22.5 g carbohydrate; 2.5 g dietary fiber; 40.3 mg cholesterol;
81 mg sodium

Ingredients

3 sweet baking apples, unpeeled, cored, and
    chopped (such as Golden Delicious)

1 cup (100 g) thickly sliced rhubarb

1 cup (200 g) Sucanat, sugar, or xylitol,
    divided

¼ cup (50 g) xylitol, optional

1 tablespoon (8 g) kudzu dissolved in
    2 tablespoons (28 ml) apple juice or
    water (or 1 tablespoon [8 g] cornstarch
    or 2 tablespoons [16 g] wheat flour)

2 eggs, separated

½ cup (40 g) rolled oats

⅓ cup (40 g) wheat flour (or whole-wheat
    pastry flour for more fiber)

¼ teaspoon salt

¼ cup (55 g) butter, softened (or coconut or
    almond oil)

¾ cup (105 g) toasted pine nuts (or toasted
    sliced almonds)

Vitamin C–Rich Sweet-Tart Apple Rhubarb Crisp

From Dr. Jonny: I'm mystified as to why more people don't know about rhubarb. A cup of the stuff has almost no calories (okay, okay, 26 if you must know), more than 100 mg of calcium, and almost as much potassium as a banana (351 mg for a cup of rhubarb versus 422 mg for a medium banana). Plus, its tart flavor makes it perfect for a dessert. This dish, which is normally supersweet, benefits beautifully from the pleasant tangy-tart complement of the rhubarb. But because it is so tart, you need a fair amount of sweetener. We recommend that at least part of that sweetness comes from xylitol, a naturally occurring sugar alcohol that has a very minor glycemic impact (it won't do anything of consequence to your blood sugar) and also has health benefits—it helps prevent bacteria from adhering to the mucous membranes. Chef Jeannette also lightened up on the usually sugary crumble topping and added nuts (fiber, minerals, and monounsaturated fats) and oats (fiber and more nutrients). Throw in two eggs for additional high-quality protein and cinnamon to help balance the impact on blood sugar. And of course, leave the peels on the apples, which is where a lot of the valuable pectin fiber is found. Fun fact: Rhubarb is classified as a vegetable, botanically speaking, but in 1947, a New York court decided to count it as a fruit for regulatory purposes. This little taxonomy sleight of hand resulted in a reduction in taxes paid. Hey, it's no worse than classifying ketchup as a vegetable.

Preheat the oven to 375°F (190°C, or gas mark 5).

In a large bowl, toss the apples and rhubarb with ½ cup (100 g) of the Sucanat, the xylitol, and the kudzu.

In a small bowl, beat the egg yolks until pale yellow and stir into the fruit. In a mixer, beat the egg whites until they form stiff peaks, and then fold into the fruit. Pour the mixture into a 9 x 9-inch (23 x 23-cm) pan and set aside.

In a medium bowl, mix together the oats, flour, remaining ½ cup (100 g) Sucanat, and salt until well combined. Add the butter and mix until it forms large crumbs. Stir in the nuts and sprinkle the mixture evenly over the top.

Cover lightly with aluminum foil and bake for 30 to 40 minutes, or until bubbly and the fruit is tender. Remove the foil to brown the topping for the last 10 minutes of cooking time, if desired.

Yield: 9 generous servings

Per Serving: 258.6 calories; 14.4 g fat (48% calories from fat); 4.2 g protein; 31.4 g carbohydrate; 2.9 g dietary fiber; 60.1 mg cholesterol; 82 mg sodium

Ingredients

Cooking oil spray

5 pounds (2.3 kg) ripe fresh peaches

⅓ cup (67 g) sugar (or Sucanat or xylitol), divided

1½ teaspoons (3.5 g) cinnamon, divided

½ teaspoon coriander

½ teaspoon nutmeg

⅓ cups (42 g) plus 1½ cups (190 g) unbleached flour, divided

½ teaspoon salt

½ teaspoon sugar

⅔ cup (150 g) butter, well-chilled

1 small egg (or ½ large, lightly beaten egg)

½ teaspoon white vinegar

2 tablespoons (28 ml) cold water

1½ cups (230 g) frozen blueberries

1 egg white, lightly beaten

Tender and Trans Fat–Free Peach and Blueberry Cobbler

From Dr. Jonny: Explaining why this peach and blueberry cobbler is much healthier for you than the usual fare requires me to give you a fast lesson in fats. But stick with me because when you know this, you will know more than most people, including some doctors, sad to say, about fats and the human body. So here goes: Trans fats are the most damaging fat on Earth. They are much worse for you than saturated fats, which actually are turning out to be nowhere near as bad as conventional medicine believes. (Want proof? Write me on my website, www.jonnybowden.com, and I'll send you the studies.) But because saturated fats have been wrongly demonized, everyone stopped using them and shifted to vegetable shortening—which is a nutritional nightmare. All of that white thick shortening is absolutely loaded with trans fats, which significantly increase the risk for heart disease and stroke. (I'll send you the studies on that, too, if you want!) Bottom line: We use butter for this cobbler. That's right, real, wholesome butter, which is a perfectly acceptable whole food containing not a mg of trans fats, some monounsaturated fat, and yes, some perfectly acceptable saturated fat. It also makes the darn thing taste amazing. Because the taste is rich and smooth, we can use a smaller amount of crust, which is as light and flaky as any you'll ever taste. We leave the skins on the peaches (rich in healthy plant compounds), add blueberries for extra antioxidants, and use about only one-third the sugar in conventional recipes. This will knock you out as a delicious and satisfying treat in the summer. Hint: Make it when the peaches are freshest—they're also cheaper then, too!

Preheat the oven to 425°F (220°C, or gas mark 7) and spray a nonstick 9 x 13-inch (23 x 33-cm) baking pan lightly with a neutral, high-heat cooking oil and set aside.

Pit the peaches and slice them thickly (eight to ten slices each, depending on the size of the peach). Place the sliced peaches into a large bowl and sprinkle with ¼ cup, or 50 g, of the sugar, ⅓ cup, or 42 g of the flour, 1 teaspoon of the cinnamon, the coriander, and nutmeg. Mix gently and set aside to rest.

In a large bowl, whisk together the remaining 1½ cups (190 g) flour, salt, and sugar.

(continued on page 152)

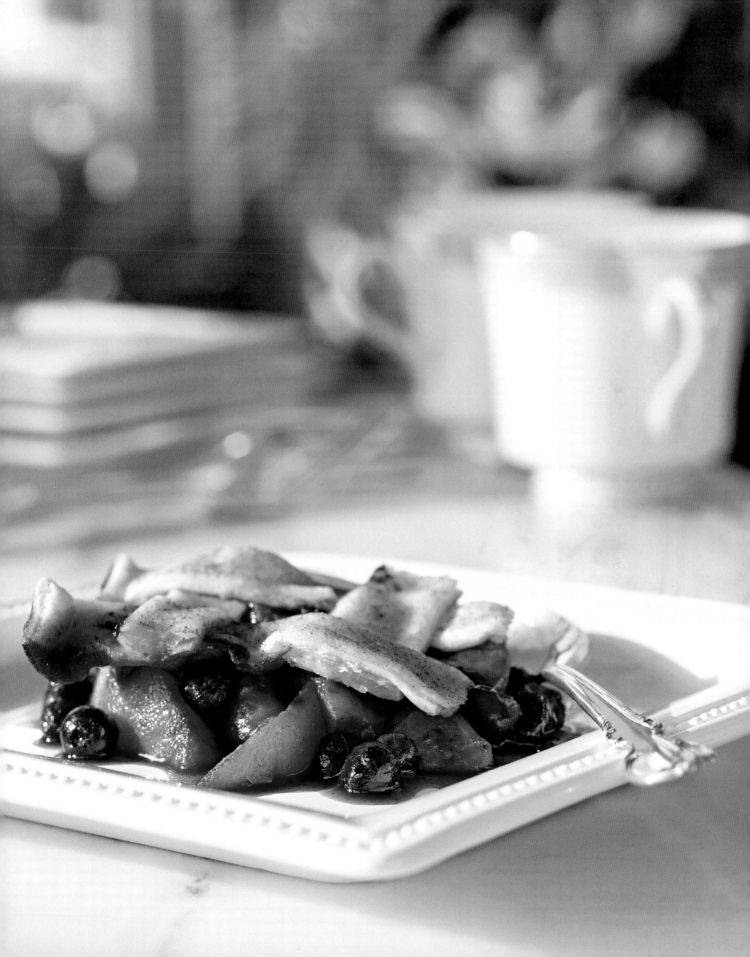

Add the cold butter to a food processor and pulse a few times to chop. Gently pour in the flour mixture and pulse until it forms moist crumbs, scraping down the sides, as necessary. Don't worry if you can still see bits of butter—that helps with the flakiness. (You can also use a pastry cutter or two knives: Dice the chilled butter into pieces—or grate by hand using a cheese grater—and cut them into the flour until the mixture forms moist crumbs.) Return the flour mixture to the large bowl.

Whisk the egg, vinegar, and water together in a small bowl and pour it into the flour crumbs. Knead with your hands just until it achieves a smooth, elastic consistency. Do not overwork the dough or it will become tough.

Flour a smooth surface (a pastry stone works the best for this) and lay the dough in the center. Pull the dough into a large rectangle. Flour a rolling pin and roll the dough into a large rectangle about ¼ inch (6 mm) thick. Slice widthwise into ¾-inch (2-cm) strips. (If the dough warms it will get sticky and harder to handle—just pop it in the refrigerator for 10 minutes and try again.)

Stir the frozen blueberries gently into the peaches and pour the mixture into the prepared pan. Gently lifting each strip from the pastry stone (using the sharp blade of a knife to help you remove it in one piece, if necessary), lay strips of the dough lengthwise across the peaches, and then lay shorter strips widthwise across the longer strips to make a crosshatch pattern. Wrap any leftover dough tightly in plastic wrap and store in the refrigerator for another use.

In a small bowl, mix the remaining 4 teaspoons (17 g) sugar and remaining ½ teaspoon cinnamon together.

Lightly brush the crust with the beaten egg white and sprinkle the cinnamon sugar evenly over the coated crust. Cover tightly with aluminum foil and bake for 30 minutes.

Reduce the oven temperature to 350°F (180°C, or gas mark 4) and bake for an additional 20 to 30 minutes, until the fruit is bubbling. Once the fruit is bubbling, remove the foil and cook for about 20 minutes longer, or until the crust is lightly browned. Let cool for at least 10 minutes before serving.

Yield: about 16 servings
Per Serving: 197.1 calories; 8.5 g fat (38% calories from fat); 3.3 g protein; 29.1 g carbohydrate; 3 g dietary fiber; 33.4 mg cholesterol; 82 mg sodium

Ingredients

1/2 cup (112 g) butter, softened

1/2 cup (115 g) packed brown sugar

1/4 cup (50 g) sugar or xylitol

1 egg

1 egg yolk

2 tablespoons (28 ml) milk (low-fat cow's, or unsweetened vanilla almond or soy milk)

1 teaspoon vanilla extract

1 cup (125 g) whole-wheat pastry flour

3/4 cup (95 g) oat flour (or unbleached flour)

2 tablespoons (14 g) wheat germ

1/2 teaspoon cinnamon

3/4 teaspoon baking soda

1/4 teaspoon salt

1 cup (175 g) high-quality dark chocolate chips

2/3 cup (73 g) chopped unsalted pecans

From Chef Jeannette

Even Healthier: If you want to cut down on the butterfat even further and add some nut or seed nutrients, leave out half the butter and replace it with 1/4 cup (65 g) of natural, no-added-sugar peanut butter or tahini. Add the seed or nut butter after creaming the 1/4 cup (55 g) butter and sugars. You may wish to add an extra tablespoon (15 g) of brown sugar as well, but that's optional.

Decadent Dark Chocolate Chip Multigrain Cookies

From Dr. Jonny: Chocolate chip cookies are another of my favorite food memories. You could always count on being able to find at least one box of Chips Ahoy in the kitchen pantry at our apartment in Jackson Heights, Queens, and at age eight or so I wasn't exactly reading ingredients labels, so all I knew was that they tasted great and were especially good dipped in milk. Then as I got older we progressed to Famous Amos (when he was still Famous Amos and not a conglomerate), Mrs. Fields, David's, and all the rest. If you weren't paying attention, you might not have noticed that as the decades went on the size of the average cookie seemed to grow . . . and grow . . . and grow. Now even the "healthy" versions of chocolate chip cookies they sell at places like Whole Foods are the size of flying saucers. Which I guess is fine if you don't mind ingesting about 900 calories a pop (I exaggerate, but I assure you, not by much). So we downsized the gigantimungus version you see in the stores, used two different kinds of whole-grain flours, and boosted the fiber content with wheat germ. We halved the sugar and cut back on the butter by a good 33 percent. And to up the health quotient we used high-quality dark chocolate for the chips (high in blood pressure–lowering antioxidants known as flavonols). Bonus health points for the pecans, rich in the same monounsaturated fat found in olive oil.

Preheat the oven to 350°F (180°C, or gas mark 4).

In a mixer beat together the butter and sugars until fluffy. Beat in the egg and egg yolk, then the milk and vanilla. In a medium bowl, whisk together the flours, wheat germ, cinnamon, baking soda, and salt. Add the dry mix to the wet and beat on low until just combined. Fold in the chocolate chips and pecans.

Using a tablespoon, scoop 1½-inch (3.8-cm) balls and arrange on a large cookie sheet (you don't have to shape the cookies—just drop batter onto the sheet). Bake for 10 to 12 minutes, or until golden brown.

Yield: about 24 cookies, serving size 1 cookie

Per Serving: 153 calories; 8.8 g fat (49% calories from fat); 2.5 g protein; 18.1 g carbohydrate; 1.7 g dietary fiber; 26.4 mg cholesterol; 93.6 mg sodium

Ingredients

²/₃ cup (150 g) butter, softened

³/₄ cup (150 g) sugar

1 egg

1 teaspoon ginger juice, prepared or
     fresh squeezed

¹/₄ cup (85 g) blackstrap molasses

1 cup (125 g) unbleached flour

³/₄ cup (95 g) whole-wheat pastry flour

1 tablespoon (5.5 g) ground ginger

1 teaspoon baking soda

Pinch of salt

From Chef Jeannette

To make ginger juice, grate 1 to 2
tablespoons (8 to 16 g) of fresh ginger
and squeeze the gratings in your hand to
release the juice.

Simple Snappy Real Ginger Cookies

From Dr. Jonny: Here's one of my vivid childhood memories: searching through the kitchen cabinet in our apartment in Jackson Heights, Queens, in hopes of finding treasure, treasure that came in three flavors, from some strange land named Nabisco. The three flavors of treasure? Chocolate-covered grahams, chocolate-covered marshmallows (Mallomars to those of you born after 1960), and gingersnaps—the latter of which tasted especially good when dipped in milk and softened. But I digress. To make this version of my childhood treasure, we used less sugar and butter than usual and included blackstrap molasses for its rich array of minerals (including iron). We also swapped out half the regular flour for a higher-fiber version. Warming and comforting like the best childhood Christmases, our gingersnaps are light and satisfying. And they get soft if you dip them in milk. (I'm just saying.)

Preheat the oven to 350°F (180°C, or gas mark 4).

In a mixer, cream the butter and sugar together until light and fluffy. Add the egg, ginger juice, and molasses and beat until well incorporated.

In a large bowl, whisk together the flours, ground ginger, baking soda, and salt. Slowly add the dry ingredients to the wet and beat on low until well mixed. Roll the dough into 1½-inch (3.8-cm) balls and place on a cookie sheet about 2 inches (5 cm) apart. Bake for 9 to 10 minutes, or until the cookies have flattened and the surfaces look dryish and lightly cracked. They should still be a little wet inside. Transfer the cookies to a cooling rack for 5 minutes or until cooled completely.

Yield: about 24 cookies, serving size 1 cookie

Per Serving: 113.9 calories; 5.4 g fat (41% calories from fat); 1.3 g protein; 15.5 g carbohydrate; 0.3 g dietary fiber; 22.3 mg cholesterol; 93.5 mg sodium

Ingredients

1/3 cup (65 g) Sucanat or brown sugar

1/3 cup (65 g) sugar or xylitol

1/3 cup (75 g) butter, softened

2/3 cup (175 g) natural peanut butter, no sugar added

1 egg

1 teaspoon vanilla extract

3/4 cup (95 g) unbleached flour

1/2 cup (40 g) quick-cooking oats

3/4 teaspoon baking soda

1/4 teaspoon salt

1/2 cup (88 g) dark chocolate chips, optional

From Chef Jeannette

Even Healthier: For more fiber and nutrients, substitute whole-wheat pastry flour for the regular unbleached flour.

Dreamy, All-Natural Choco–Peanut Butter Cookies

From Dr. Jonny: Cookies have to be on everyone's top-five list of comfort foods, and it's remarkably easy to make this old favorite a bit healthier than the usual fare. All you have to do is cut back a bit on the butter and sugar and use natural peanut butter. It's not widely known, but most commercial peanut butters—and you know who I'm talking about Mr. Jif/Skippy—have a significant amount of added sugar and, even worse, trans fats. Just look at the label and you'll see sugar as the second ingredient and hydrogenated vegetable oils as the third. (Hydrogenated and partially hydrogenated oils are trans fats!) So go with peanut butter that is as close as possible to what comes out of the grinder when you put in a bunch of peanuts—in fact, many grocery stores now have grinders for just that purpose and you can "roll your own" right there in the store. We also substituted oats, with their rich concentration of phytonutrients, for part of the flour to boost the fiber content. Dark (cocoa-rich) chocolate guarantees a nice helping of those plant compounds called flavonols that have made chocolate into the latest health food!

Preheat the oven to 375°F (190°C, or gas mark 5).

Combine the Sucanat, sugar, and butter in a large bowl and beat with a mixer until light and fluffy. Add the peanut butter and beat until creamy. Add the egg and vanilla and beat to incorporate.

In a medium bowl, whisk together the flour, oats, baking soda, and salt. Add the dry ingredients to the wet and mix by hand until incorporated. Stir in the chocolate chips. Make 1½-inch (3.8-cm) balls and arrange on a nonstick cookie sheet (or use a regular baking sheet lined with parchment paper). Moisten a fork with water and flatten the cookies slightly with a crisscross pattern. Bake for 7 to 9 minutes, or to desired doneness.

Yield: about 20 cookies, serving size 1 cookie

Per Serving: 126.7 calories; 2 g fat (13% calories from fat); 3.5 g protein; 14.2 g carbohydrate; 1.2 g dietary fiber; 11.3 mg cholesterol; 83.8 mg sodium

Ingredients

1 teaspoon cardamom seeds (or ¾ teaspoon ground cardamom or 1 teaspoon ground cinnamon)

¼ cup (55 g) butter, softened

¾ cup (150 g) plus 1 tablespoon (13 g) sugar, divided

2 tablespoons (28 ml) almond oil

1 teaspoon vanilla extract

2 eggs

1 cup (125 g) unbleached flour

½ cup (63 g) whole-wheat pastry flour

½ teaspoon baking soda

¼ teaspoon salt

From Chef Jeannette

Even Healthier: To increase protein and fiber, exchange ⅓ cup (40 g) of the unbleached flour (not the pastry flour) for ⅓ cup (40 g) blanched almond flour. This will give your cookies a satisfyingly dense consistency as well.

Spiced, Lower-Sugar Cookies

From Dr. Jonny: How do you make one of the ultimate comfort foods—sugar cookies—better for you? After all, they're sugar cookies, for goodness sake! Well, you're not going to turn sugar cookies into the nutritional equivalent of a grass-fed burger with a side of carrots, but you can definitely improve them by lowering the amount of sugar and using whole-wheat flour (which gives you at least some fiber!). Use cardamom to spice things up, and the end result is a unique and puffy sugar cookie that will have everyone in the house drifting to the kitchen to discover the source of that incredible aroma. (Note: Substitute cinnamon for the cardamom for a nice twist on an old favorite.) Fun fact: Cardamom is frequently mentioned in *The Arabian Nights* and was considered a catalyst for romance. It also improves digestion and is used as a breath freshener, for which it's terrifically effective.

Preheat the oven to 350°F (180°C, or gas mark 4).

In a small saucepan, toast the cardamom seeds over medium heat for 3 to 4 minutes or until very fragrant. Remove from the heat and grind them to a powder (a designated coffee grinder or spice grinder works well for this).

In the mixer, cream together the butter, ¾ cup (150 g) of the sugar, almond oil, and vanilla until fluffy. Add the eggs and beat at medium speed until incorporated. Set aside.

In a medium bowl, whisk together the flours, baking soda, and salt. Spoon the creamed mix into the dry mix and stir together until well incorporated. Form 1-inch (2.5-cm) balls and place on 2 cookies sheets with space between each cookie, flattening slightly.

In a small bowl, mix together the remaining 1 tablespoon (13 g) sugar and ground cardamom. Sprinkle each cookie with a pinch or two of the cardamom sugar, to taste, and bake for 8 to 9 minutes, or until just lightly browned on the bottoms.

Yield: about 20 cookies, serving size 1 cookie

Per Serving: 104.9 calories; 4.1 g fat (35% calories from fat); 1.6 g protein; 15.4 g carbohydrate; 0.3 g dietary fiber; 27.1 mg cholesterol; 68.1 mg sodium

Decadent Better-Fat Walnut Brownies

Ingredients

Neutral cooking oil spray

4 ounces (115 g) high-quality unsweetened chocolate (such as Scharffen Berger, Dagoba, or Callebaut)

3 tablespoons (45 g) butter

3 tablespoons (45 g) coconut oil

4 eggs

1¹⁄₃ cups (265 g) sugar

³⁄₄ cup (180 g) natural applesauce (no sugar added)

1 teaspoon vanilla extract

¹⁄₄ teaspoon salt

¹⁄₂ teaspoon cinnamon, optional

1 cup (125 g) unbleached flour

¹⁄₃ cup (40 g) chopped toasted walnuts or pecans

From Chef Jeannette

Even Healthier: For more fiber and nutrients, substitute whole-wheat pastry flour for the regular flour.

From Dr. Jonny: Both Chef Jeannette and I are in agreement: Brownies are a food group. They're not? Well, they should be. Seriously folks, it's hardly unusual to see a recipe for brownies that calls for two sticks of (nonorganic) butter and two cups of white sugar. That's a ton of calories—and you can do better. Just replace some of the butter with applesauce and use less sugar. Don't worry—the brownie still has that rich mouthfeel, only it comes from a mix of butter and coconut oil (rich in antimicrobial fatty acids) plus the fat in heart-healthy walnuts (also rich in fiber and minerals such as potassium, calcium, phosphorus, and magnesium). Don't forget to use dark chocolate—it's the only kind that contains flavonols, plant compounds that help lower blood pressure and do double duty as antioxidants. The four eggs add plenty of protein, and the optional cinnamon (delish if you ask me) may help blunt the impact of the brownie on your blood sugar.

Preheat the oven to 350°F (180°C, or gas mark 4). Lightly spray a 9 x 13-inch (23 x 33-cm) pan with oil.

Melt the chocolate, butter, and coconut oil in a medium pan over medium heat, whisking to incorporate. As soon as it is melted and mixed, remove from the heat and allow to cool.

Combine the eggs and sugar and beat with a mixer until well mixed. Add the applesauce, vanilla, and salt and beat to incorporate. Add the cooled chocolate mixture and beat to mix well.

In a separate bowl, combine the salt, cinnamon, and flour. Add the flour mixture to the chocolate mixture and beat on low just until incorporated. Fold in the nuts and pour into the pan. Bake for 20 to 25 minutes, or until the center springs back when lightly pressed.

Yield: 24 brownies, serving size 1 brownie

Per Serving: 142 calories; 7.9 g fat (48% calories from fat); 2.5 g protein; 17.7 g carbohydrate; 1.2 g dietary fiber; 39.3 mg cholesterol; 37.6 mg sodium

Ingredients

1 cup (235 ml) light coconut milk, divided

¼ cup (50 g) sugar

3 tablespoons (45 g) brown sugar or Sucanat

¼ cup (30 g) high-quality cocoa

3 tablespoons (24 g) kudzu (or cornstarch, but cook it for a couple of minutes longer to dissipate the starchy taste)

1 teaspoon cinnamon

Pinch of salt

1 cup (235 ml) milk (low fat cow's, or unsweetened chocolate almond or soy)

4 ounces (115 g) high-quality semisweet chocolate (such as Scharffen Berger, Dagoba, or Callebaut), broken into small pieces

1½ teaspoons (7.5 ml) vanilla extract

Jonny's Fudgy Chocolate Antioxidant Pudding

From Dr. Jonny: Chocolate pudding was one of my favorite childhood treats. However, my mother was—bless her heart—not the greatest cook in the world. So we wound up with a bowl of pudding made from a mix that featured a thin film on top that I absolutely loved but found out later meant that she burned it. Oh, well. It's still my favorite comfort food, and in honor of my childhood memories, Chef Jeannette has whipped up this version. It's lighter on the sugar and higher on the protein. It's also waaaay richer than the stuff that comes in the box! The dark chocolate in cocoa is brimming with plant compounds called flavonols, which are powerful antioxidants and also have the ability to lower blood pressure. Cinnamon does double duty by adding a terrific spiced flavor to the end result while slightly lowering the impact on your blood sugar. Fun fact: Kudzu is now being researched at Harvard for its potential in reducing alcohol cravings. And because of the plant's tendency to grow at the rate that rabbits reproduce, it's earned the nickname "mile-a-minute vine."

Place ½ cup (120 ml) of the coconut milk, the sugars, cocoa, kudzu, cinnamon, and salt in a narrow bowl with high sides and blend with an immersion blender until well mixed and the thickener is dissolved (or use a regular blender). Set aside.

In a medium pan over medium heat, bring the milk and remaining ½ cup (120 ml) coconut milk almost to a boil (you will see the steam increasing and tiny bubbles beginning to form). When you see the milk starting to steam, stir the cold mixture and, just before the milk boils, pour the cold mixture into the hot milk in the pan and whisk until it thickens and comes to a boil. Remove the pan from the heat, stir in the semisweet chocolate and vanilla, let sit for about 30 seconds, then whisk until melted and well incorporated. Pour into 4 to 6 dessert bowls or glasses.

Serve warm or chilled.

Yield: 4 to 6 servings

Per Serving: 219 calories; 8.8 g fat (33% calories from fat); 2.9 g protein; 36.8 g carbohydrate; 3 g dietary fiber; 3.3 mg cholesterol; 37.5 mg sodium

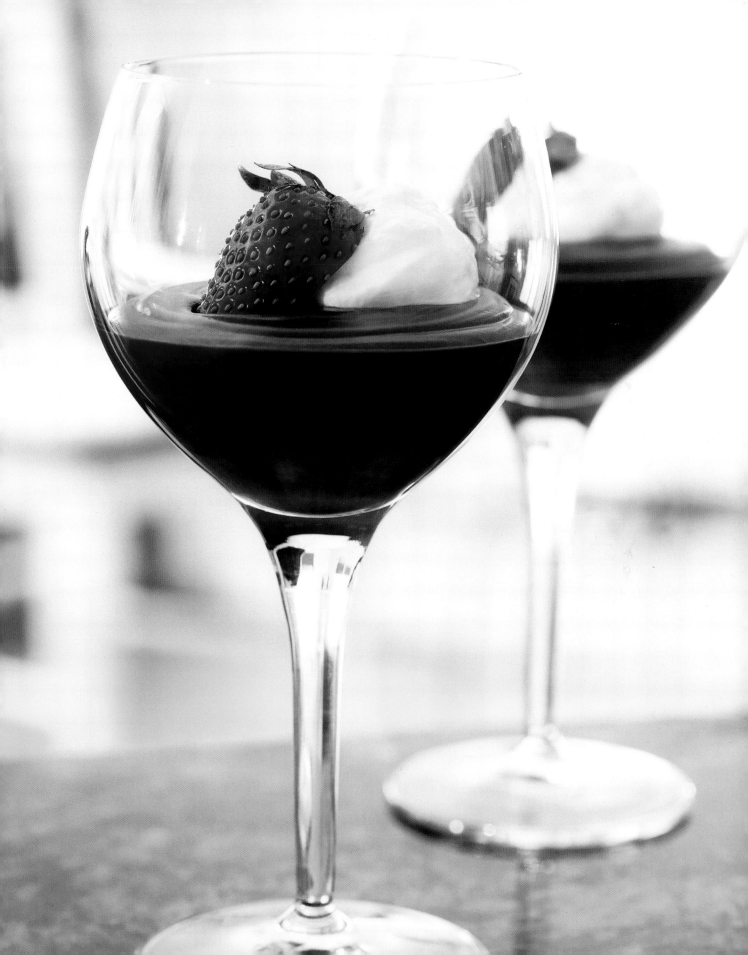

Creamy and Nutritious Coconutty Rice Pudding

Ingredients

1 can (14 ounces, or 425 ml) light coconut milk

Water to make total liquid content (including coconut milk) just over 2³/₄ cups (650 ml)

1 cup (190 g) short-grain brown rice

¼ cup (20 g) dried shredded coconut, unsweetened

³/₄ teaspoon vanilla extract

3 to 4 tablespoons (45 to 60 ml) 100 percent maple syrup, preferably grade B (or xylitol for no-added-sugar version), to taste

³/₄ teaspoon cinnamon, optional

½ teaspoon nutmeg

¹/₃ cup (40 g) toasted slivered almonds (or toasted and chopped pistachios or pecans), optional

From Chef Jeannette

Time-Saver Tip: To save on the cooking time, replace the short-grain rice with parboiled brown rice. Combine 2³/₄ cups (650 ml) total liquid (versus 3 cups with short-grain rice) with 1 cup (190 g) parboiled rice, cook for 35 minutes or until creamy, add the remaining ingredients as described, and serve or let chill.

From Dr. Jonny: Along with chocolate graham crackers, chocolate pudding, gingerbread cake, and ice cream, rice pudding is one of my all-time favorite desserts, almost high enough on my list to give it the coveted "kryptonite" rating. I'm just kidding (about the kryptonite, not the rice pudding). Regular old rice pudding is typically made with white rice (not a nutrient in sight), cow's milk, and a ton of sugar. Make it a healthier comfort food by subbing out the white rice for brown, increasing nutrients and fiber, and swapping the cow's milk for coconut milk and water. Coconut milk? Yep. Coconut is a true health food, containing all sorts of goodies such as antimicrobial lauric acid and a type of fat the body doesn't like to put on your hips (it's called MCTs if you want to impress your friends). Sweeten with a small amount of mineral-rich grade-B maple syrup, cinnamon (which helps modulate blood sugar), and nuts for monounsaturated fat, fiber, and minerals. Little fun fact: Two major studies found that just 5 ounces, or 140 g, of nuts per week was associated with a 35 to 50 percent reduction in the risk of coronary heart disease and death!

Combine the coconut milk, water, rice, and coconut in a medium, heavy-bottomed saucepan and bring to a boil over high heat. Stir, reduce the heat to low, cover, and simmer for about 50 minutes, or until the rice is tender and creamy. Stir in the vanilla, maple syrup, cinnamon, and nutmeg until well combined, cover, remove from the heat, and let stand for 10 minutes. Top with the nuts. Serve hot or cold.

Yield: 4 to 6 servings

Per Serving: 228.8 calories; 8.6 g fat (32% calories from fat); 3.5 g protein; 38.1 g carbohydrate; 4 g dietary fiber; 0 mg cholesterol; 37.8 mg sodium

Ingredients

8 small high-quality, all-natural chocolate
    cookie snaps (such as MI-DEL)
1 pint (490 g) vanilla frozen yogurt (or ice
    milk or low-fat ice cream)
2 scoops unsweetened, undenatured vanilla
    whey protein powder, softened
3 tablespoons (48 g) natural peanut butter,
    no added sugar
3/4 cup (175 ml) milk (low-fat cow's,
    unsweetened vanilla soy or almond)
1 teaspoon vanilla extract

From Chef Jeannette

Even Healthier: To reduce the calories
and sugar even more, omit the cookies
and add 1 heaping tablespoon (8 g)
raw cacao powder or 2 teaspoons (5 g)
cocoa powder.

Chocolate Peanut Butter Protein-Power Milkshakes

From Dr. Jonny: Here's a great way to make a milkshake healthier: Use frozen yogurt and real peanut butter. The classic milkshake is really high in calories because of the premium ice cream and chocolate syrup. No one loves ice cream more than I do, but in combination with pure chocolate syrup, it is lethal from a sugar and calorie point of view. Frozen yogurt lowers the calories and using real peanut butter is an inspired touch, adding healthy fat, some protein, and a ton of flavor without breaking the calorie bank. (And with lots less sugar than the "classic" version.) The added nuts and protein powder will not only lower the glycemic impact (the impact on your blood sugar) but will also beef up the protein and keep you satisfied much longer.

Crush the cookies into small pieces in a resealable plastic bag with a rolling pin or in a food processor. Add the crushed cookies, frozen yogurt, protein powder, peanut butter, milk, and vanilla to a high-powered blender and blend until mostly smooth.

Yield: 4 servings
Per Serving: 321 calories; 5 g fat (14% calories from fat); 24.5 g protein; 32.4 g carbohydrate; 2.2 g dietary fiber; 9.8 mg cholesterol; 189.6 mg sodium

Light and Groovy Sorbet and Homemade Soda Floats

Ingredients

4 teaspoons (16 g) sugar, xylitol, or
    erythritol, or to taste

1 lemon, quartered

1 cup (125 g) fresh raspberries, optional

About 4 cups (933 ml) chilled lemon seltzer
    (no sugar or artificial ingredients)

4 scoops low-sugar, all-fruit raspberry
    sorbet

1 teaspoon lemon zest, optional

From Chef Jeannette

Variation: Customize these floats to meet
your own personal tastes. Try muddling
1 cup (30 g) lightly crushed mint leaves
with the sugar and adding plain seltzer
and chocolate sorbet for a cooling
chocolate-mint treat. Or mix 4 cups
(946 ml) plain seltzer with 2 cups
(475 ml) 100 percent pineapple juice
(not from concentrate) and use coconut
sorbet for a piña colada float.

From Dr. Jonny: Back in the day, I was a big fan of Archie comics. (Does anyone remember Archie? And the perpetual, almost biblical, allegory of good versus evil in the form of sweet-as-pie Betty and luscious Veronica? But I digress.) So in Archie world, teenagers were always going to "Le Sweet Shoppe" for ice cream floats, which meant I had to do the same thing. Talk about comfort food! Here's a way to make it better. Use lower-in-sugar, lower-in-fat sorbet instead of ice cream. And here's the fun part: Make your own soda. Nope, it's not hard at all—just some lemon seltzer and lemon zest will do the trick. Add fresh fruit such as raspberries and, as my mother used to say, "You're cookin' with gas!" We like this "soda" sweetened with erythritol, one of the safest and best of the "artificial" sweeteners (it's really a natural sugar alcohol, but let's not get technical). Its cooling properties are perfect for this recipe. Light, refreshing, and tangy, this really hits the spot on a hot summer night! (Note: Erythritol is available everywhere at supermarkets under the brand name Truvia.)

Spoon 1 teaspoon of sugar into each of 4 tall glasses. Squeeze the juice from ¼ lemon into each glass and mix with the sugar. Spoon ¼ cup (30 g) raspberries into each glass. Gently (and slowly, to prevent fizzing over!) add lemon seltzer to fill each glass to two-thirds full, stirring gently to combine. Gently place 1 scoop of sorbet into each glass and top with ¼ teaspoon of the zest.

Yield: 4 servings

Per Serving: 237.4 calories; 0.3 g fat (1% calories from fat); 0.7 g protein; 60.7 g carbohydrate; 423.4 g dietary fiber; 0 mg cholesterol; 1.2 mg sodium

Choose the Right Drink for Comfort—and Health

If you think drinking diet soda has no effect on your health, think again. Mounting evidence has shown that diet soda will not only not help you lose weight, it may also help you gain weight.

Unpleasant fact: A 2005 study at the University of Texas Health Science Center found a 41 percent increase in the risk for being overweight for every single can of diet soda a person consumed daily.

There's more. Researchers studied the dietary information of more than 9,500 people over nine years to determine how diet might affect metabolic syndrome—the collection of risk factors for cardiovascular disease and diabetes that includes abdominal obesity, high cholesterol and blood glucose levels, and elevated blood pressure—a well-known energy drainer. Not surprisingly, they found those who ate a diet high in refined grains, fried foods, and red meat had a higher risk—18 percent higher—for metabolic syndrome. Those who ate the most red meat increased their risk by 25 percent more than those who ate the least.

But here's the kicker—people who drank one can of diet soda a day had a whopping 34 percent higher risk of developing metabolic syndrome than those who drank none. That's one can of diet soda per day. Sweetened beverages such as juices and regular soda carried no extra risk.

So, you might well ask, how can something with no calories increase the risk for obesity and heart disease?

Sugar Cravings and the Pavlovian Response

One theory, the one I hold dear, has to do with Pavlov's dogs. You may remember from high school that Pavlov fed his dogs steak at the same time as he rang a bell. Eventually, the mere ringing of the bell caused the dogs to salivate, even though there was no meat in sight. Pavlov named this a "conditioned response."

My long-held theory has been that the sweet taste of diet soda works in the brain to create a conditioned response, and the body responds as it usually does to normal sugar—with insulin, the fat-storing hormone. Those circuits in the brain are pretty primitive, and they don't immediately recognize chemical fakery; as far as your brain is concerned, sweet means sugar. It's entirely possible that physiologically, you would respond to artificial sweeteners in the same way as you would to table sugar.

Now Josephine M. Egan, M.D., and Robert F. Margolskee, M.D., Ph.D., of the National Institutes of Health and Mount Sinai School of Medicine, respectively, have published research that offers a variation on my explanation. They write, "Apparently, the gut 'tastes' sugars and sweeteners in much the same way as does the tongue and by using many of the same signaling elements. Taste receptors and other taste signaling elements in the gut may be contributors to obesity, diabetes, metabolic syndrome, and other diet-related disorders." Our body can't tell the difference between real and artificial sweeteners.

Another theory is that the taste of something sweet—even if it's fake—creates the same cascade of cravings in a carb addict that real sugar does. Cravings lead to refrigerator raids and an overload of food, which leads to obesity. Then there's the diet soda and ice cream sundae theory. Some people believe that by drinking diet beverages they're "saving" calories, which subconsciously gives them "permission" to eat more.

Ingredients

Cooking oil spray

2 ounces (55 g) high-quality unsweetened chocolate (such as Scharffen Berger, Dagoba, or Callebaut)

$\frac{1}{2}$ cup (120 ml) water

$\frac{1}{3}$ cup (75 g) coconut oil, softened, but not completely melted (or butter)

1$\frac{1}{4}$ cups (250 g) sugar

3 eggs

1 teaspoon vanilla extract

1 teaspoon baking soda

2 cups (250 g) unbleached flour

1 cup (230 g) plain low-fat Greek yogurt

From Chef Jeannette

Even Healthier: For a sugar-free, lower-glycemic option, replace the sugar with xylitol.

Lower-Cal, Moist Mock Sour Cream Chocolate Cake

From Dr. Jonny: I love sour cream, and truth be told I don't think it's all that bad for you. But it's got 444 calories per cup, which means that any dessert you make with sour cream is going to be a caloric nightmare. Add butter, and you've pretty much broken the calorie bank. But that doesn't mean you can't have the rich moistness that you want in a dessert. Just substitute Greek yogurt for sour cream—it's higher in protein than regular yogurt. We use coconut oil because it's rich in immune-supporting ingredients such as lauric acid. (Highly recommended: Barlean's organic unrefined coconut oil.) We also use a little less sugar (you'll never miss it) and dark chocolate for its rich assortment \o plant compounds known as flavonols, which have multiple health benefits. (One study showed that eating about one square of dark chocolate a day lowered blood pressure by a couple of points!) Chocolatey, moist, and satisfying on its own, this cake doesn't need icing—a huge calorie- and sugar-saving bonus.

Preheat the oven to 325°F (170°C, or gas mark 3). Lightly spray a 9 x 13-inch (23 x 33-cm) baking pan with neutral cooking oil and set aside.

In a small saucepan over medium heat, combine the chocolate and water. Heat, whisking occasionally, until the chocolate is fully melted and mixed with the water until smooth. Set aside to cool.

In a mixer, cream together the coconut oil and sugar until light and fluffy. Add the eggs and vanilla and beat until well incorporated.

In a medium bowl, whisk the baking soda into the flour. Add half the flour mixture and the yogurt to the sugar mixture and beat on low until just combined. Add the rest of the flour mixture and the cooled chocolate and beat or mix by hand until just combined. Spoon the batter into the prepared pan and bake for 35 to 40 minutes, or until a toothpick inserted into the center comes out clean.

Yield: about 15 servings

Per Serving: 211.5 calories; 8.3 g fat (34% calories from fat); 4.3 g protein; 31.7 g carbohydrate; 1.1 g dietary fiber; 43.2 mg cholesterol; 109.9 mg sodium

Ingredients

Cooking oil spray

½ cup (120 ml) almond oil (or other neutrally flavored oil)

¼ cup (60 ml) walnut oil

½ cup (125 g) applesauce, unsweetened

1 cup (200 g) Sucanat or sugar

¼ cup frozen apple juice concentrate, thawed

4 eggs

2 cups (220 g) grated carrots

1 can (8 ounces, or 225 g) crushed pineapple in water or juice, partially drained

¾ cup (65 g) dried shredded coconut, unsweetened

½ cup (60 g) chopped walnuts

2 cups (250 g) unbleached flour

1½ teaspoons (7 g) baking soda

1 teaspoon baking powder

2 teaspoons (4.6 g) cinnamon

½ teaspoon cardamom, optional

½ teaspoon salt

1 recipe Rich and Creamy Lower-Cal Cream Cheese Frosting (page 166)

From Chef Jeannette

Even Healthier: For more fiber, nutrients, and a slightly denser texture, replace half or all of the flour with whole-wheat pastry flour.

Dense and Dreamy Fruit 'n Nut–Filled Carrot Cake

From Dr. Jonny: People eat carrot cake for two reasons. The first is obvious—it's delicious. The second is more subtle—we tell ourselves it can't be "bad" because, after all, it's made with carrots. The trouble with commercial carrot cake is that it's got too much sugar and too many calories. Try using delectable pineapple for its natural sweetness, which considerably reduces the need for additional sugar. Use applesauce instead of butter for the mouthfeel of fat without the additional calories. Walnuts and walnut oil are a great source of plant-based omega-3 fats, and the carrots give you fiber, calcium, potassium, beta-carotene, and vitamin A. Fun fact: According to an ancient philosophy called "The Doctrine of Signatures," foods that resemble certain organs can be used to benefit that same organ; according to the Doctrine, walnuts—which actually look like a little brain with a right and left hemisphere and wrinkles just like those on the neocortex—are considered "brain food."

Preheat the oven to 375°F (190°C, or gas mark 5). Lightly spray two 8-inch (20-cm) round cake pans with oil. Dust lightly with flour, tap to remove the excess, and set aside.

In a mixer, beat the oils, applesauce, Sucanat, and apple juice concentrate together until combined. Add the eggs and beat until well mixed. Stir in the carrots, pineapple, coconut, and walnuts until well incorporated. In a medium bowl, whisk together the flour, baking soda, baking powder, cinnamon, cardamom, and salt. Add the dry ingredients to the wet in batches, mixing gently until incorporated.

Pour the batter evenly into the 2 pans and bake for 30 to 35 minutes, or until a toothpick inserted into the center comes out clean. Cool for at least 10 minutes and carefully turn out onto wire racks. Cool completely and frost thinly as a layer cake with the frosting.

Yield: 9 servings

Per Serving: 588.1 calories; 35.9 g fat (53% calories from fat); 10.1 g protein; 59.7 g carbohydrate; 3.8 g dietary fiber; 113 mg cholesterol; 550 mg sodium

Rich and Creamy Lower-Cal Cream Cheese Frosting

Ingredients

1 package (8 ounces, or 225 g)
    Neufchâtel cheese, slightly softened
    (or ⅓ reduced-fat cream cheese)
1 cup (100 g) confectioners' sugar
1 teaspoon vanilla extract
¾ teaspoon orange or lemon zest, optional

From Dr. Jonny: Cream cheese frosting tastes great, no doubt about it. But it's made with two basic ingredients, cream cheese and sugar, which translates into a ton of calories and (obviously) a lot of sugar, both of which you don't really need. Chef Jeannette reduced the calories by substituting Neufchâtel cheese and cut the sugar in half. The result is so good you'll never miss the extra sugar! Tip: Use that optional lemon or orange zest to punch up the flavors even more, and create a good-looking presentation!

In a mixer, beat together the Neufchâtel, confectioners' sugar, vanilla, and zest until very smooth. Use or store in the refrigerator.

Yield: about ¾ cup (150 g), 9 servings
Per Serving: 109.7 calories; 5.7 g fat (47% calories from fat); 2.5 g protein; 11.9 g carbohydrate; 0.02 g dietary fiber; 19 mg cholesterol; 99.9 mg sodium

Real Fresh, Real Fruit Strawberry Ice Cream

From Dr. Jonny: If there were no consequences to doing so, I'd probably eat ice cream every night. It's one of my absolute favorite treats. So when I'm able to find ice cream that's not so bad for me, I jump on it. Chef Jeannette's take on strawberry ice cream is a heck of a lot healthier than the commercial stuff, which has way too much sugar and fat and often a ton of artificial ingredients and chemicals to boot. Chef Jeannette cleaned it up a bit with organic cream and milk and went light on the sugar. The result? A near-perfect, pink, sweet, cool comfort treat for a hot summer afternoon—or for any other time! For best results choose strawberries at the peak of their summer season—the flavor is a lot better. And choose organic strawberries. According to the Environmental Working Group, strawberries are one of the "dirty dozen" fruits and vegetables that are most exposed to pesticides and chemicals.

Ingredients

3 cups (435 g) stemmed and halved or quartered fresh, ripe strawberries

²/₃ cup (130 g) sugar

2 tablespoons (28 ml) fresh-squeezed lemon juice

6 egg yolks

1 cup (235 ml) heavy cream (choose half-and-half to reduce calories)

½ cup (120 ml) cow's milk (choose low-fat to reduce calories)

1 teaspoon vanilla extract

Heat the berries, sugar, and lemon juice in a large saucepan over medium-low heat. Bring the mixture to a boil and continue to cook for about 20 minutes, stirring often (reduce the heat to low if it gets too sputtery). Using an immersion wand, purée the mixture until mostly smooth (you can also do this with caution in a blender or food processor). Cool the purée in the refrigerator.

In a mixer, beat the egg yolks together until smooth and creamy, and set aside.

Whisk the cream and milk together in a large, heavy-bottomed saucepan and heat over medium heat until it is just about to boil—you will see steam rising and tiny bubbles just beginning to form around the edges—but do not let it actually boil. Remove from the heat and stir in the vanilla.

Temper the yolks by slowly adding about ¼ cup (60 ml) of the steaming cream mixture to the yolks while beating them in the mixer. Whisking constantly to incorporate them (versus cooking the yolks in the hot cream), pour the tempered yolks slowly into the cream pan.

Place the pan over low heat and cook, stirring constantly, until the mixture thickens (it should reach about 175°F, or 80°C).

Fill your sink with a low ice bath and place the saucepan into the bath. Stir it a few times until it is cool. In a glass storage container, combine the cooled cream mixture and the cooled strawberry mixture, mixing well. Cover and chill overnight in the refrigerator.

The next day, stir to recombine, and prepare the mixture in the ice cream maker of your choice, according to its directions.

Yield: 8 to 12 servings (about 4 cups, or 560 g)

Per Serving: 120.7 calories; 6.2 g fat (45% calories from fat); 2.1 g protein; 14.9 g carbohydrate; 0.7 g dietary fiber; 116.8 mg cholesterol; 12.4 mg sodium

Ingredients

4 cups (580 g) stemmed and sliced fresh, ripe strawberries

6 tablespoons (75 g) sugar, divided

½ cup (115 g) low-fat sour cream, plain low-fat Greek yogurt, or low-fat buttermilk

1 egg

1 cup (125 g) whole-wheat pastry flour

1 cup (125 g) unbleached flour (or 1 additional cup whole-wheat pastry flour for more fiber)

1½ teaspoons (7 g) baking powder

½ teaspoon baking soda

4 tablespoons (55 g) butter, frozen

¼ cup (60 g) Neufchâtel cheese, chopped into small pieces and chilled in the freezer for 5 to 10 minutes

1 teaspoon lemon zest

2 cups (475 ml) fresh, whipped cream (see our recipe for Lightly Sweetened Fresh Whipped Cream, page 171)

From Chef Jeannette

Even Healthier: To reduce the calorie count and add a refreshing tang (plus a nice hit of protein) to the whipping cream, reduce the whipped cream by ⅓ cup (80 ml) and whisk in ⅓ cup (77 g) plain Greek yogurt in its place.

Time-Saver Tip: Substitute halves of 4 warmed, prepared whole-grain biscuits in place of the fresh scones.

Magnificent Madeover Strawberry Shortcake

From Dr. Jonny: There are a million ways to make shortcake (technically a crumbly, biscuit-y affair), but all of them involve flour, sugar, salt, butter, cream (or milk), and—occasionally—eggs. Pile on the ice cream and strawberries swimming in a bath of sticky sugar syrup, add gobs of whipped cream (or worse, whipped "topping"), and you've pretty much got half your calories for the day (and that's assuming you're a 6-foot-tall, athletically inclined male!). Try our version. We start with lots of the freshest strawberries and use just a hint of sugar to help them release their natural juices. A whole-grain scone substitutes for the traditional shortcake, with a bunch of lemon zest and delicious Neufchâtel cheese replacing half the butter (to reduce calories and bump up the protein). Finish it off with just a dollop of real—repeat, real—whipped cream and you've got a knockout of a dessert.

Place the middle cooking rack in the lower middle position and preheat the oven to 400°F (200°C, or gas mark 6). Line a large cookie sheet with parchment paper (or lightly spray with cooking oil) and set aside.

Place the prepared strawberries in a large bowl and sprinkle with 2 tablespoons (25 g) of the sugar. Toss gently to combne. Set aside to rest at room temperature while you make the scones. They will start to get juicy and form a light syrup—the fresher and riper they are, the faster that will happen.

In a small bowl, whisk the sour cream and egg together until well combined. Set aside.

In a large bowl, whisk together the flours, remaining ¼ cup (50 g) sugar, baking powder, and baking soda.

Pulse the frozen butter in a food processor to coarsely chop (or quickly grate it by hand with a cheese grater) and add to the flour mixture. Add the Neufchâtel and quickly work the butter and cheese into the flour using a pastry cutter or your hands until it forms small crumbs. Stir in the zest, then add the sour cream and egg mixture. Stir until the mixture just forms a dough, and transfer it to a floured surface. Gently knead it a few times and press it into a thick circle about 8 inches (20 cm) in diameter. Slice the circle into 8 thin wedges like a pie and place the wedges on the prepared cookie sheet with space between each piece. Bake for 15 to 16 minutes, until lightly browned. Allow to cool for about 10 minutes, then slice each piece in half and top with ¼ cup (40 g) prepared strawberries and ¼ cup (60 ml) whipped cream (or less for fewer calories). Serve immediately.

Yield: 8 servings

Per Serving: 483.4 calories; 34 g fat (59% calories from fat); 5.7 g protein; 43.4 g carbohydrate; 2.3 g dietary fiber; 131.7 mg cholesterol; 237.9 mg sodium

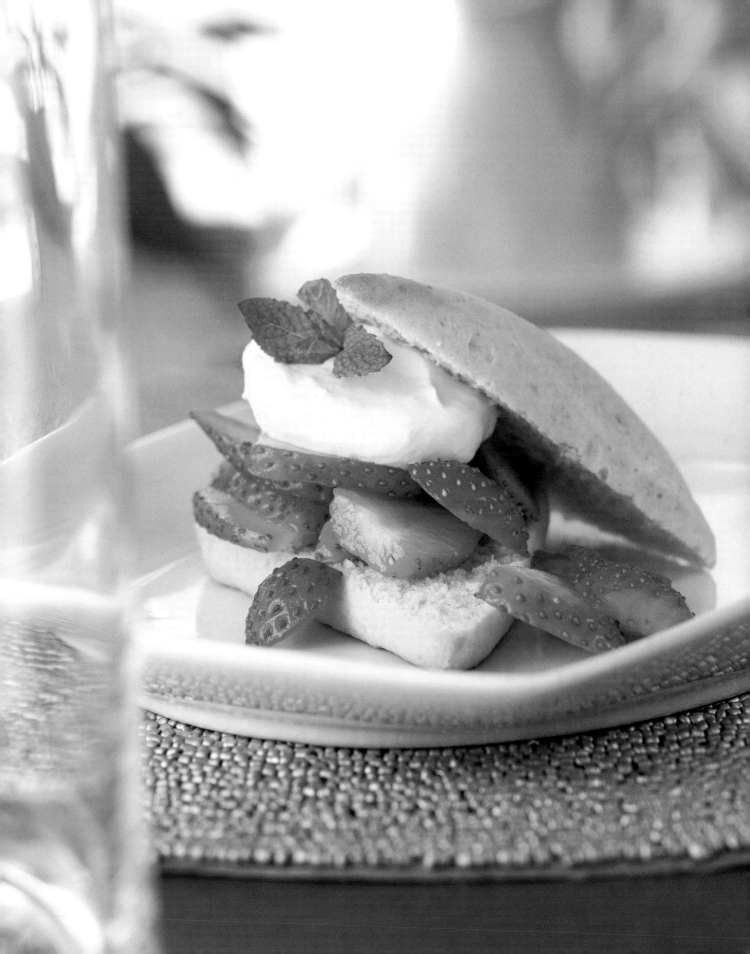

Ingredients

Cooking oil spray

1 tablespoon (14 g) butter

2 ripe baking pears (such as D'Anjou or Bartlett), cored and sliced, unpeeled

2 teaspoons (9 g) Sucanat, brown sugar, or xylitol

2 tablespoons (28 ml) Poire William liqueur or pear brandy (or apple cider)

½ cup (170 g) blackstrap molasses, unsulphured

½ cup (120 ml) water

½ teaspoon baking soda

⅓ cup (65 g) Sucanat or brown sugar

2 tablespoons (28 g) butter, softened

2 tablespoons (30 g) applesauce

1 egg

½ cup (65 g) wheat flour

½ cup (65 g) whole-wheat pastry flour

1½ teaspoons (7 g) baking powder

1 teaspoon cinnamon

1 teaspoon ground ginger

¼ teaspoon ground cloves

2 tablespoons (12 g) minced crystallized ginger, optional

Iron-Strong Gingerbread Cake with Poire William

From Dr. Jonny: Gingerbread is my kryptonite. They sell a great version at Whole Foods down the street from me, and periodically the manager puts out a huge tray of samples, and on those days it's best for me to stay away from the store. With just a few tweaks you can make this "A-list" comfort food pretty healthy, or at least not so bad for you! Just add pears and leave the skins on (that's where many of the nutrients are, as well as the wonderful fiber pectin), dump the extra sugar, use blackstrap molasses (rich in iron and B vitamins), and replace most of the butter with applesauce to reduce calories. Simple, right? One more easy fix: Replace half the regular flour with whole-wheat pastry flour. Dark, spicy, and warming, this baby needs no whipped cream to make it great! (But if you must, use real cream [page 171]. At least it's a real food, not that foamy chemical stuff that comes out of a can!)

Preheat the oven to 350°F (180°C, or gas mark 4). Spray an 8 x 8-inch (20 x 20-cm) baking pan with neutrally flavored oil and set aside.

In a large skillet or Dutch oven, melt the butter over medium heat. Add the pears, cover, and cook for 5 to 7 minutes, until they begin to soften (this will take longer if they aren't fully ripe). Sprinkle the Sucanat over the pears and pour in the liqueur, stirring to combine. Cook for 4 to 5 minutes, or until pears are very soft and beginning to brown. Spoon the pears evenly into the bottom of the prepared baking pan and set aside.

While the pears are cooking, whisk the molasses and water together in a medium saucepan and bring to a boil over high heat. When it boils, remove from the heat and stir in the baking soda. It will foam up. Pour into a bowl and set aside to cool.

In a mixer, combine the sweetener, butter, and applesauce and beat until nearly smooth. This takes a couple of minutes if using Sucanat. Add the egg and beat until well incorporated. Set aside.

In a large bowl, whisk together the flours, baking powder, cinnamon, ginger, and cloves. Add the creamed butter to the dry ingredients, mix gently, and add the cooled molasses. Fold together and mix well. Add the crystallized ginger and gently fold in. Pour the batter evenly over the pears in the prepared pan and bake for about 35 minutes, or until you can easily pull the cake away from the pan corners and it springs back to a light touch in the middle.

Let it rest for at least 10 minutes before serving.

Yield: about 9 servings

Per Serving: 151 calories; 4.6 g fat (27% calories from fat); 2.4 g protein; 26.2 g carbohydrate; 2.1 g dietary fiber; 33.5 mg cholesterol; 189.6 mg sodium

Ingredients

1 pint (475 ml) organic whipping cream

1 teaspoon vanilla extract

2 to 3 tablespoons (26 to 39 g) sugar, or to taste

From Chef Jeannette

Even Healthier: Help balance the glycemic impact of the small amount of sugar used by mixing ¾ teaspoon cinnamon into the sugar before adding to make cinnamon whipped cream. Or mix in 1 teaspoon sifted high-quality cocoa powder instead for an antioxidant boost.

The Real Deal: Lightly Sweetened Fresh Whipped Cream

From Dr. Jonny: Excuse me for asking, but what exactly is Cool Whip? Other than using it for "tricking" during Halloween, I can't think of a single purpose for this imitation whipped cream. Real whipped cream, on the other hand, is an actual food. Sure, it's high in calories, but it's made from real food and has tiny amounts of actual nutrients (calcium, magnesium, monounsaturated fat) and zero amounts of unpronounceable chemicals. We used far less sugar than normal (just a hint really, because truth be told you don't need a lot). Add a little high-quality vanilla and you've got a dream topping that is incredible over seasonal fresh fruit. (Try just dipping the fruit with a light coating of the cream—you won't need much to make the flavor combo really pop!)

Chill the bowl and beater from your mixing bowl in the freezer for 20 minutes.

Remove the whipping cream from the refrigerator just before you plan to use it so the cream and all the tools are ice cold—this will help it stiffen properly.

Add the cream and vanilla to the bowl and beat on medium-high until it begins to thicken. Increase the beater speed to high and gradually sprinkle in the sugar, to taste, while continuing to beat until soft peaks form. Use immediately or chill in the refrigerator.

Yield: about 3 cups, or 710 ml (1 serving is about 3 tablespoons, or 45 ml)
Per Serving: 106 calories; 11.9 g fat (93% calories from fat); 0 g protein; 1.7 g carbohydrate; 0 g dietary fiber; 39.6 mg cholesterol; 9.9 mg sodium

Ingredients

Cooking oil spray

2 cups (475 ml) unsweetened almond milk

1/4 cup (50 g) Sucanat, sugar, or xylitol, optional

8 ounces (225 g) high-quality dark chocolate chips

1 package (12.3 ounces, or 350 g) soft silken tofu

1 teaspoon vanilla extract

4 cups (200 g) 3/4-inch (1.9-cm) day-old whole-grain bread cubes

1/2 cup (63 g) dried tart cherries

Tart Cherry Chocolate Whole-Grain Bread Pudding

From Dr. Jonny: Bread pudding is so delicious my salivary glands start working overtime as soon as I even think about it, let alone eat it. And it's a real challenge to make this comfort food favorite even moderately healthy because the basic recipe calls for a ton of heavy cream, nutritionally useless white bread, and way too much sugar. But really, that's the whole point, isn't it? Maybe not. We made a couple of changes that—surprisingly—don't diminish the joy of this dish one iota. We started with a whole-grain bread base (light years better than white bread), added dark chocolate (rich in antioxidants, magnesium, and plant compounds called flavonols, which may lower blood pressure), reduced the total sugar content (you'll never miss it), and replaced the heavy cream with protein-rich (and much lower-calorie) almond milk and silken tofu. Bingo, you're in bread pudding heaven. Fun fact: Tart cherries are loaded with plant compounds called anthocyanins, which give cherries their deep red color. Anthocyanins are powerful anti-inflammatory agents (which may account for why cherries are so effective against the pain of gout). Research from the University of Michigan Cardiovascular Center demonstrated that rats receiving whole tart cherry powder had significantly lower levels of molecules that indicate the kind of inflammation that's linked to diabetes and heart disease.

Spray an 8 x 8-inch (20 x 20-cm) baking pan lightly with cooking oil and set aside.

Combine the almond milk and Sucanat in a large saucepan over medium-high heat and bring just to a boil, stirring frequently. Remove from the heat and stir in the chocolate chips until melted. Set aside to cool slightly.

Combine the tofu and vanilla in a food processor and process until very smooth. Add the chocolate mixture and process until smooth and well combined. Put the bread cubes and the cherries into a large bowl and pour the chocolate mixture over all. Mix gently to combine.

Pour the mixture into the prepared baking pan, press the bread cubes under the liquid mixture, cover with a lid or tightly sealed plastic wrap, and let rest at room temperature for 20 to 30 minutes.

Preheat the oven to 350°F (180°C, or gas mark 4), remove the covering, press the bread under the chocolate mixture, and bake for 35 to 45 minutes, until thick and hot throughout.

Yield: 9 servings

Per Serving: 234.8 calories; 10.1 g fat (35% calories from fat); 7.2 g protein; 32.5 g carbohydrate; 3.2 g dietary fiber; 0 mg cholesterol; 110.6 mg sodium

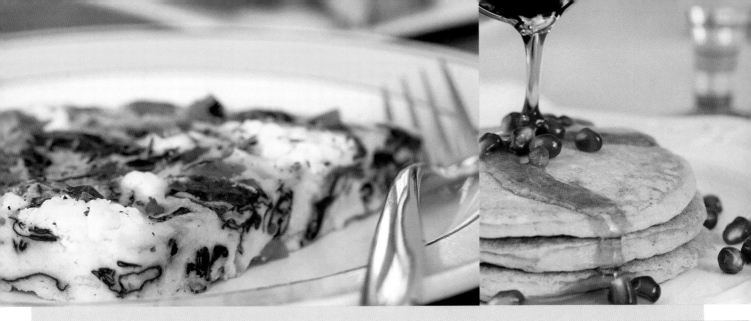

Breakfasts

Breakfast seems to be one of the most difficult healthy meal decisions. People don't have time, aren't hungry, or have no idea what to substitute for the usual eggs, potatoes, toast, and juice. Well, wonder no more. There are some absolutely scrumptious ideas in this section, and we've upped the nutrition on all of them, taken out the worst ingredients, substituted better choices, and come up with some killer recipes that taste amazing.

Corn-Rich Whole-Grain Jonnycakes

Warm, Lower-Sugar Apple Cranberry Compote

Satisfying Real-Food Pumpkin Pancakes

Hearty High-Fiber Baked Cinnamon French Toast

Homemade Heart-Healthy Nutty Ginger Granola

Open-Your-Eyes Orange High-Fiber Waffles

Nutritious Real-Deal Oatmeal

Clean and Cheesy Apple Turkey Sausage

Two-Cheese Fit and Flavorful Frittata

High-Protein Smoked Chicken Quiche Dijon

Lighten Up Cheesy Mediterranean Egg Scramble

Savory Baked-Not-Fried Hash Browns

Whole-Wheat Chili Biscuit Breakfast Pie

Fiber-Full Sweet Potato Mini-Muffins

Low-Fat, Light, and Luscious Banana Muffins

Lemony Light and Bright Breakfast Fruit Salad

Banana-Sweet Strawberry Breakfast Bread

Nutty Antioxidant Power Cran-Orange Bread

Portobello Benedict with Sundried Tomato Pesto

Two Better Omelets

Gourmet Whole-Grain Breakfast Burrito

Luscious, Lighter Almond Coffee Cake

Delicious Low-Sugar Choco-Banana Smoothie

Corn-Rich Whole-Grain Jonnycakes

From Dr. Jonny: We renamed this early American comfort food in honor of, well, me! The classic johnnycake was actually a cornmeal flatbread made from fried gruel or cornmeal mixed together with milk or hot water. Johnnycakes ('scuse me, Jonnycakes) come in all shapes and sizes (and spellings, apparently) and can be made sweet (with lots of butter and maple syrup, like a pancake) or savory (highly salted and seasoned with pepper). Chef Jeannette took a slightly different approach, blending fresh corn and milk with regular cornmeal, which adds a rich and moist feel to what is too often a dry dish. She also swapped the butter for unrefined corn oil, which deepens the corn flavor. She calls these "three-corn Jonnycakes." You'll call them "fantastic!"

Ingredients

1⅓ cups (185 g) stone-ground cornmeal, fine grind
½ teaspoon baking powder
Pinch of salt
¼ teaspoon fresh-ground black pepper (for savory) OR 2 teaspoons (9 g) Sucanat, sugar, or xylitol (for sweet)
1 cup (130 g) frozen corn, thawed
1½ cups (355 ml) milk (low-fat cow's or plain, unsweetened soy or almond)
1 egg, separated
2 tablespoons (28 ml) unrefined corn oil (or other neutral vegetable oil or melted butter)
High-heat cooking spray or stick of butter

In a medium bowl, whisk together the cornmeal, baking powder, salt, and either pepper or Sucanat.

In a blender or food processor, blend the thawed corn and milk together until well puréed.

In a large bowl, whisk the egg yolk and oil until well blended. Pour the corn and milk purée into the yolk and oil and whisk to mix well. Add the cornmeal mix to the dry mix and stir until just combined.

In a small bowl, whisk the egg white until frothy, and gently mix into the batter.

To cook, heat a nonstick griddle over medium-high heat until a drop of water skitters across the surface. Oil the surface lightly with a high-heat spray or run a stick of butter briefly over the surface of the pan. Using a ¼-cup (60-g) measuring cup or ladle, drop enough batter to make a 3- to 4-inch (7.5- to 10-cm) pancake—the pancake should be thin. Cook for a couple of minutes until bubbles form on the pancake surface, then flip and cook for a couple minutes more until cooked through and lightly browned on both sides (pancakes will stop steaming when cooked through on the second side).

Yield: 4 servings

Per Serving: 313.9 calories; 11.3 g fat (32% calories from fat); 9.2 g protein; 46.3 g carbohydrate; 4.2 g dietary fiber; 60.2 mg cholesterol; 211.9 mg sodium

From Chef Jeannette

If you let the batter rest for 10 or 15 minutes before cooking, the cornmeal will absorb some of the liquids and soften. I personally prefer that little cornmeal crunch so I cook 'em right away.

Serving Suggestions: Serve these Jonnycakes savory with more fresh-ground pepper and salt, to taste, plus a light smear of butter and a couple shots of hot sauce. Or serve them sweet with the Warm, Lower-Sugar Apple Cranberry Compote (page 175) or simply with fresh berries (high-season raspberries or blueberries are amazing!) and a bit of warmed applesauce or 100 percent grade B maple syrup.

Warm, Lower-Sugar Apple Cranberry Compote

From Dr. Jonny: So if you've made the fantastic light pumpkin pancakes (page 176) and Jonnycakes (page 174) in this chapter, you already know a pancake can taste delicious without being a health disaster. But even a great pancake can be ruined with the addition of tons of butter and syrup, especially when the syrup is the runny, fake-flavored high-fructose corn syrup served in most restaurants. (Note: The butter doesn't ruin anything from a health perspective, but it does add a substantial number of unnecessary calories. And margarine does ruin it from a health perspective by adding loads of trans fats and artificial junk.) So why not enhance the health value of those delicious pancakes you just made by using a compote made with healthy fruit and just a bit of sweetener? Our version is made from apples and cranberries—two of the richest fruits in antioxidant power—plus just the gentlest hint of sweetener from real, genuine maple syrup. Use this compote and it will turn even plain pancakes (or French toast, come to think of it) into the best kind of comfort food treat—one that comes without any guilt!

Ingredients

3 fresh, sweet cooking apples (Golden Delicious or Jonagold work well), peeled, cored, and chopped
¼ cup (25 g) fresh or frozen cranberries
¼ cup (30 g) dried, juice-sweetened cranberries
¼ cup (60 ml) apple cider (or water)
3 tablespoons (45 ml) 100 percent maple syrup
¼ teaspoon cinnamon

Place the apples, cranberries, cider, and syrup into a medium saucepan over medium heat and cover to bring to a simmer. When the mixture is simmering, sprinkle in the cinnamon and mix well to combine. Reduce the heat to medium-low, cover, and cook, stirring periodically, until the apples have broken down and the berries have softened, about 20 minutes. If the mixture gets too thick, add a little more cider to keep it wet. Stir well or use an immersion blender to achieve the desired consistency and serve warm, at room temperature, or chilled, over pancakes, waffles, French toast, or plain Greek yogurt.

Yield: 6 servings
Per Serving: 86.7 calories; 0.2 g fat (2% calories from fat); 0.2 g protein; 22.2 g carbohydrate; 2.1 g dietary fiber; 0 mg cholesterol; 4.5 mg sodium

From Chef Jeannette

Even Healthier: For more fiber and nutrients, leave the skins on the apples when you cook them.

Ingredients

1 tablespoon (15 ml) apple cider vinegar

1 cup (235 ml) whole milk (choose cow's or unsweetened plain soy milk)

3 eggs

1/4 cup (60 ml) milk (whole or low-fat cow's or plain, unsweetened soy or almond)

1/4 cup (60 g) applesauce

3 tablespoons (45 g) coconut oil, melted and cooled

1 teaspoon vanilla extract

1/2 cup (125 g) pumpkin purée (unsweetened)

1/2 cup (125 g) part-skim ricotta cheese (fresh if you can find it)

1 1/4 cups (155 g) flour (use unbleached, whole-wheat pastry, or a combination)

2 tablespoons (28 g) baking powder

2 teaspoons (9 g) sugar or xylitol

1 1/2 teaspoons (3.5 g) pumpkin pie spice (or 1 teaspoon cinnamon with 1/8 teaspoon each allspice, nutmeg, and clove)

1/4 teaspoon salt

Cooking oil spray

From Chef Jeannette

Serving Suggestions: To serve these, top with a small amount of warmed 100 percent maple syrup (choose grade B for more flavor and nutrients with less expense), a few juice-sweetened dried cranberries, and a sprinkling of chopped toasted pecans, or our Warm, Lower-Sugar Apple Cranberry Compote (page 175).

Satisfying Real-Food Pumpkin Pancakes

From Dr. Jonny: There's a famous restaurant on the Upper West Side of New York City—my old stomping grounds—that's known for serving pancakes that no human on Earth can finish, unless you're a professional Sumo wrestler. You can see the expressions on the tourists' faces when the waitperson brings the dish—absolutely humongous, ridiculous pancakes that look like gym mats—easily a good 12 inches (30 cm) in diameter, hanging over the plate, and stacked about five high. Although the portion size might be ridiculous, fact is that in most restaurant pancakes are white flour affairs with fake, maple-flavored syrup that bears about as much resemblance to real food as "processed cheese food" bears to aged cheese. But we love our pancakes! So Chef Jeannette duplicated the flavor and texture of the junky kind by using whole milk and cider vinegar in place of calorie-heavy buttermilk, and used ricotta cheese for more protein. Plus we replaced most of the oils typically used with low-calorie applesauce. These unusual pancakes are light and creamy, almost custard-y in quality, with subtle hints of pumpkin and spice—delicious and satisfying! (And by the way, if you visit New York City—stay away from any restaurant whose pancakes could be used as Frisbees!) Fun fact: Apple cider vinegar has been used for centuries as a general tonic and, when made the old-fashioned way, contains valuable enzymes and nutrients that help alkalize the system!

In a small bowl, whisk the cider vinegar into the whole milk and set aside for 5 minutes.

In a mixer, beat the eggs. Add the milk, applesauce, coconut oil, vanilla, and vinegar-milk, and beat until well incorporated. Add the pumpkin and ricotta and beat on low until well mixed.

In another large bowl, add the flour, baking powder, sugar, pumpkin pie spice, and salt, and whisk lightly until combined. Slowly add the dry mix to the wet and beat on low until just combined; do not overmix.

Spray a griddle pan or cast-iron skillet with oil and heat over medium heat until a drop of water added to the pan sizzles. Reduce the heat to medium-low. Pour small puddles of batter (3- to 4-inch, or 7.5- to 10-cm, rounds) and cook until bubbles begin to form on the top surface. Flip once and cook for another 2 to 3 minutes, or until the other side is cooked through (they'll stop steaming).

Yield: about thirty 3-inch (7.5-cm) pancakes (5 or 6 servings)

Per Serving: 276.8 calories; 13.5 g fat (14% calories from fat); 10.1 g protein; 29.4 g carbohydrate; 1.5 g dietary fiber; 117.1 mg cholesterol; 675.2 mg sodium

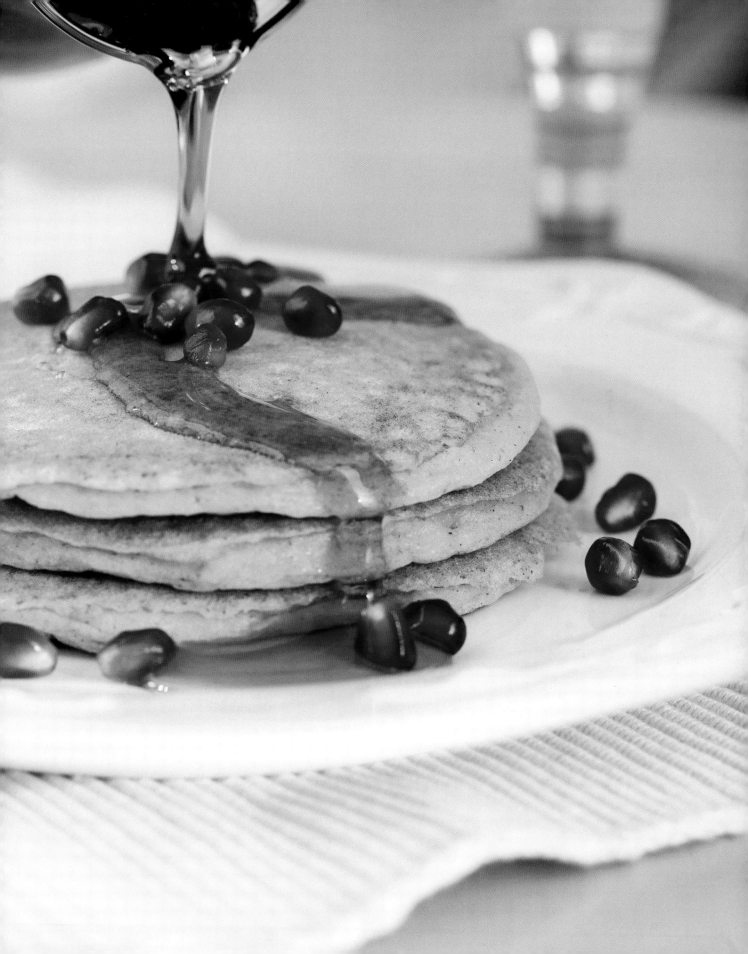

Hearty High-Fiber Baked Cinnamon French Toast

Ingredients

Cooking oil spray

6 eggs

1²/₃ cups (395 ml) milk (low-fat cow's, evaporated skim, or unsweetened vanilla almond or soy)

3 to 4 tablespoons (39 to 52 g) dry sweetener of your choice, to taste (Sucanat, xylitol, etc.)

1 teaspoon vanilla extract

1 tablespoon (7 g) cinnamon

¹/₂ teaspoon nutmeg

3 tablespoons (27 g) raisins, optional (or dried, juice-sweetened cranberries)

3 tablespoons (21 g) sliced almonds, optional

8 thick slices high-fiber, multigrain bread, slightly stale, sliced into thirds (or use multigrain raisin bread, omit the raisins, and reduce the sweetener by 1 tablespoon)

1¹/₂ tablespoons (11 g) toasted wheat germ

1¹/₂ tablespoons (10 g) ground flaxseed

From Dr. Jonny: When I was a kid we took family vacations for a week or so every August. My parents were very into "togetherness," so we went to family resorts like Sacks Lodge near Woodstock, New York. The kids would eat at separate tables in the children's camp area, and we were all really excited when French toast was served for breakfast. Years later, I learned to make my own healthier version of this comfort food favorite using whole-grain or sprouted-grain bread, eggs, and a fruit compote instead of maple syrup. So I was curious to see what Chef Jeannette's take would be on this delicious breakfast treat. As usual, she did not disappoint. For this version, use a multigrain bread as your base, and lose the Aunt Jemima–type syrup, which is little more than maple-flavored corn syrup, really. Soften the effect on your blood sugar by adding plenty of protein from the eggs and milk, and use a light hand on the sweetener. (Hint: Grade B maple syrup is a better choice if you're going that route because it's much higher in minerals and somewhat less refined than grade A.) Use cinnamon for its rich array of antioxidants, and boost the nutritional wallop even higher with (optional) dried fruits and mineral-filled almonds. Finish with high-fiber wheat germ and flaxseed and you're good to go! Fun fact: Almonds contain calcium and magnesium in the perfect 1:1 ratio. One ounce (28 g) contains about 75 mg of each mineral.

Spray a 9 x 13-inch (23 x 33-cm) shallow roasting pan (or use a high-heat casserole dish) lightly with cooking oil and set aside.

In a mixer, combine the eggs, milk, sweetener, vanilla, cinnamon, and nutmeg, and beat until smooth and well incorporated.

Sprinkle the raisins and almonds evenly over the bottom of the pan.

Arrange the strips of bread in a layer over the raisins and nuts to cover the bottom of the pan. Pour the liquid mixture evenly over the bread to cover. Cover with a lid or tightly sealed plastic wrap and let soak in the refrigerator overnight (up to 24 hours).

Remove the baking dish from the refrigerator and preheat the oven to 425°F (220°C, or gas mark 7).

Sprinkle the wheat germ evenly over the surface of the French toast and bake for 25 to 30 minutes, or until lightly browned and set. Sprinkle on the flaxseed just before serving.

Yield: about 8 servings

Per Serving: 199.2 calories; 7.9 g fat (35% calories from fat); 11.1 g protein; 21.8 g carbohydrate; 3.4 g dietary fiber; 162.7 mg cholesterol; 183.7 mg sodium

Ingredients

1 cup (80 g) whole rolled oats

¼ cup (36 g) raw almonds (crushed lightly or whole)

¼ cup (25 g) raw cashews or pecans (crushed lightly or whole)

¼ cup (55 g) raw pumpkin seeds

¼ cup (55 g) raw sunflower seeds

¼ cup (36 g) raw sesame seeds

¼ cup (36 g) flaxseed

¼ cup (21 g) dried, unsweetened coconut

¼ cup (28 g) wheat germ or oat bran

¼ cup (32 g) powdered milk

¼ cup (32 g) whole-wheat flour

¼ cup (60 ml) almond oil

¼ cup (60 ml) 100 percent grade B maple syrup (or honey), or more to taste

2 teaspoons (3.6 g) ground ginger

1 teaspoon cinnamon

2 to 4 tablespoons (12 to 24 g) finely chopped crystallized ginger, to taste (or ¼ cup, or 33 g, finely chopped dried apples or unsulphured apricots or unsweetened dried cherries)

From Chef Jeannette

Double or even triple the ingredients to make a larger batch, if desired.

If you like your granola well toasted, turn the heat off after 35 minutes, stir, and leave the granola in the oven until it cools off.

Homemade Heart-Healthy Nutty Ginger Granola

From Dr. Jonny: One of the oldest books in my health library is a long out-of-print paperback called *The Natural Breakfast Book*, and it's where I first learned that you could actually make homemade granola! We love granola because it's yummy and sweet, but unfortunately it's one of the highest-calorie selections in the breakfast cereal aisles. And much of the packaged stuff is made to look all healthy and "granola-y" but is in fact not much more than another sugary cereal with low-quality fat and little to recommend it except some clever packaging. (I've even seen "healthy granolas" with high-fructose corn syrup as one of the first ingredients!) For this much-better homemade version we used almond oil, which is mostly heart-healthy monounsaturated fat (the same kind found in olive oil), and only a small amount of pure maple syrup to sweeten. The rich-tasting spices (cinnamon and ginger) really pop the flavors so you don't need as much sugar. The powdered milk adds calcium to the mix. Try it over plain yogurt (Greek or regular) with fresh berries or other seasonal fruit.

Preheat the oven to 250°F (120°C, or gas mark ½).

In a large bowl, mix together the oats, nuts, seeds, coconut, wheat germ, powdered milk, and flour.

In a medium bowl, whisk together the almond oil, syrup, ginger, and cinnamon until well blended. Pour the liquid mixture over the dry and mix well until lightly coated. Spread the mixture thinly and evenly over the bottom of a large, shallow roasting pan and bake for 30 to 40 minutes, stirring every 15 minutes, until lightly browned.

Stir in the crystallized ginger, cool, and store in an airtight container in the refrigerator.

Yield: about 3½ cups, or 385 g (serving size ⅓ cup, or 37 g)

Per Serving: 250.7 calories; 15 g fat (50% calories from fat); 8.2 g protein; 72.5 g carbohydrate; 4 g dietary fiber; 4.3 mg cholesterol; 32.5 mg sodium

Open-Your-Eyes Orange High-Fiber Waffles

Ingredients

Waffles

1 cup (235 ml) unsweetened vanilla soy or almond milk
1 tablespoon (15 ml) apple cider vinegar
1/4 cup (20 g) rolled oats
1 1/3 cup (42 g) whole-wheat pastry flour
3 tablespoons (27 g) stone-ground corn-meal, fine grind
1 tablespoon (6.5 g) ground flaxseed
1 1/2 tablespoons (20 g) Sucanat, sugar, or xylitol
3/4 teaspoon baking powder
1/2 teaspoon baking soda
1/4 teaspoon nutmeg
Pinch of salt
1 egg, separated
2 teaspoons (10 ml) almond oil (or other vegetable oil)
1 teaspoon vanilla extract
1 teaspoon orange zest
Cooking oil spray

Topping

2 cups (460 g) low-fat plain Greek yogurt
1/4 cup (60 ml) fresh-squeezed orange juice
2 tablespoons (85 g) raw honey, warmed to liquid, if necessary, or more to taste
1 1/2 teaspoons (3 g) orange zest

From Dr. Jonny: I love waffles as much as you do, but they're flabby and white and they're served with too much butter and way too much syrup. Eat them for breakfast and you're looking at a ride on the blood sugar roller coaster for the rest of the day—not exactly a great way to rev up your metabolism. We improve on the old standby by using three different types of whole grains and throwing in a nice dose of flaxseed for its extra fiber, omega-3s, and cancer-fighting lignans. And—get this—we replaced the butter and syrup with a light, bright, and tangy protein-rich orange topping that will keep you out of blood sugar hell but leave you with the creamy feel and taste of a dessert waffle. Extra nutrition points for the rolled oats, a low-glycemic carb with plenty of fiber. Enjoy!

To make the waffles: In a small bowl, combine the milk and vinegar and stir to mix well. Add the oats and let the mixture rest at room temperature for 10 to 15 minutes.

In a medium bowl, whisk together the flour, cornmeal, flaxseed, Sucanat, baking powder, baking soda, nutmeg, and salt.

In a small bowl, whisk the egg white until frothy.

In large bowl, whisk together the egg yolk, almond oil, vanilla, and zest. Add the milk and oat mixture and whisk to combine. Add the dry mix to the wet mix and stir until just combined. Fold in the egg white and stir to incorporate.

Lightly spray a waffle iron with cooking oil and preheat. Using a cup measure, pour enough batter into the center to cover the iron to about 1 1/2 to 2 inches (3.8 to 5 cm) from the outer edge. Close and cook for about 4 minutes, or until the waffle is golden brown. Repeat with the remaining batter.

To make the topping: While the waffles are cooking, in a medium bowl whisk together the yogurt, orange juice, honey, and zest until thoroughly mixed. Top the hot waffles with orange yogurt, to taste.

Yield: about 4 servings
Per Serving: 308.1 calories; 7.4 g fat (21% calories from fat); 10.9 g protein; 50.6 g carbohydrate; 2 g dietary fiber; 59.9 mg cholesterol; 351.7 mg sodium

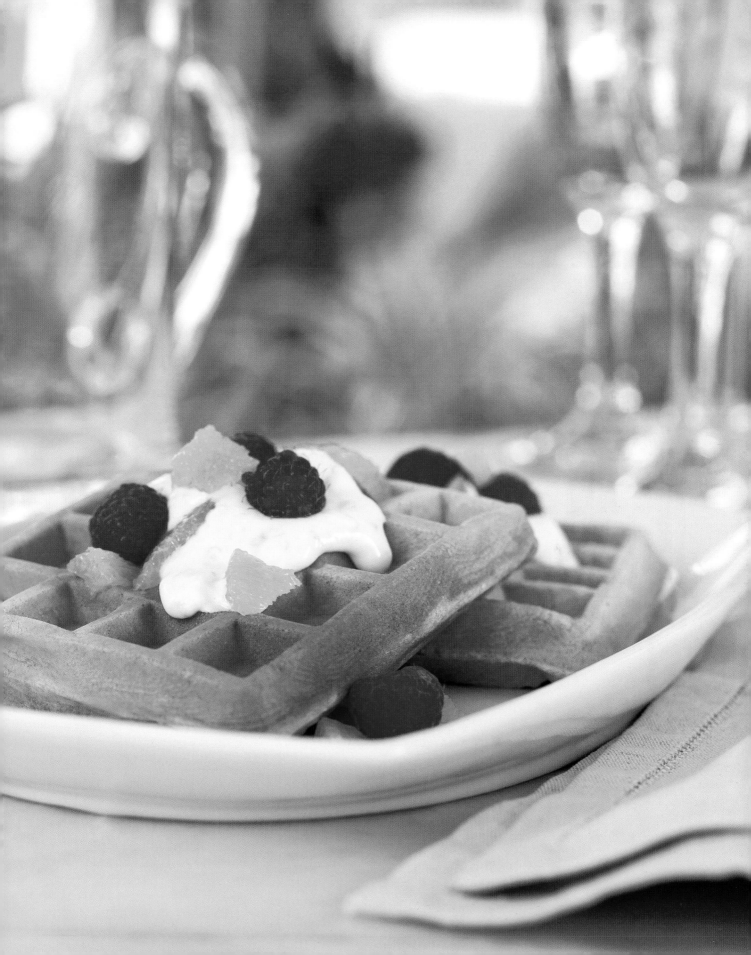

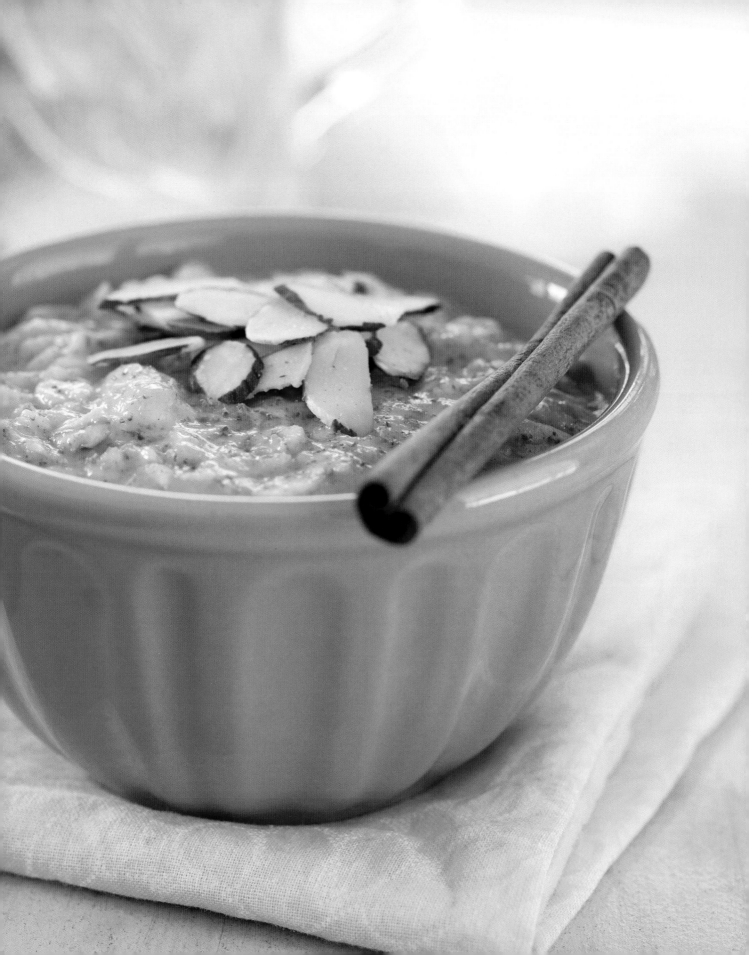

Nutritious Real-Deal Oatmeal

From Dr. Jonny: Back in the days when I lived in the gym, oatmeal was the favorite food of bodybuilders and fitness buffs everywhere. When I'd recommend oatmeal to clients they'd often say, "But it takes so long to make!" That brought up the subject of instant oatmeal. Which is terrible. It's got tons of artificial ingredients and loads of sugar, and isn't nearly as nutritious or fiber-rich as the real deal. And here's the thing—the real stuff doesn't take long to make at all! In fact, it doesn't even need to be cooked—Swiss muesli (one of the original "healthy" cereals) is just raw oats with dried fruit and nuts! You can even make regular oatmeal by simply pouring boiling water on it and letting it soften (a great trick for travel), or you can cook it up normally in a pan in a short time. Either way, you get all the wonderful benefits of oats—fiber, protein, and a special compound called beta-glucan, which has been found to lower cholesterol and protect the prostate! Use the oatmeal as the basis for a fabulous, comforting breakfast and punch up the nutritional values by trying one of the following ideas.

Ingredients

2 cups (475 ml) milk (low-fat cow's or unsweetened, plain almond or soy)

1 to 3 teaspoons (4 to 13 g) Sucanat, xylitol or brown sugar, to taste

1 cup (80 g) whole rolled oats

Pinch of salt

1 small ripe banana, mashed to the consistency of yogurt

$\frac{1}{2}$ teaspoon cinnamon

$\frac{1}{4}$ teaspoon nutmeg

$\frac{1}{3}$ cup (48 g) toasted slivered almonds

2 tablespoons (14 g) toasted wheat germ

Sweet Nutty Banana Oats

To up the protein in this dish, we used a milk base. We lowered the sugar and used banana to sweeten it. (If you like it sweeter, try starting with just a sprinkle of Sucanat and then increase it at the end if you need to.) Nutmeg and cinnamon actually add to the sense of sweetness. Wheat germ adds vitamin E and almonds add minerals and mono-unsaturated fat, plus the nutty flavor we're "bananas" for . . . get it?

In a large saucepan, whisk together the milk, Sucanat, oats, and salt over medium heat. Bring to a low boil, whisking frequently. Reduce the heat and cook for about 10 minutes, or until the oats are tender, whisking frequently. In the last 5 minutes of cooking time, whisk in the mashed banana, cinnamon, and nutmeg. Stir in the almonds and wheat germ just before serving.

Yield: 3 to 4 servings

Per Serving: 244.3 calories; 10.2 g fat (32% calories from fat); 10.4 g protein; 153.7 g carbohydrate; 4.7 g dietary fiber; 9.8 mg cholesterol; 52.3 mg sodium

Ingredients

1 cup (235 ml) milk (low-fat cow's, or
    unsweetened, plain almond or soy)

1 cup (235 ml) water

2 eggs

1 cup (80 g) whole rolled oats

¼ teaspoon each salt and fresh-ground
    black pepper, or to taste

¼ cup (26 g) ground flaxseed

½ cup (50 g) sliced scallion, optional

⅓ to ½ cup (40 to 60 g) grated Cheddar or
    feta cheese, to taste

From Chef Jeannette

Whisking the eggs into the cold liquids,
heating slowly, and continuing to whisk
frequently throughout cooking will keep
the eggs incorporated. The oats will be
extra-rich, light, and creamy, and there
will be no visible bits of cooked egg in
your oatmeal.

Protein-Powered Cheesy Onion Oats

Savory breakfast oats? Try it—you'll like it! We added two eggs to
the mix for ultra protein, plus cheese for a rich, creamy flavor (and, of
course, calcium). The flaxseeds are a great touch—we use Barlean's
Forti-Flax (it's the best). Why? Because fresh organic flaxseeds, including Forti-Flax, add fiber, some omega-3s, and best of all, healthy plant
compounds called lignans, which have been found to have anticancer
activity in a number of published studies. The scallions provide warm
flavor undertones and go surprisingly well with this unusual, tasty dish.
Not only does this oatmeal really hit the spot on a cold winter's morning, but it's not bad for dinner, either!

In a large saucepan, whisk together the milk, water, and eggs until well
blended. Whisk in the oats and bring to a low boil over medium to medium-
high heat, continuing to whisk frequently.

Reduce the heat, cover, and cook for 10 minutes or until the oats reach
the desired tenderness, whisking frequently. Season with salt and pepper,
fold in the flaxseed and scallions, sprinkle on the cheese, remove from the
heat, and serve.

Yield: 3 or 4 small servings
Per Serving: 207.3 calories; 9.8 g fat (37% calories from fat); 10.7 g
protein; 143.6 g carbohydrate; 4.1 g dietary fiber; 119.5 mg cholesterol;
322 mg sodium

Ingredients

1 pound (455 g) leanest ground turkey

¹⁄₃ cup (38 g) shredded Cheddar cheese

¹⁄₃ cup (80 ml) apple cider (or low-sodium chicken broth)

1 teaspoon coriander

¹⁄₂ teaspoon sage, crumbled, optional

¹⁄₂ teaspoon ground fennel

¹⁄₂ teaspoon thyme

¹⁄₄ teaspoon nutmeg

¹⁄₄ teaspoon basil

¹⁄₂ teaspoon salt

¹⁄₄ teaspoon cayenne pepper, optional

Clean and Cheesy Apple Turkey Sausage

From Dr. Jonny: Having a craving for good, old-fashioned sausage? I know the feeling. Here's a great no-grease way to satisfy that craving and not feel guilty. Skip the factory-farmed pork (you don't even want to know about that one), and go for the low-fat ground turkey. The cider in this recipe gives the sausage a delightful sweetness (and a nice little shot of vitamin C just for good measure). Spices including basil and thyme give the end result a great mouthfeel and, best of all, there's not a nitrate in sight. The result is a low-sugar "clean-eating" treat that's lower in calories than the commercial kind and just as comforting!

In a large mixing bowl, combine all the ingredients and mix with your hands until well combined—the mixture will be sticky. Form into 8 to 12 thin patties. Spray a griddle or large skillet lightly with olive oil and heat over medium heat. Cook the patties for 3 to 4 minutes per side, or until cooked through.

Yield: 6 to 8 servings

Per Serving: 110.8 calories; 6.4 g fat (52% calories from fat); 11.2 g protein; 1.6 g carbohydrate; 0.2 g dietary fiber; 49.9 mg cholesterol; 228.9 mg sodium

Two-Cheese Fit and Flavorful Frittata

Ingredients

8 eggs

⅓ cup (80 ml) milk (low-fat cow's or unsweetened, plain soy or almond)

⅓ cup (33 g) fresh-grated Parmesan cheese

¼ teaspoon each salt and fresh-ground black pepper

2 tablespoons (28 ml) olive oil

1 medium sweet onion, diced

2 large cloves garlic, minced

1 bag (5 ounces, or 140 g) baby spinach

2 large prepared roasted red pepper halves, chopped (about ⅔ cup, or 120 g)

3 ounces (85 g) chèvre

2 tablespoons (8 g) minced fresh parsley, optional

From Chef Jeannette

Even Healthier: For more nutrients and freshness, roast your own peppers. Preheat the oven to high broil. Halve, stem, and seed one large red bell pepper (or make extra for use in sandwiches and salads). Lay the pepper halves facedown on a broiling sheet. Broil for about 10 to 15 minutes until they are charred all over. Remove from the heat and place in a bowl, covering tightly with plastic wrap for about 10 minutes, until they are cool enough to handle. Slip the skins off with your hands and they are ready for use or storage in the refrigerator.

From Dr. Jonny: Frittatas are a staple where I live in Southern California, but they can often be spoiled by being cooked in puddles of poor-quality fat and filled with even worse-quality sausage and smothered in too much cheese. In this recipe, we use olive oil for its healthy monounsaturated fat and rich assortment of olive phenols (healthy plant compounds that support immunity). And we limit the amount of cheese we use. The vibrantly flavored Parmesan cheese is not nearly as fattening as you think, by the way. Two tablespoons (10 g) have only 42 calories and provide quite a bit of calcium—more than 125 mg! And goat cheese contains more than 5 grams of protein per ounce (28 g) of cheese. We add spinach for taste and color (and an abundance of nutrients including iron and calcium) and red peppers for their vitamin C. Fun fact: The difference between an omelet and a frittata comes down to sequence: In an omelet you cook the eggs and then add the fillings in (or vice versa!), using the eggs to envelope the added ingredients; in a frittata you just mix all the stuff together and then cook it all at once.

Preheat the oven to broil.

In a large bowl, whisk together the eggs, milk, Parmesan cheese, salt, and pepper.

Heat the oil in a 10-inch (25-cm) cast-iron skillet over medium heat. Swirl the oil to coat the entire inner surface of the pan, including the sides (use a paper towel and wipe the sides to oil completely). Add the onion and cook for 4 to 5 minutes, stirring occasionally. Add the garlic, spinach, and peppers and cook for 2 to 3 minutes, stirring frequently, until the spinach is wilted. (Covering the pan will speed the wilting.) Drain excess liquids from the pan, return to the heat, and gently pour the prepared eggs evenly over the top of all. Stir gently to allow the eggs to run through everything. Dot the top evenly with pieces of the goat cheese. Cover and cook for about 6 to 7 minutes, or until the outer edges are cooked, the frittata is mostly solid, but the center is still a little wet. Place under the broiler and cook for about 1 minute, or until the center is set and the surface is firm.

Sprinkle with the parsley and serve.

Yield: 3 or 4 small servings

Per Serving: 305.7 calories; 21.9 g fat (65% calories from fat); 18.9 g protein; 9.3 g carbohydrate; 2.1 g dietary fiber; 436.1 mg cholesterol; 387 mg sodium

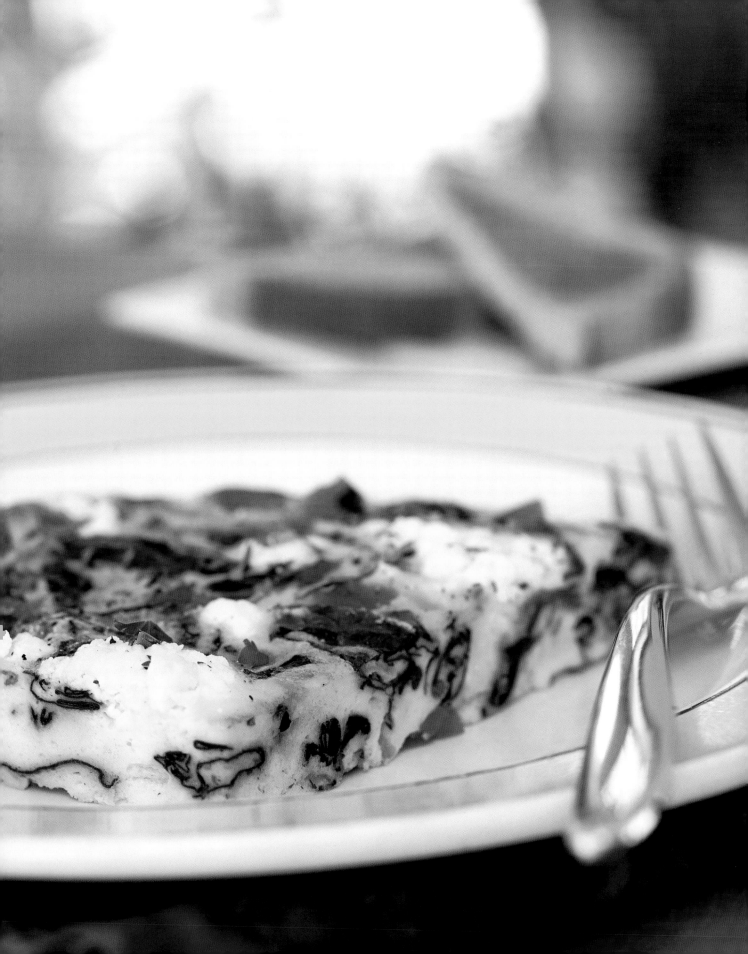

High-Protein Smoked Chicken Quiche Dijon

Ingredients

2 teaspoons (10 ml) olive oil

1 yellow onion, chopped

Sprinkling of garlic salt

6 eggs

1/2 cup (120 ml) evaporated skim milk (or low-fat cow's, or plain, unsweetened almond or soy)

1/4 cup (60 g) low-fat sour cream

2 tablespoons (30 g) Dijon mustard

1/4 teaspoon each salt and fresh-ground black pepper

1/2 teaspoon sweet paprika (or Hungarian hot)

3/4 cup (90 g) shredded Gruyère cheese

1 1/2 cups (338 g) smoked shredded chicken

1 lightly baked 9-inch (23-cm) piecrust (try our Satisfying Real-Food Piecrust, page 137)

2 tablespoons (6 g) minced chives, optional

From Chef Jeannette

Even Healthier: Reduce the overall calories in this dish by preparing your quiche without a crust. "Naked" quiche holds together beautifully, and its only carbs are from the veggies—a high-protein delight! Just spray the pie plate lightly with olive oil before adding the fillings and bake it the same way.

From Dr. Jonny: The concept of quiche is really smart. It's basically an egg pie, which means you get protein, nutrients such as choline (good for the brain), lutein, and zeaxanthin (good for the eyes), and everything else that's good about the whole egg. But too often quiche is just a cream pie with a few eggs thrown in and the crust, unfortunately, is loaded with trans fats. Our version uses a much-healthier trans fat–free crust and brings the eggs center stage with evaporated skim milk for that creamy texture we all find so comforting. We use just a bit of sour cream for a tangy richness that goes perfectly with the "smoke" of the chicken. A reasonable amount of delicious Gruyère cheese rounds out the package. (Note: See Chef Jeannette's tip for "going naked" and making the whole shebang even healthier!) Fun fact: Trans fats are made when manufacturers add hydrogen to vegetable oil, a process known as hydrogenation or partial hydrogenation. A comprehensive review of studies on trans fats published in the *New England Journal of Medicine* in 2006 estimated that between 30,000 and 100,000 cardiac deaths per year in the United States alone are attributable to the consumption of trans fats.

Preheat the oven to 375°F (190°C, or gas mark 5).

Heat the oil in a large skillet over medium heat. Add the onion, sprinkle with the garlic salt, and sauté until softened, but not browned, 5 to 6 minutes. Set aside to cool slightly.

In a large mixing bowl, combine the eggs, evaporated milk, sour cream, Dijon, salt, pepper, and paprika, and beat together. Stir in the cheese and chicken.

Spread the cooked onions over the bottom of the crust and gently pour the egg mixture over all. Sprinkle the chives over the top. Bake for 35 to 40 minutes, or until the filling is set in the center and the top is lightly browned.

Yield: 6 servings

Per Serving: 470.2 calories; 29.1 g fat (55% calories from fat); 25.5 g protein; 27 g carbohydrate; 1.3 g dietary fiber; 273.3 mg cholesterol; 773.1 mg sodium

Ingredients

6 eggs

1 teaspoon water

¼ teaspoon oregano

¼ teaspoon each salt and fresh-ground
   black pepper

¼ cup (38 g) crumbled feta cheese

2 teaspoons (10 ml) olive oil

4 cups (120 g) chopped fresh spinach

2 ripe plum tomatoes, seeded and chopped

¼ cup (10 g) sliced fresh basil

1 to 2 tablespoons (5 to 10 g) fresh-grated
   Parmesan cheese, optional, to taste

Lighten Up Cheesy Mediterranean Egg Scramble

From Dr. Jonny: Scrambles are one of my go-to dishes when I need to whip up something really fast. They can be amazingly healthy affairs, quick and easy, and nutrient-packed, not to mention a great source of highly absorbable protein. But restaurant scrambled eggs, or, even worse, the buffet versions, aren't the best. For one thing, they use a ton of cheese, contain more eggs than you really need, and are stir-fried in inferior oil. To make a healthier dish we recommend choosing free-range chicken eggs (less likely to be contaminated and more likely to contain omega-3 fats) and small amounts of strongly flavored cheese so you can get by with less. (Examples: Feta cheese, 1 ounce [28 g] of which has 4 grams of protein and 140 mg of calcium, or Parmesan, 2 tablespoons [10 g] of which has almost 4 grams of protein and 125 mg of calcium.) The result is a delicious dish with a hint of the Mediterranean made all the better with the addition of flavor-rich basil. Scrambles are easy yet deeply satisfying. Fun fact: Basil contains a strongly scented volatile oil composed of plant chemicals known as terpenoids. It's been a culinary herb in Europe and Central Asia since before the written word!

In a medium bowl, add the eggs, water, oregano, salt, and pepper, and beat lightly. Stir in the feta and set aside.

Heat the oil in a large skillet over medium heat and add the spinach, stirring to coat.

Cover for 1 to 2 minutes to speed the wilting. Uncover, stir, and add the tomatoes, cooking until the spinach has cooked down and the tomatoes are hot. Pour the eggs over all and cook, turning occasionally. When the eggs are nearly solid, stir in the basil and cook until softly set. Sprinkle on the Parmesan to taste and serve hot.

Yield: 4 servings

Per Serving: 178.2 calories; 12.4 g fat (62% calories from fat); 12.8 g protein; 5 g carbohydrate; 1.6 g dietary fiber; 326.8 mg cholesterol; 402.8 mg sodium

Ingredients

Olive oil cooking spray

2½ (8 g) teaspoons organic chicken Better Than Bouillon

⅔ cup (160 ml) evaporated skim milk

1 cup (230 g) plain low-fat Greek yogurt

2 tablespoons (28 ml) melted butter

4 ounces (115 g) extra-sharp Cheddar cheese, shredded

¾ cup (75 g) sliced scallion

1 pound (455 g) Yukon gold potatoes (about 2 large), unpeeled and grated

½ teaspoon sweet paprika, optional

From Chef Jeannette

Time-Saver Tip: To save on grating time, use precut hash brown potatoes from the refrigerator section, or frozen hash brown potatoes, thawed for 30 minutes.

Even Healthier: If you want to boost the nutrient content and lower the glycemic impact of this dish even further, substitute grated sweet potatoes for half or all of the white potatoes.

Savory Baked-Not-Fried Hash Browns

From Dr. Jonny: Hash browns, that old favorite at diners everywhere, usually means straight white potatoes fried in heavy, reused oils. It's the worst possible combo: starchy potatoes and damaged fats. The only thing worse is French fries. However, all is not lost! Here's how to do a quick hash brown upgrade: Add cheese for calcium and protein, use evaporated skim milk for even more protein, and finally, bake them instead of frying them. Presto, you've got a delicious hash brown dish that's substantially better than diner fare. We used just a tiny amount of butter for flavor richness and substituted high-protein Greek yogurt for the much more caloric sour cream. And no surprise: We left the skins on the potato for all the usual reasons, more fiber being at the top of the list. These hashies are dense and satisfying, not to mention very quick and easy to prepare! Enjoy!

Preheat the oven to 375°F (190°C, or gas mark 5). Spray an 8 x 8-inch (20 x 20-cm) baking dish lightly with olive oil. Set aside.

In a large bowl, whisk the bouillon paste into the milk. Stir in the yogurt, butter, and cheese until well incorporated. Stir in the scallions and fold in the potatoes to evenly coat. Spoon into the prepared baking dish and sprinkle evenly with the paprika.

Bake for 40 to 50 minutes, or until set, browned on top, and the potatoes are tender. It will continue to set as it cools.

Yield: about 9 servings

Per Serving: 143.9 calories; 7.3 g fat (44% calories from fat); 7.7 g protein; 14 g carbohydrate; 1.3 g dietary fiber; 22.5 mg cholesterol; 242.7 mg sodium

Ingredients

Olive oil cooking spray

1 cup (125 g) whole-wheat pastry flour

2 teaspoons (9 g) baking powder

¼ teaspoon salt

⅓ cup (75 g) butter, chopped into small pieces and chilled in the freezer for 10 minutes

½ cup (115 g) plain low-fat Greek yogurt

1 teaspoon lime zest

2 teaspoons (10 ml) olive oil

1 yellow onion, chopped

1 pound (455 g) leanest ground beef (or turkey)

1 teaspoon chili powder

½ teaspoon cumin

½ teaspoon each salt and fresh-ground black pepper

¾ cup (185 g) tomato sauce

1 cup (130 g) frozen corn, thawed

1 egg

½ cup (115 g) low-fat sour cream

¼ cup (4 g) chopped fresh cilantro

½ cup (58 g) shredded high-quality Cheddar cheese

Whole-Wheat Chili Biscuit Breakfast Pie

From Dr. Jonny: One of Bob Newhart's standup routines involved imitating a hapless airline pilot on the public address system saying, "In just a few moments, ladies and gentlemen, you will be looking at the beautiful skyline of either Buenos Aires . . . (long pause) . . . or San Francisco." I was reminded of that routine when Chef Jeannette sent me this recipe, which is either a biscuit sandwich . . . (long pause) . . . or a mild breakfast chili. Either way, it makes a dense and satisfying breakfast. We dumped the typical shortening in favor of much healthier butter (yes, I said that—butter is a real whole food and shortening is a trans fat–laden nightmare). Whole-wheat pastry flour boosts the fiber, and the beef is lean. The sour cream and cheese add just the right amount of cheesy richness without breaking the calorie bank. Fun fact: Cheese is as good a calcium source as milk. One half cup (58 g) of Cheddar (the amount in this recipe) delivers well over 400 mg of this important mineral!

Preheat the oven to 375°F (190°C, or gas mark 5). Lightly spray a 9½-inch (24-cm) deep-dish pie plate with olive oil and set aside.

In a large bowl whisk together the flour, baking powder, and salt. Using a pastry cutter or two knives, cut the chilled butter pieces into the flour until the mixture is holding together in pea-size pieces. Add the yogurt and zest and stir just until the mixture forms a dough. Turn the dough out onto a floured surface and gently knead it a few times. Roll it out into a roughly 9½-inch (24-cm) circle and, using a biscuit cutter or the rim of a juice glass, cut it into 9 thin 3-inch (7.5-cm) biscuits. Set aside.

Heat the oil in a large skillet over medium-high heat. Add the onion and cook for about 3 minutes. Add the beef and break it up. Cook until no pink remains, about 5 to 6 minutes, and drain off any oils. Add the chili powder, cumin, salt, pepper, tomato sauce, and corn, and stir to mix. In a small bowl, whisk the egg, add the sour cream, and whisk together until well combined. Stir in the cilantro. Stir the sour cream mixture into the beef mixture until combined and heat for about 2 minutes. Pour the beef mixture into the prepared pie plate. Sprinkle the cheese evenly over the top. Lay the biscuits in a single layer on top of the beef. Bake for 20 to 25 minutes, or until cooked through and the biscuits are golden brown (top loosely with aluminum foil if the biscuits are browning too quickly).

Yield: 9 servings

Per Serving: 272 calories; 15 g fat (49% calories from fat); 16.5 g protein; 17.9 g carbohydrate; 1.4 g dietary fiber; 85.3 mg cholesterol; 590.5 mg sodium

Ingredients

Cooking oil spray

4 tablespoons (55 g) butter, softened

½ cup (100 g) sugar (or Sucanat)

2 large eggs

1 teaspoon vanilla extract

1 cup (245 g) applesauce

1½ cups (188 g) oat flour (or whole-wheat pastry flour to increase the fiber)

1 teaspoon baking soda

½ cup (56 g) toasted wheat germ

¼ cup (26 g) ground flaxseed

¼ teaspoon salt

1 teaspoon ground cardamom

1 teaspoon ground cinnamon

3 cups (330 g) grated sweet potato

From Chef Jeannette

Cool and seal any leftovers in an airtight resealable plastic bag for a fresh-tasting breakfast, snack, or dessert anytime.

Fiber-Full Sweet Potato Mini-Muffins

From Dr. Jonny: I'll never forget how, during the idiotic low-fat craze of the '80s, people would routinely scarf down these humongous "no-fat" bran muffins thinking they were consuming healthy fare when in fact they were consuming 500 calories of heavily sugared processed carbs that turned out to be way more of a health hazard than fat ever was. What a fiasco. (And it's still going on today, but don't get me started.) Classic bakery muffins are typically loaded with sugar, not to mention high-calorie (but perfectly acceptable) butter, and rarely do any of them contain much fiber. In fact, muffins are pretty much the dictionary definition of a high-calorie, low-nutrient food. But not so with these gems. They're high in fiber and other nutrients from the sweet potatoes, and there's only ½ cup (100 g) of sugar in the entire recipe. Best of all, the taste is out of this world—sweet and spicy at the same time. Making "mini" muffins can also help with portion control. This is comfort food that makes sense!

Preheat the oven to 375°F (190°C, or gas mark 5) and spray a large mini-muffin tin (makes 24 mini-muffins) with cooking oil. Set aside.

In a mixer, cream the butter and sugar together. Add the eggs, vanilla, and applesauce, and beat until smooth.

In a medium bowl, whisk together the flour, baking soda, wheat germ, flaxseed, salt, cardamom, and cinnamon. Add the dry mix to the wet mix, fold in the sweet potato, and mix by hand until just incorporated. Pour the batter into the tins and bake for 20 to 25 minutes, or until a toothpick inserted into the center of a muffin comes out clean.

Yield: 24 mini-muffins (12 servings)

Per Serving: 203.18 calories; 7.38 g fat (32% calories from fat); 5.35 g protein; 29.91 g carbohydrate; 3.46 g dietary fiber; 45.1 mg cholesterol; 185.3 mg sodium

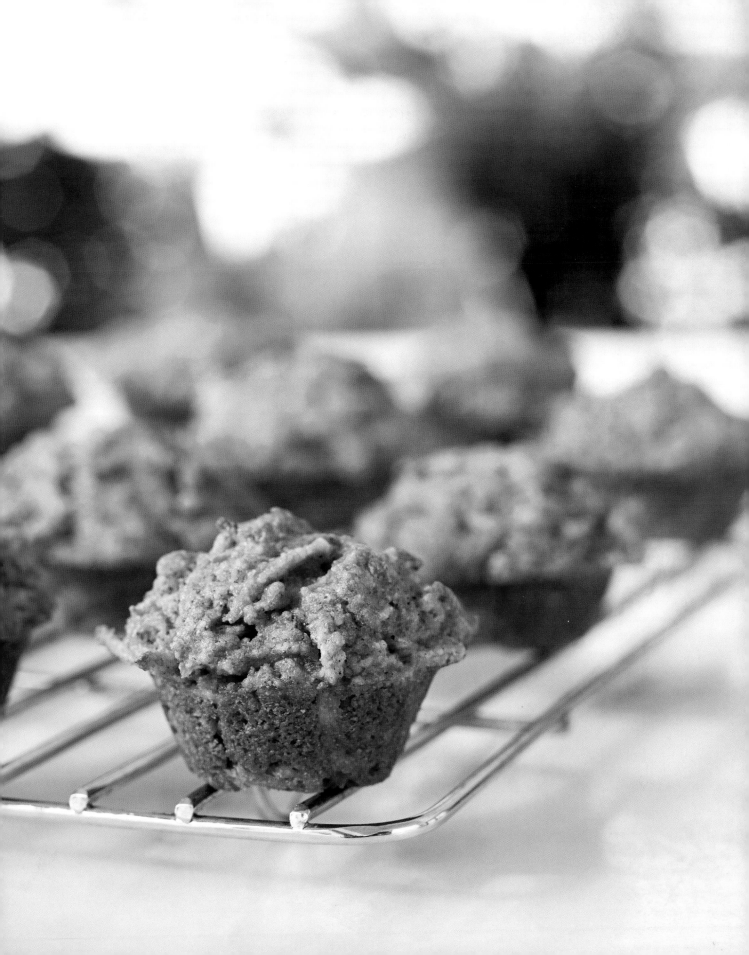

Ingredients

4 large ripe bananas

1/3 cup (65 g) Sucanat, sugar, or xylitol

1 egg

1/3 cup (80 g) melted butter, Earth Balance
     (or other nonhydrogenated buttery
     spread), and/or applesauce (use any one
     or a blend of butter and applesauce)

1 teaspoon baking soda

1 teaspoon baking powder

1/2 teaspoon salt

1 1/2 cups (188 g) whole-wheat pastry flour

From Chef Jeannette

Even Healthier: To make this muffin
with no added sugar and additional fiber,
sweeten with 1/4 cup (50 g) xylitol and
1/4 cup (50 g) MoreFiber stevia baking
blend from NuNaturals in place of the
1/3 cup (65 g) Sucanat.

Low-Fat, Light, and Luscious Banana Muffins

From Dr. Jonny: On what planet is a sweet, moist, delicious banana muffin not a comfort food? Not on any planet I've lived on lately! These light muffins are sweetened mostly with bananas and are so soft and juicy they give new meaning to the phrase "melt in your mouth." If you're not familiar with xylitol, it's a sugar alcohol that actually has some health benefits (it helps discourage bacteria from sticking to moist surfaces, such as those in the mouth). It also has minimal impact on blood sugar, while cooking, baking, and tasting exactly like sugar. Hint: If you want to minimize calories even more, try using applesauce instead of butter!

Preheat the oven to 350°F (180°C, or gas mark 4). Spray a 12-muffin tin lightly with cooking oil.

Beat the bananas with a mixer until mostly smooth. Beat in the sweetener, egg, and butter/applesauce mix. Set aside.

In a separate bowl, whisk together the baking soda, baking powder, salt, and flour.

Pour the wet ingredients into the dry and mix gently until just combined. Spoon into the muffin tins and bake for about 20 minutes, or until a toothpick inserted into the center of a muffin comes out clean.

Yield: 12 muffins

Per Serving: 158.5 calories; 6.3 g fat (35% calories from fat); 3.2 g protein; 24.8 g carbohydrate; 3.1 g dietary fiber; 32 mg cholesterol; 250.2 mg sodium

Lemony Light and Bright Breakfast Fruit Salad

From Dr. Jonny: Fruit for breakfast is as American as apple pie, but you want to eat it with some protein, as you'll stay full for longer and get a much better start to your day. So we added lemon-spiked, high-protein yogurt plus a honey sweetener to coat this delectable assortment of fresh, crisp fall fruits. Add almonds for their rich array of minerals including calcium, iron, and potassium and generous amount of heart-healthy monounsaturated fat. (The almonds also help slow the entrance of sugar into the bloodstream so that you have less of a spike of energy followed by a long, energy-draining fall!) Throw in a little wheat germ for extra fiber and vitamin E. (Hint: You can also sprinkle on Barlean's Forti-Flax for extra crunchiness, fiber, cancer-fighting lignans, and omega-3s to boot.) This'll help wake you right up in the morning—and it comes together in a flash!

Ingredients

1 cup (230 g) plain low-fat yogurt

2 tablespoons (40 g) raw honey, warmed to liquid, if necessary, or 100 percent maple syrup, or to taste

1 tablespoon (15 ml) fresh-squeezed lemon juice

1 teaspoon lemon zest

$\frac{1}{2}$ teaspoon ground ginger, optional

1 Granny Smith apple, unpeeled, cored, and chopped

1 crisp sweet red apple, unpeeled, cored, and chopped (try Red Delicious or Braeburn)

1 crisp sweet ripe pear, unpeeled, cored, and chopped

1 large navel orange, peeled, sliced widthwise "around the equator," and slices quartered

2 tablespoons (15 g) juice-sweetened dried cranberries

$\frac{1}{3}$ cup (37 g) slivered almonds

1 tablespoon (7 g) toasted wheat germ, optional

In a large bowl, whisk together the yogurt, honey, lemon juice, lemon zest, and ginger Add the prepared apples, pear, orange, cranberries, and almonds and toss gently to coat. Sprinkle with the toasted wheat germ before serving.

Yield: 4 servings

Per Serving: 230.7 calories; 1 g fat (22% calories from fat); 6.2 g protein; 42.5 g carbohydrate; 6.4 g dietary fiber; 3.5 mg cholesterol; 43.9 mg sodium

From Chef Jeannette

Time-Saver Tip: To save time coring and slicing, invest in a good corer-slicer. It's a round tool with blades like spokes on a wheel. You simply push it down over the top of an apple and it will remove the core and leave you with neat, even slices. You still have to chop if you want bite-size pieces, but this little tool comes in very handy for pies and cobblers and it's very inexpensive—worth the small investment for a speedy, whole-foods kitchen where we leave the fiber-rich skins on the apples!

Banana-Sweet Strawberry Breakfast Bread

From Dr. Jonny: At my local Whole Foods, the bakery department is known for putting out samples of all kinds of delicious goodies. (Thank you, bakery department!) One of my faves is banana bread. Love this stuff! (Who doesn't, really?) But while the good bakers at Whole Foods tend to be careful about their ingredients, most everyday banana bread can wind up being a carb-fest with little fiber and a ton of sugar. You can do better with Chef Jeannette's version (and it's still as sweet as ever). We bumped up the nutrition by using two things: whole-wheat pastry flour (not perfect, but a lot better than the useless white stuff) and . . . drumroll please . . . ground flaxseed. The flax adds a nutty note as well as providing fiber and plant compounds called lignans, which have been found to have significant anticancer activity. (Highly recommended: Barlean's Forti-Flax, available at health food or grocery stores.) The sweetness—did I mention there's plenty of that?—comes primarily from the banana itself (plus just a little sugar or xylitol). Fun fact: Research from Harvard Medical School found that strawberries may offer cardiovascular disease protection. In an analysis of data from the Women's Health Study, those who reported eating the most strawberries experienced lower blood levels of C-reactive protein, a biomarker for inflammation in the blood vessels.

Ingredients

Cooking oil spray
3 ripe bananas
½ cup (120 ml) milk (low-fat cow's or vanilla unsweetened almond or soy)
1 egg
3 tablespoons (45 ml) almond oil
2 cups (250 g) whole-wheat pastry flour
2 tablespoons (13 g) ground flaxseed
½ cup (100 g) sugar or xylitol
2 teaspoons (9 g) baking powder
¼ teaspoon baking soda
½ teaspoon salt
¼ teaspoon allspice
1 cup (85 g) sliced fresh strawberries (or frozen, thawed)

From Chef Jeannette

Variation: Add ½ cup (88 g) dark chocolate chips when you add the strawberries for a rich dessert-y feel and a shot of magnesium to boot!

Preheat the oven to 350°F (180°C, or gas mark 4). Spray a standard loaf pan with cooking oil.

In a medium bowl, mash the bananas until they are the consistency of yogurt.

In another medium bowl, whisk together the milk, egg, and oil. Add the mashed banana and mix to combine.

In a large bowl, whisk together the flour, flaxseed, sweetener, baking powder, baking soda, salt, and allspice. Pour the wet mix into the dry and mix until just combined. Gently fold in the strawberries. Pour the mixture into the prepared loaf pan and bake for about 1 hour, or until a toothpick inserted into the center comes out clean.

Cool for at least 5 minutes in the pan, then turn out and cool completely on a wire rack.

Yield: about 9 slices
Per Serving: 254.3 calories; 6.9 g fat (24% calories from fat); 5 g protein; 44.4 g carbohydrate; 2.3 g dietary fiber; 24.5 mg cholesterol; 287.4 mg sodium

Ingredients

Cooking oil spray

1 cup (100 g) fresh cranberries

1 cup (125 g) whole-wheat pastry flour

1 cup (125 g) unbleached flour

2 teaspoons (9 g) baking powder

1/4 teaspoon baking soda

1/4 teaspoon salt

2 eggs

2/3 cup (130 g) sugar

3 tablespoons (45 ml) almond oil

Juice and zest of 2 large navel oranges (between 2/3 and 3/4 cup, or 160 and 175 ml, juice)

1 teaspoon vanilla extract

2/3 cup (75 g) sliced toasted almonds

From Chef Jeannette

Variation: You can also substitute the almond oil and almonds for walnut oil and chopped toasted walnuts (unsalted).

Nutty Antioxidant Power Cran-Orange Bread

From Dr. Jonny: Here's a bread that's a comfort food classic, but we took the liberty of loading it up with antioxidants. (Hope you don't mind!) We also did some damage control on the carb and calorie front by reducing the sugar and removing the butter. For added fiber, which, trust me, we all need, we made a mix of whole-wheat pastry flour and the regular kind. We used almond oil (with its high concentration of heart-healthy monounsaturated fat) and almonds for additional fiber and a rich assortment of minerals (including calcium, magnesium, potassium, and iron). The result is not too sweet, with hits of real tang from the cranberries and a subtle background of orange notes. Is your mouth watering yet? Fun fact: Although many Americans think of cranberries only when Thanksgiving comes around, these berries are among the highest in antioxidant phenols (plant compounds with health benefits) of any commonly eaten fruit. According to Joe Vinson, Ph.D., research chemist at the University of Scranton, "Cranberries are loaded with antioxidants and should be eaten more often."

Preheat the oven to 350°F (180°C, or gas mark 4). Spray a standard loaf pan with oil and set aside.

Add half the cranberries to a food processor and pulse a few times just until very coarsely chopped—you don't want them minced. Remove and repeat with the remaining cranberries. Set aside.

In a large bowl whisk together the whole-wheat pastry flour, unbleached flour, baking powder, baking soda, and salt.

In a medium bowl, lightly whisk the eggs. Add the sugar, almond oil, orange juice, zest, and vanilla, and whisk until well combined. Pour the wet mixture into the dry and mix until just incorporated. Gently fold in the cranberries and almonds. Bake for 50 to 55 minutes, or until a toothpick inserted into the center comes out clean. Cool for at least 5 minutes in the pan, then turn out and cool completely on a wire rack.

Yield: about 9 slices

Per Serving: 277.8 calories; 10.2 g fat (32% calories from fat); 6.2 g protein; 41.4 g carbohydrate; 2.3 g dietary fiber; 47 mg cholesterol; 222.2 mg sodium

Portobello Benedict with Sundried Tomato Pesto

Ingredients

High-heat cooking oil spray

4 large portobello mushroom caps, stemmed and gills removed

1 tablespoon (15 ml) olive oil

2 cloves garlic, minced (or 1 teaspoon prepared minced garlic)

1 bag (10 ounces, or 280 g) baby spinach

1 bag (10 ounces, or 280 g) baby arugula

Salt and fresh-ground black pepper, to taste

½ teaspoon salt (omit if eggs are very fresh)

1 teaspoon apple cider vinegar (omit if eggs are very fresh)

4 very fresh, extra-large eggs

½ large, ripe Hass avocado, thinly sliced optional

1 large heirloom tomato, cut into 4 thick slices, optional

4 teaspoons (20 g) prepared high-quality sundried tomato pesto, or to taste

From Dr. Jonny: I know, I know—you're worried about the fat in those four extra-large eggs. And—gasp—the avocado! Won't that fat put on weight? Actually, no. According to the most respected nutrition epidemiologist of our time, Walter Willett, M.D., Ph.D., of Harvard University, "We have found virtually no relationship between the percentage of calories from fat and any important health outcome." And that includes obesity. That doesn't mean calories, type of fat, and type of carbs don't matter, but it does mean that you can relax about the eggs. The good fats in avocado, eggs, and pesto will satisfy your hunger, calm your cravings, and set you up for sustained energy throughout the day. The protein will stimulate your metabolism. And if you reduce cravings, guess what? You're less likely to overeat!

Preheat the broiler and lightly spray a broiler pan with high-heat cooking oil. Place the prepared portobellos top-down on the broiler pan and broil for 7 to 8 minutes, or until tender. Watch closely to prevent scorching.

While the mushrooms are cooking, heat the oil in a large sauté pan (5-quart, or 4.7-L, works well). Add the garlic and sauté for 1 minute. Add the spinach and arugula, and cover for 1 minute to wilt slightly. Remove the cover, season with salt and pepper to taste, turn gently for even cooking, and continue to sauté for another 2 minutes, or until the greens are wilted to the desired tenderness.

While the greens are wilting, fill a medium sauté pan about half full with water, add the salt and vinegar, and bring the water just to a simmer (not a full boil). Break the eggs one at a time into a small bowl and slide gently into the simmering water. Try to slide them against the edge of the sauté pan to help them keep their shape. Simmer the eggs for about 4 minutes, or until the whites are cooked through but the yolks are still soft. Using a slotted spoon, remove the eggs from the pan and set them aside to drain.

While the eggs are draining, place 1 broiled portobello cap on each of 4 plates. Lay one-fourth of the avocado slices evenly over each mushroom, top with one-fourth of the prepared greens, 1 tomato slice, and 1 poached egg.

Spoon 1 teaspoon (5 g) pesto (or to taste) over the egg and serve immediately.

Yield: 4 servings

Per Serving: 248.7 calories; 15.4 g fat (54% calories from fat); 15.8 g protein; 17.7 g carbohydrate; 7.1 g dietary fiber; 213 mg cholesterol; 484.7 mg sodium

From Chef Jeannette

This Benedict eschews puddles of classic hollandaise in favor of fresh, raw pesto. Not only is it simple to make from scratch (while hollandaise is notoriously fussy), but it has the anti-inflammatory benefits of olive oil as well. Using portobellos to replace white English muffins not only reduces calories and poor-quality carbs, but also improves the overall flavor of the dish while providing some great-for-you nutrients such as B vitamins and potassium.

To stem the portobellos, gently pinch and grip the stem firmly at the base with one hand, and slowly twist the cap with the other hand until the stem separates. To remove the gills, scoop them out with a teaspoon, leaving hollowed-out shells.

The freshest eggs have very firm whites and yolks, and so tend to retain their shape better when cooking—yet another reason to buy right from the source! If you didn't buy your eggs at a farm stand, use the salt and vinegar to help them hold their shape when poaching.

Even Healthier: When you have the time, you can make flavorful, nutrient-rich, fresh pesto yourself. This can easily be prepared in advance because it keeps for a week tightly sealed in the refrigerator. Extra sundried tomato pesto is excellent spooned over grilled fish or chicken, too.

½ cup (55 g) julienned sundried tomatoes in oil, drained
3 tablespoons (45 ml) olive oil, plus extra if needed
1 tablespoon (15 ml) balsamic vinegar
1 clove garlic, crushed
2 tablespoons (18 g) toasted pine nuts
¼ cup (10 g) basil leaves
¼ cup (25 g) fresh-grated Parmesan cheese
¼ teaspoon each salt and fresh-ground black pepper

In the food processor, pulse together the tomatoes, olive oil, vinegar, garlic, pine nuts, basil, Parmesan, salt, and pepper until smooth, scraping down the sides as necessary. Drizzle in extra olive oil, 1 teaspoon at a time, if the mixture is too dry.

Yield: Entire recipe, ⅔ cup (173 g)

Per Serving: 754.4 calories; 68.7 g fat (79% calories from fat); 16.6 g protein; 26.4 g carbohydrate; 8.1 g dietary fiber; 22 mg cholesterol; 1,119 mg sodium

Two Better Omelets

From Dr. Jonny: There's a local diner in my area where I often go when I'm having a breakfast meeting, and here's what I've noticed about its omelets: they're huge. As in enormous. As in humongous. As in no one should be able to finish them. And it's not just my local diner—apparently, omelets with six eggs are not uncommon, and they're also usually drowning in butter and salt. But omelets are a great dish—just cut back to a more reasonable portion size (two eggs works!), use less oil or butter, and fill them with delectable healthy treats. Presto! A high-calorie nightmare turns into a really healthy comfort food. Note: If you want the most health out of your eggs, get them from pasture-raised hens. Much like pasture-raised cows, these hens actually eat the diet they were meant to eat, so their eggs are far better. Some are even omega-3 enriched.

Ingredients

2 eggs

1 teaspoon water

1 tablespoon (7.5 g) grated Gruyère cheese (or Parmesan)

¼ teaspoon each salt and fresh-ground black pepper

Olive oil cooking spray

2 slices nitrate-free turkey bacon, sliced into bite-size pieces

2 tablespoons (16 g) grated apple

⅓ cup (10 g) chopped fresh baby spinach

Protein-Packed Green Eggs and Bacon Omelet

From Dr. Jonny: To boost this omelet, we've added extra protein with lower-calorie nitrate-free turkey bacon, used olive oil instead of butter for the olive phenols that are so good for you, and added mushrooms and spinach. (The spinach provides iron, calcium, potassium, vitamin K, vitamin A, fiber, and the superstars of eye nutrition, lutein and zeaxanthin.) Satisfying and as healthy as Jack LaLanne. And it's not just for breakfast—it works great as an "anytime" meal!

In a small bowl, lightly whisk the eggs, water, cheese, salt, and pepper.

Spray a small, light skillet (or a 7-inch, or 18-cm, omelet pan) with olive oil and heat over medium heat. Add the bacon and apple and cook until the bacon is crispy. Add the spinach, stir to combine and wilt, increase the heat to medium-high, and pour the egg mix gently over the contents of the pan.

Do not disturb for about 30 seconds, then, using your spatula, lift the edges of the omelet up and allow the runny egg on top to seep underneath and cook until the whole thing is firm enough to turn. Gently lift and tuck one side of the omelet, keeping the filling inside. Flip if you need to cook it further, and slide it off onto a plate.

Yield: 1 omelet

Per Serving: 254.3 calories; 17.9 g fat (63% calories from fat); 19.5 g protein; 4.2 g carbohydrate; 0.7 g dietary fiber; 456.2 mg cholesterol; 1,123.3 mg sodium

Ingredients

2 eggs

1 teaspoon water

1 tablespoon (5 g) fresh-grated Parmesan or
mozzarella cheese

1/4 teaspoon each salt and fresh-ground
black pepper

2 teaspoons (10 ml) olive oil

2 tablespoons (20 g) minced onion

2 tablespoons (20 g) minced green bell
pepper

1 large mushroom, thinly sliced, optional

1/2 teaspoon dried oregano

3 tablespoons (15 g) tomato sauce
(use plain or spaghetti sauce), warmed

Pizza Omelet

From Dr. Jonny: The Whole Foods near my house in Southern California sells a "breakfast pizza" and they tell me it's next to impossible to keep up with the demand. I like this version better. It's a healthy twist on the pizza idea and it makes a superb breakfast. Instead of the standard crust made of flour, the "crust" is made of eggs. Onions, peppers, and mushrooms provide a nice mix of healthy vegetables, the grated cheese provides calcium (and delicious taste), and the warm tomato sauce gives it that pizza "feel." Fun fact: The "pizza capital of the world" is not in Italy, but in Brazil! Sao Paulo has 6,000 pizza establishments, and Brazilians in that city alone consume 1.4 million pizzas on a daily basis!

In a small bowl, lightly whisk the eggs, water, cheese, salt, and pepper.

Coat a small, light skillet (or a 7-inch, or 18-cm, omelet pan) with the olive oil and heat over medium heat (you can swipe it with a paper towel to evenly coat). Add the onion, bell pepper, mushroom, and oregano. Cook until the mushroom has released its juices and all the veggies are tender. Increase the heat to medium-high and pour the egg mix gently over the contents of the pan.

Do not disturb for about 30 seconds, then, using your spatula, lift the edges of the omelet up and allow the runny egg on top to seep underneath and cook until the whole thing is firm enough to turn. Gently lift and tuck one side of the omelet, keeping the filling inside. Flip if you need to cook it further, and slide it off onto a plate. Top with the warm tomato sauce and serve.

Yield: 1 omelet

Per Serving: 268.2 calories; 20.8 g fat (69% calories from fat); 15.9 g protein; 5.8 g carbohydrate; 1.5 g dietary fiber; 427.4 mg cholesterol; 879.4 mg sodium

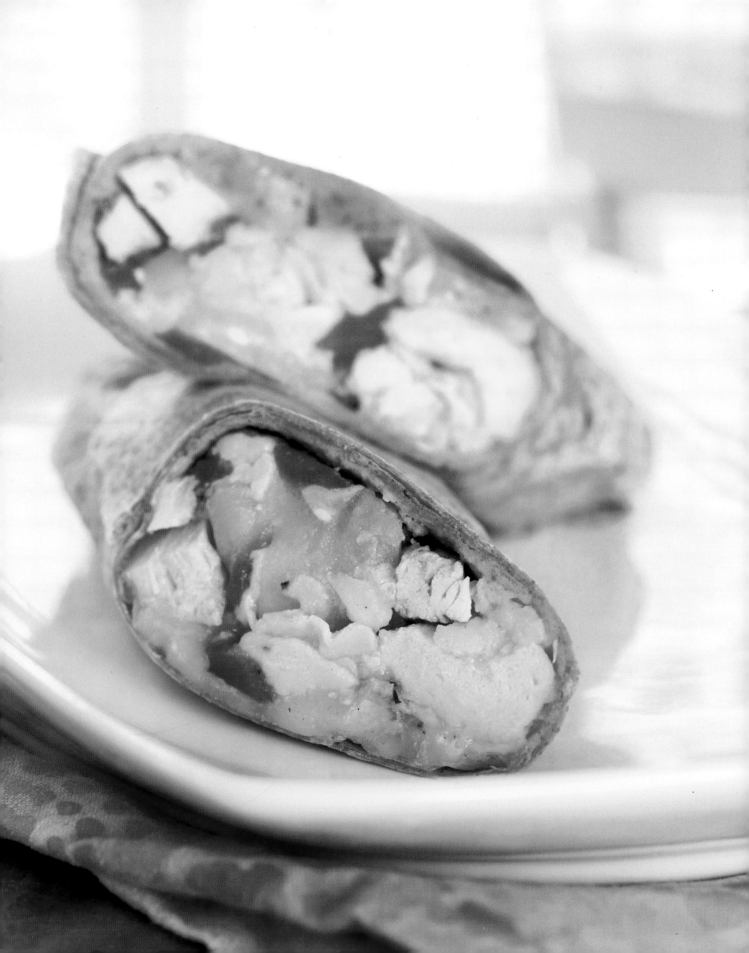

Gourmet Whole-Grain Breakfast Burrito

From Dr. Jonny: I'm a big fan of "unconventional" breakfast foods, such as salmon, burgers, salads, and . . . wait for it . . . burritos! After all, why not? It's only convention that says we have to eat cereal and orange juice! But even if you don't eat this burrito for breakfast it can still make a terrific one-pot meal. We improved on the usual restaurant fare by loading it up with a bunch of protein from eggs, smoked chicken, and Greek yogurt, which replaces the sour cream (less than half the calories, four times the protein, and a thick and creamy texture to boot). Greek yogurt has way more protein than standard yogurt as well as significantly fewer carbs. We added roasted red peppers to the mix for color, flavor, and high levels of vitamins C and A, and used whole-grain wraps for more fiber.

Ingredients

Olive oil cooking spray

4 eggs

1 large Yukon gold potato, unpeeled, boiled, and cut into bite-size pieces

1 roasted red bell pepper, cut into bite-size pieces

3 tablespoons (45 g) plain low-fat Greek yogurt

Salt and fresh-ground black pepper, to taste

Four 10-inch (25-cm) whole-grain tortillas

3 ounces (85 g) nitrate-free smoked chicken, cut into bite-size pieces

⅓ cup (37 g) shredded fontina cheese

Preheat the oven to 375°F (190°C, or gas mark 5).

Spray a large skillet with the olive oil and place over medium heat. Lightly beat the eggs and pour into the hot skillet, stirring frequently for a few minutes until the eggs are just set. Remove from the heat.

In a large bowl, gently mix the scrambled eggs, potato, bell pepper, yogurt, salt, and pepper until combined.

Lay out the tortillas and place one-fourth of the egg mixture into the center of each wrap. Top with one-fourth of the chicken and one-fourth of the cheese. Fold the top edge up and over the filling, tuck in the sides, and roll toward you, leaving the seam-side down.

Wrap each burrito in aluminum foil, place the wrapped burritos on a baking sheet, and bake for about 15 minutes, or until hot throughout and the cheese is melted.

Yield: 4 burritos

Per Serving: 270.1 calories; 9 g fat (30% calories from fat); 18.2 g protein; 32.2 g carbohydrate; 5.2 g dietary fiber; 222.9 mg cholesterol; 254.3 mg sodium

Ingredients

Cooking oil spray
1½ cups (188 g) unbleached flour
½ cup (100 g) xylitol (or sugar)
1 teaspoon baking powder
½ teaspoon baking soda
¼ teaspoon salt
¾ cup (45 g) plain low-fat Greek yogurt
½ cup (120 ml) milk (low-fat cow's, or un-
    sweetened vanilla soy or almond milk)
⅓ cup (80 ml) almond oil
1 teaspoon vanilla extract
1 cup (110 g) toasted slivered almonds
1½ teaspoons (3.5 g) cinnamon
⅓ cup (65 g) sugar
2 tablespoons (28 g) butter, softened

From Chef Jeannette

Even Healthier: For more fiber and nutrients, replace half or all of the regular flour in this dish with whole-wheat pastry flour.

Luscious, Lighter Almond Coffee Cake

From Dr. Jonny: Recently I went on vacation with my girlfriend Michelle—my first (vacation, not girlfriend!) in three years! When I returned, my beloved housekeeper and dog wrangler, Jessica, had left a little "welcome home" treat for me in the refrigerator: coffee cake. Since this is an old favorite of mine, and something I have conscientiously avoided for about two decades, and because Jessica was nice enough to go out and get it for me, I decided to indulge. And two thoughts hit me right away: One, this is delicious—no wonder it's a top comfort food. Two—this could be made so much less unhealthy with just a few tweaks. Tweak number one: Replace full-fat sour cream with lower-fat (and higher-protein) Greek yogurt. Tweak number two: Reduce the sugar content just enough so that it's still tasty. (Hint: You can reduce the added sugar even more by swapping sugar for the healthy xylitol, a terrific sugar alcohol that has fewer calories and virtually no impact on blood sugar.) Three, replace the butter (or nearly all of it) with nut oil for its healthy fat content. Bingo—you've got a moist and cinn-nutty (not-so-bad-for-you) version of this perennial favorite. Include a protein (such as eggs over easy) and enjoy guiltlessly on a Sunday morning with the weekend papers.

Preheat the oven to 350°F (180°C, or gas mark 4). Lightly spray an 8 x 8-inch (20 x 20-cm) baking dish with oil and set aside.

In a large bowl, whisk together the flour, xylitol, baking powder, baking soda, and salt. In a medium bowl, whisk together the yogurt, milk, oil, and vanilla. In a small bowl, mix together the almonds, cinnamon, and sugar.

Work the butter into the flour mixture until combined and crumbly. Add the wet ingredients to the flour mixture and stir until just combined. Spoon into the prepared baking pan and top with the nut mixture in an even layer. Bake for about 35 minutes, or until a toothpick inserted into the center comes out clean.

Yield: 9 servings
Per Serving: 313.1 calories; 17.8 g fat (49% calories from fat); 5.7 g protein; 38.3 g carbohydrate; 2.2 g dietary fiber; 8.2 mg cholesterol; 200 mg sodium

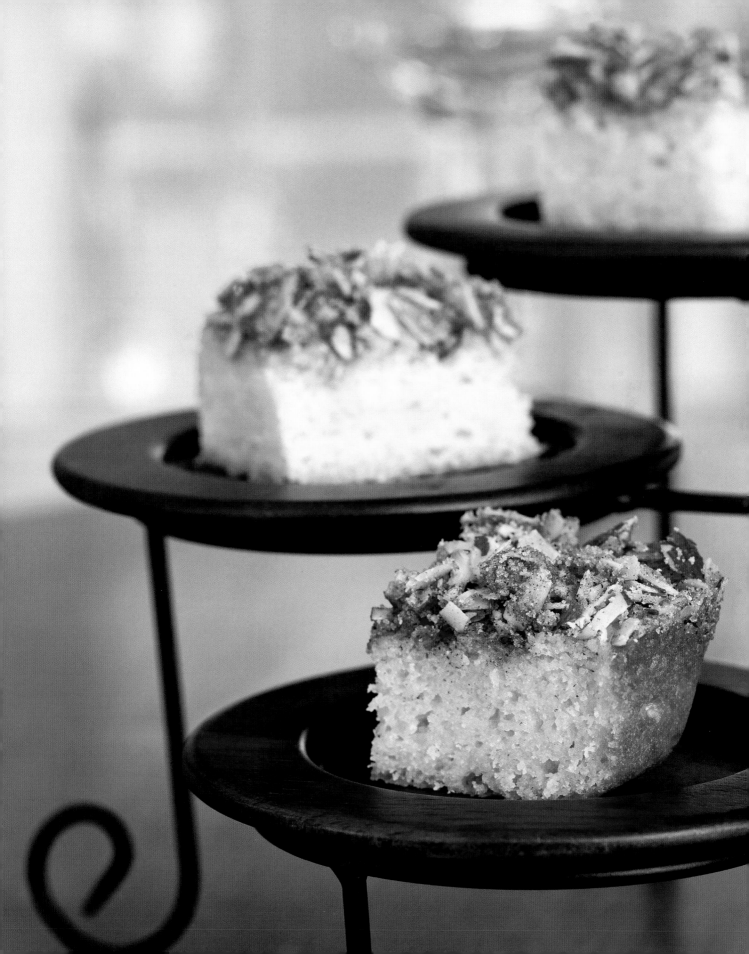

Delicious Low-Sugar Choco-Banana Smoothie

Ingredients

1½ cups (355 ml) milk (low-fat cow's, unsweetened chocolate almond, or soy milk)

½ cup (120 ml) light coconut milk (or omit and use 2 cups, or 475 ml, milk)

2½ tablespoons (35 g) raw cacao powder (or 1½ tablespoons, or 21 g, cocoa powder)

2 scoops unsweetened, undenatured whey protein powder

2 frozen bananas

2 to 4 ice cubes, optional

From Dr. Jonny: There are a lot of reasons why smoothies are so popular. For one thing, you can make them in a flash, so they fit nicely into today's busy lifestyle. For another, there is an endless variety of ways to make them. Then there's the fact that a lot of people just aren't hungry at breakfast, even though they know it's "the most important meal of the day." But even someone who can't stomach the thought of food in the morning can always manage to drink a smoothie. Now the question is, how do you make it delicious and nutritious? Easy. Lose all the extra sugar that you don't need, sweeten with bananas, and use one of the milks we suggest (instead of juice!) to up the protein and cut down on sugar even more. Raw cacao powder gives it a rich chocolate taste while adding valuable flavonols, which lower blood pressure. Enjoy!

In a powerful blender, add all the ingredients and blend until smooth. Use 2 to 4 ice cubes (or freeze the coconut milk in an ice cube tray) for a frostier milkshake consistency.

Yield: 2 smoothies

Per Serving: 376.4 calories; 10.3 g fat (23% calories from fat); 36.4 g protein; 49.1 g carbohydrate; 9.3 g dietary fiber; 14.6 mg cholesterol; 171.5 mg sodium

From Chef Jeannette

Even Healthier: For added fiber and omegas, add 2 tablespoons (10 g) whole rolled oats and 2 teaspoons (10 ml) high-lignin flaxseed oil with the rest of the ingredients.

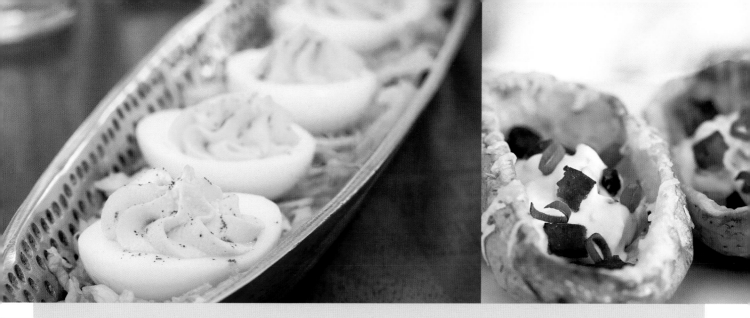

Appetizers, Snacks, and Drinks

Appetizers get your salivary juices going so you can better enjoy the meal to come. And you could make a whole meal out of a number of the following selections! But what about snacks? Many people find that they can keep their energy on an even keel by eating more frequently than three meals a day. That's where snacks and drinks come in. These won't break your daily caloric budget, but will keep you going through the day.

APPETIZERS
Lower-Cal Loaded Potato Skins

Creamy, Stuffed, Potassium-Packed Portobellos

Healthier, High-Quality Almond Cheese Puffs

Higher-Protein 2-Cheese Chicken Quesadilla with Cranberry

Best Broiled Buffalo Wings

Lean and Classic Game Night 3-Layer Mexi-Dip

Cheesy, Iron-Rich Spinach Squares

SNACKS/DRINKS
Warm and Soft Lower-Sodium Pretzels

Lower-Sugar Shrimp Cocktail with a Kick

Heart-Lovin' Spicy and Sweet Nuts

Better-for-You Cinnamon Applesauce

Fiberlicious Sweet 'n Smoky Baked Beans Dip

Heavenly Omega-Boosted Deviled Eggs

Calorie-Light Caramelized Onion Dip

All-Natural Spicy Salsa Guacamole

Lower-Cal Instant Tropical Frozen "Rice Cream"

Pure and Simple Spiced Cider

Fresh and Fruity Coconut Lime Mojito

Sweet and Spicy Antioxidant Hot Chocolate

Ingredients

4 russet potatoes

2 teaspoons (10 ml) olive oil

Salt and fresh-ground black pepper, to taste

3 tablespoons (15 g) shredded Parmesan cheese

4 strips nitrate-free turkey bacon

¼ cup (60 g) Greek yogurt

1 clove garlic, minced

¼ teaspoon salt

⅓ cup (33 g) sliced scallion

Lower-Cal Loaded Potato Skins

From Dr. Jonny: Did you ever wonder how and when potato skins first became popular as a comfort food? Glad you asked. It was in the days when we first figured out that a lot of the fiber—or as my grandmother used to call it, "roughage"—was found in the skins and that throwing them out was a big nutritional waste. Around that time folks also figured out that the white stuff inside wasn't all that great nutritionally, offering not much more than a bunch of calories and carbs. (As it turns out, potatoes do have some nutrients in them, but that's a whole other discussion.) So the era of the potato skin as a stand-alone side dish was born. The concept was good, but the execution . . . not so much. Gobs of dripping cheese and bacon with oil running down your fork as you spear a piece. And don't even ask about the calories! (But since you asked, a typical 12-ounce [340-g], eight-skin restaurant serving is estimated to be safely over 1,000 calories.) What to do? Simple. Dump the starchy innards and replace that mystery yellow "cheese food" with reasonable amounts of wholesome Parmesan cheese. Swap fatty pork bacon for low-cal turkey bacon. Try high-protein Greek yogurt instead of sour cream and presto, you've got a savory, delicious appetizer perfect for game night! (Just try not to eat twelve of them in one sitting!)

Preheat the oven to 400°F (200°C, or gas mark 6).

Scrub the potatoes well and slice them in half lengthwise. Using a melonballer or short paring knife and trying not to cut the skin, gently scoop or cut out the potato centers of each half, leaving about ¼ inch (6 mm) of potato on the hollowed-out skins. (For large potatoes, quarter them before removing the flesh. Use the flesh for another recipe, such as our Creamy Low-Fat Mashed Potatoes, page 122, or discard.) Add the skins to a large bowl, drizzle with the olive oil, and toss gently to coat all the surfaces, inside and out. Sprinkle to taste with salt and pepper, toss again, and arrange faceup on a baking sheet. Sprinkle just over 1 teaspoon of Parmesan cheese evenly into each half and bake for about 25 minutes, or until tender and lightly browned.

While the potatoes cook, fry the turkey bacon in a dry skillet over medium heat for 8 to 10 minutes, or until very crispy. Set aside to drain on paper towels.

In a small bowl, mix together the yogurt, garlic, and salt until well combined. Fold in the scallion. Remove the potatoes from the oven, crumble ½ bacon strip into each potato half, and top with a generous dollop of the yogurt mixture just before serving.

Yield: 8 servings

Per Serving: 112.7 calories; 3.2 g fat (26% calories from fat); 4.2 g protein; 17.2 g carbohydrate; 2.1 g dietary fiber; 8.3 mg cholesterol; 205 mg sodium

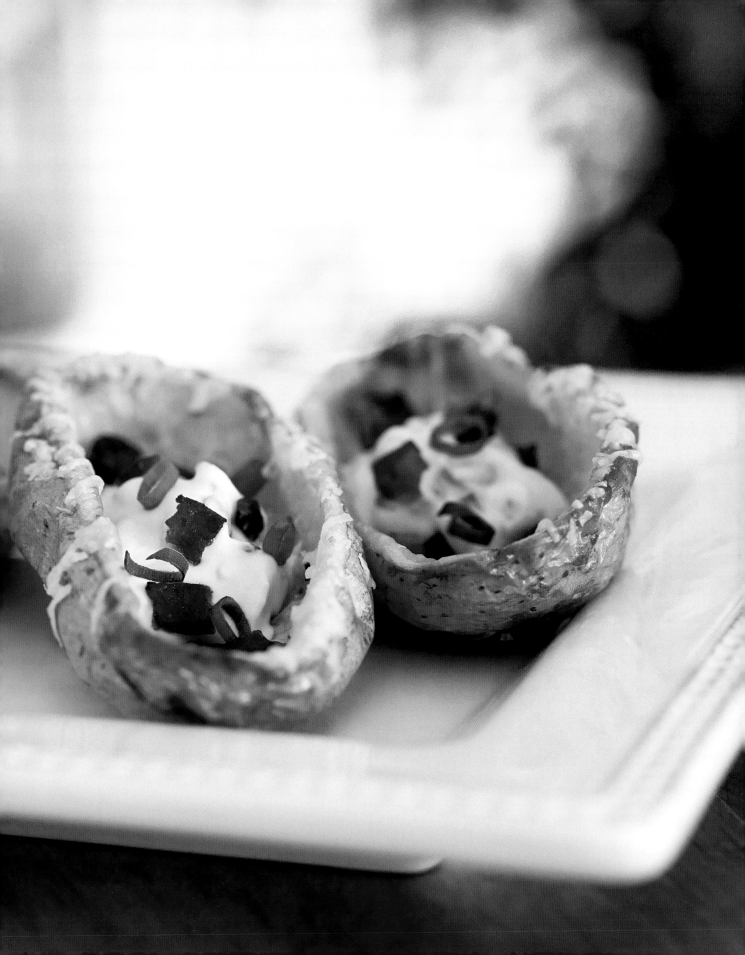

Creamy, Stuffed, Potassium-Packed Portobellos

Ingredients

4 portobello mushrooms, cleaned

1 tablespoon (15 ml) olive oil, divided

1 teaspoon butter

1 small onion, finely chopped

4 cloves garlic, minced

2 tablespoons (28 ml) dry sherry

Olive oil cooking spray

4 ounces (115 g) Neufchâtel cheese

1/4 teaspoon each salt and fresh-ground black pepper

2 tablespoons (10 g) fresh-grated Parmesan cheese

From Dr. Jonny: Here are a few things I'll bet you didn't know about portobello mushrooms. One, they're pretty high in protein (about 5 grams per cup of diced mushrooms). Two, they're ridiculously high in potassium (more than 300 mg for the same amount). Three, they contain all kinds of exotic compounds (like beta-glucans) that exhibit anticancer properties. So portobellos make a great snack and are pretty irresistible when you combine them with cheese stuffing. Neufchâtel is the perfect choice; it tastes great and has protein, calcium, potassium, and vitamin A. Both onions and garlic are vegetable superstars from the allium family, which contain beneficial compounds that support cardiovascular health. Since the bulk of the volume from this dish comes from the low-cal portobellos, you don't have to worry about the small amount of butter and olive oil.

Preheat the oven to 425°F (220°C, or gas mark 7).

Grasp the stem of each mushroom close to the cap and gently twist the cap away until the stem comes off (or slice the stems off). Reserve the stems. Using a sharp knife, lightly score the skin on the cap side of each of the portobello caps in a tic-tac-toe pattern (this will help the mushrooms release some of their juices while roasting). Drizzle 1 teaspoon of the olive oil over the 4 scored caps and place on the broiling rack, gill sides up. Roast for 12 minutes and set aside.

Lower the oven temperature to 375°F (190°C, or gas mark 5).

While the mushrooms are roasting, trim any tough ends off of the reserved mushroom stems and finely chop them.

Heat the remaining 2 teaspoons (10 ml) of the olive oil plus the butter in a large skillet over medium heat. Add the onion and mushroom stems and cook, stirring occasionally, for 7 to 8 minutes, or until the mushrooms have released their liquid and the vegetables are soft. Add the garlic and cook for 1 minute. Add the sherry and cook, stirring frequently, until all the liquid has evaporated, 2 to 3 minutes. Remove from the heat and allow the mixture to cool to warm, not hot.

Lightly spray a baking sheet with olive oil and place the 4 roasted mushroom caps on it, gill sides up.

Stir the Neufchâtel, salt, and pepper into the mushroom stems and onion mixture and mix gently until well combined. Spoon equal portions of the mixture into the 4 mushroom caps. Sprinkle with the Parmesan and bake for about 10 to 15 minutes, or until hot throughout.

Yield: 4 caps (serves 4 to 8)

Per Serving: 86.5 calories; 6 g fat (61% calories from fat); 3.3 g protein; 4.8 g carbohydrate; 0.9 g dietary fiber; 13.3 mg cholesterol; 150.3 mg sodium

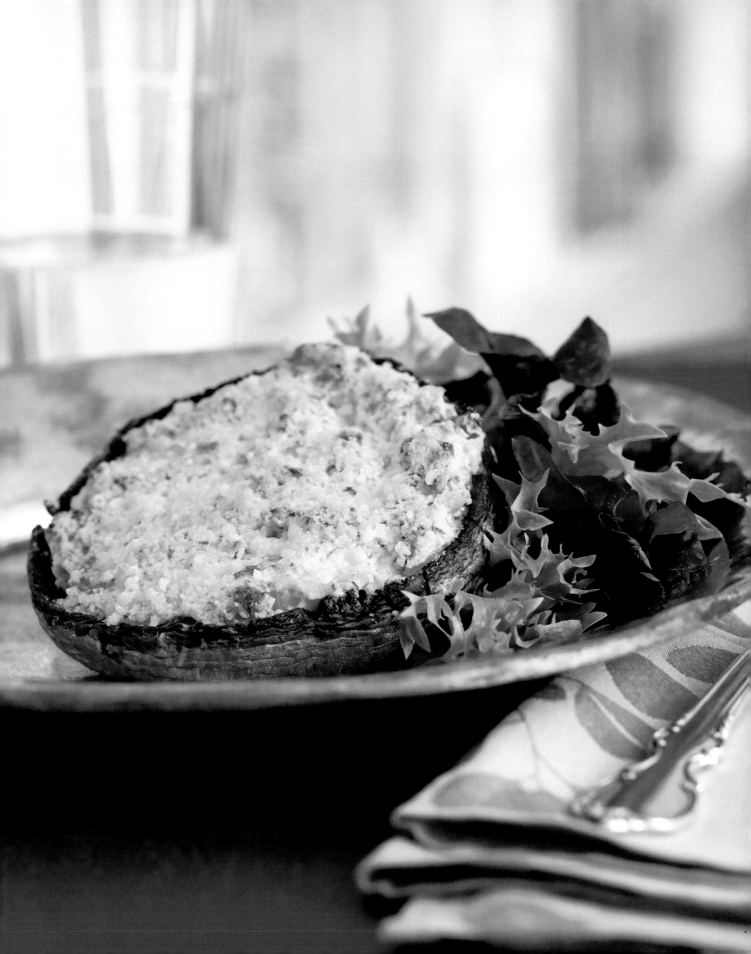

Healthier, High-Quality Almond Cheese Puffs

Ingredients

3 tablespoons (45 g) butter, at room temperature

¾ cup (90 g) grated Cheddar cheese

¼ cup (38 g) feta cheese

½ cup (63 g) whole-wheat pastry flour

¼ teaspoon salt

4 dashes hot sauce, or more to taste

12 whole roasted unsalted almonds

From Dr. Jonny: You can't turn cheese puffs into a health food. No can do. But you can make them better! Switching to whole-wheat flour adds a bit of fiber and makes them denser and heavier, more like a rich mini-biscuit. Use the highest quality cheese you can get your hands on (more on that in a moment). Keep the butter organic and add an almond for some extra minerals and good fat. I know, I know—these babies can break the caloric bank, but hey, you've got to have an indulgence once in a while, right? Make them with high-quality ingredients and don't overindulge and you've got a great, once-in-a-blue-moon treat. As for cheese, remember that even though it's high in calories, it is quite nutritious. Cheddar has a ton of calcium and vitamin A and a fair amount of protein, and if you get organic it's even better! The feta is lower in total calories than Cheddar, and gives a nice little protein boost and pleasing tang.

Preheat the oven to 425°F (220°C, or gas mark 7).

Combine the butter, cheeses, flour, salt, and hot sauce in a food processor and process just until the mixture forms a dough (it will begin to hold together), less than 1 minute. Pinch off 12 sections of the dough and wrap each around 1 almond to form twelve 1¼-inch (3.2-cm) balls. Arrange on a baking sheet and cook for 8 to 9 minutes, or until lightly browned.

Yield: 12 cheese puffs

Per Serving: 91.7 calories; 6.9 g fat (66% calories from fat); 3.2 g protein; 4.5 g carbohydrate; 0.3 g dietary fiber; 18.8 mg cholesterol; 154.7 mg sodium

Ingredients

1 teaspoon olive oil

4 packed cups (120 g) baby arugula or spinach

2 teaspoons (10 ml) balsamic vinegar

3 tablespoons (about 1 ounce, or 28 g) chèvre (soft goat cheese)

3 tablespoons (48 g) part-skim ricotta cheese

3 tablespoons (60 g) juice-sweetened prepared cranberry sauce (such as R. W. Knudsen), divided

1 cup (225 g) shredded cooked chicken or turkey breast

Two 10-inch (25-cm) whole-grain wraps

Higher-Protein 2-Cheese Chicken Quesadilla with Cranberry

From Dr. Jonny: Mexican food was a complete mystery to me when I first arrived in Southern California. Tacos, tostados, quesadillas, burritos—I was about as equipped to tell you the difference among them as I was to translate Plato from the original Greek. But I've come to love and enjoy Mexican food, and I especially appreciate the healthier versions of these dishes that Chef Jeannette has consistently devised. And now for my newfound knowledge: Quesadillas are a versatile dish because you can fill them with almost anything. But most of the restaurant versions use white flour tortillas dripping with some kind of imitation cheese food, which has an awful lot more orange and yellow in it than any "natural food" (if you get my drift). We made a lighter, lower-cal version with real food: a combo of high-protein ricotta and goat cheeses, a sweet splash from cranberries, and lots of chicken to boost the protein. Fun fact: Goats were among the first domesticated animals, and the art of making goat cheese has been around for thousands of years. It actually began in the Eastern Mediterranean where goat cheese to this day remains a staple of the Mediterranean diet.

Heat the oil in a large sauté pan over medium heat. Add the arugula, sprinkle with the vinegar, and cover for 1 minute to quickly wilt. Remove the lid and stir, cooking down until the greens are soft and the liquids have released. Transfer the cooked greens to a double-mesh sieve to drain well, pressing lightly to remove excess liquids.

In a small bowl, mix the goat cheese, ricotta cheese, and 1 tablespoon (20 g) of the cranberry sauce until well blended.

In a small bowl, mix the chicken and remaining 2 tablespoons (40 g) cranberry sauce until well mixed.

In a large sauté pan, dry toast 1 wrap over medium heat until lightly toasted. Flip and quickly spread half the cheese mixture, half the chicken, and half the drained greens over half the quesadilla. Fold the other half over the top and press to seal. Cook, flipping once, until hot throughout. Set aside in a warm toaster oven and repeat with the remaining ingredients. Cut each quesadilla into quarters and serve hot.

Yield: 4 servings

Per Serving: 193 calories; 6.7 g fat (31% calories from fat); 22.6 g protein; 10.2 g carbohydrate; 2.1 g dietary fiber; 56.6 mg cholesterol; 108.9 mg sodium

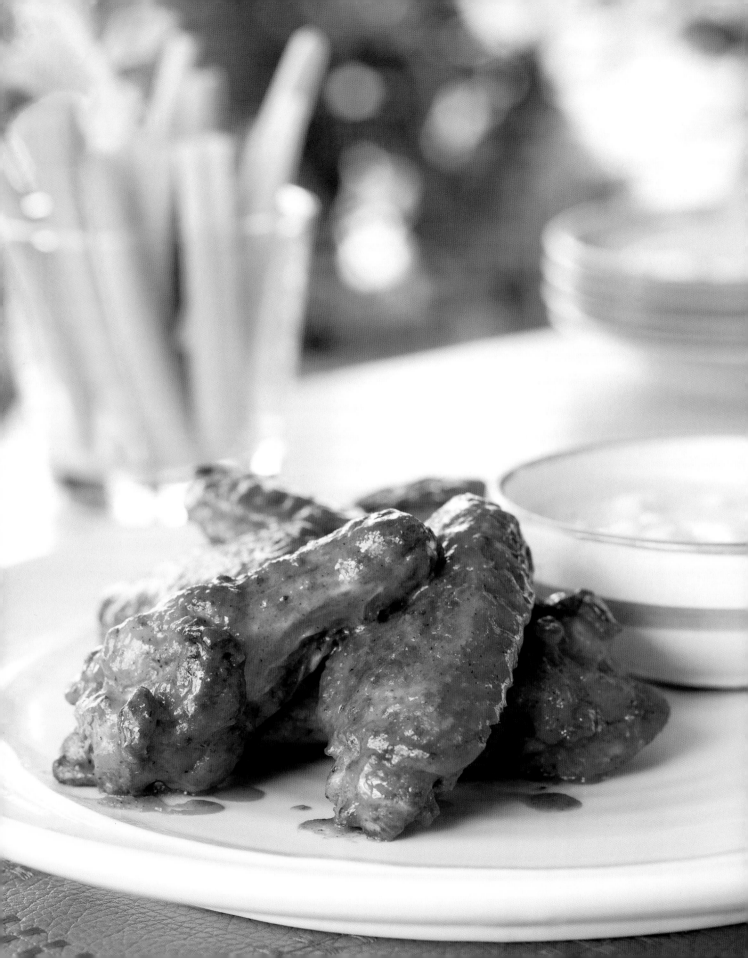

Ingredients

2 pounds (905 g) chicken wings (about 12),
   cut and prepared as directed (see below)

Salt, fresh-ground black pepper, and
   cayenne pepper, to taste

3 tablespoons (45 g) butter

¼ cup (60 ml) high-quality hot sauce (such
   as Benito's Old Bricktucky or Frank's
   RedHot Original Cayenne Pepper)

2 teaspoons (5 g) sweet paprika

¼ teaspoon each salt and fresh-ground
   black pepper

½ cup (120 ml) high-quality blue cheese
   dressing, optional

1 to 2 cups (150 to 300 g) sliced celery
   sticks

1 to 2 cups baby carrots

From Chef Jeannette

Basic Wing Prep: Choose wing cuts from high-quality, pasture-raised chickens for the best nutrition and flavor. A full wing has three different parts to it, each section separated by a joint. To prepare wings, snip off the bony tip and discard, and snip or cut the other two pieces at the other joint. You will be left with an upper wing section that looks like a tiny drumstick (it's sometimes called a drumette) and a middle section with two thin bones that is what we classically refer to as the wing in this comfort food dish. So for each full wing, you should end up with two smaller pieces to work with in the recipes. Some people prefer the wing cut, and some prefer the drumette cut, but for the purposes of these recipes, they are interchangeable.

Best Broiled Buffalo Wings

From Dr. Jonny: If a dish shows up in just about every restaurant in America, it's got to be classified as a comfort food. Ergo, chicken wings are a comfort food—big time. But how do you make a fried food healthier? Especially one that is traditionally made with way too much salt and poor-quality meat? Simple. Use higher-quality chicken (i.e., free-range with no added hormones) and you're already way ahead of the game. Then marinate, which accomplishes two things, both of which are important. Number one, it replaces the heavy flour and breading typical of a wing dish. And number two, several studies have now shown that marinating meat slashes levels of cancer-causing compounds. These compounds, called heterocyclic amines, are particularly high in fried meats (or meats grilled at very high temperatures). Plus the marinade tastes delicious and certainly better than a bunch of flour and bread! Finally, grill, broil, or bake (as we did with these dishes), all of which offer a profound improvement on deep-frying. All three delicious versions of this wildly popular dish will tickle your taste buds but with far less sugar, salt, and unnecessary calories.

Preheat the oven to broil.

Sprinkle the chicken pieces with the salt and peppers (remember, a little cayenne goes a long way!). Arrange on a broiler sheet and broil for 8 to 10 minutes per side, or until cooked through and golden.

While the wings are broiling, in a small pan over medium heat, mix together the butter, hot sauce, paprika, salt, and pepper. When the butter has melted, whisk the sauce until well combined. Toss the hot wings with the sauce, to taste, and serve with the dressing and celery and carrot sticks.

Yield: 4 to 6 servings

Per Serving: 658.4 calories; 50.6 g fat (69% calories from fat); 41 g protein; 8.5 g carbohydrate; 1.5 g dietary fiber; 141.8 mg cholesterol; 726.8 mg sodium

Ingredients

3 tablespoons (45 ml) sesame oil

3 tablespoons (45 ml) low-sodium tamari
 (or low-sodium soy sauce)

3 tablespoons (45 ml) fresh-squeezed lime
 juice

4 cloves garlic, minced

2 pounds (905 g) chicken wings (about 12),
 cut and prepared as directed (see page
 215)

⅓ cup (92 g) Thai sweet chili sauce

2 tablespoons (28 ml) unseasoned brown
 rice vinegar

¼ cup (60 ml) low-sodium chicken broth (or
 water)

1 teaspoon sugar or xylitol

2 teaspoons (4 g) minced fresh ginger

2 teaspoons (5.4 g) kudzu plus 1 tablespoon
 (15 ml) cold chicken broth or water
 (or 1½ teaspoons, or 4 g, cornstarch
 and simmer a little longer to cook off
 starchy flavor)

¼ cup (25 g) sliced scallion

¼ cup (4 g) chopped fresh cilantro

Sweet and Sassy Thai-Glazed Baked Wings

In a glass storage container, whisk together the oil, tamari, lime juice, and garlic. Place the prepared wings in the container and toss gently to coat. Marinate the wings in the refrigerator for 1 hour to overnight, turning occasionally to recoat (the longer the marinating time, the stronger the flavor).

Preheat the oven to 350°F (180°C, or gas mark 4).

Remove the chicken from the marinade and arrange on a baking sheet. Bake for about 30 minutes, or until cooked through.

While the chicken is cooking, in a small pan over medium-high heat, whisk together the chili sauce, vinegar, broth, sugar, and ginger, and bring to a boil. Dissolve the kudzu in the broth or water and add to the boiling sauce. Boil for 1 to 2 minutes, or until thickened. Remove from the heat and cool slightly. Stir in the scallion and cilantro and glaze the cooked wings to taste just before serving.

Yield: about 6 servings

Per Serving: 598.5 calories; 40.4 g fat (61% calories from fat); 40.9 g protein; 13.8 g carbohydrate; 0.4 g dietary fiber; 122.2 mg cholesterol; 620.6 mg sodium

Ingredients

1 tablespoon (7 g) smoked paprika (or
    Hungarian hot paprika for fiery wings)

1 teaspoon Sucanat or brown sugar

1/2 teaspoon onion powder

1/2 teaspoon garlic powder

1/2 teaspoon dry mustard

1/2 teaspoon each salt and fresh-ground
    black pepper

1/4 teaspoon cayenne pepper

2 pounds (905 g) chicken wings (about 12),
    cut and prepared as directed (see page
    215)

3 tablespoons (45 ml) low-sodium tamari
    (or low-sodium soy sauce)

2 tablespoons (28 ml) dark rum

1 1/2 tablespoons (30 g) blackstrap molasses

Clean and Lean Smoky Blackstrap Rum Grilled Wings

Preheat the grill to medium-low.

In a small bowl, combine the paprika, Sucanat, onion powder, garlic powder, dry mustard, salt, and peppers and mix well. Sprinkle evenly over the wings to coat. Grill for about 15 minutes, or until cooked through, turning halfway through the cooking time. If the wings are blackening too fast, reduce the heat to low.

While the chicken is grilling, in a small pan over medium-high heat, whisk together the tamari, rum, and molasses and bring to a low boil. Reduce the heat and simmer for 2 minutes, stirring frequently to prevent a boilover. Baste the chicken with the rum mixture 7 minutes into grill time and again just before removing from the heat.

Yield: 4 to 6 servings

Per Serving: 522.3 calories; 33.6 g fat (58% calories from fat); 40.7 g protein; 9 g carbohydrate; 0.7 g dietary fiber; 122.2 mg cholesterol; 668.5 mg sodium

Ingredients

1¼ pounds (565 g) leanest ground beef

1 small yellow onion, chopped

1 packet (1 ounce, or 28 g) high-quality taco seasoning (we like Simply Organic Southwest Taco Seasoning)

1 can (14 ounces, or 400 g) high-quality nonfat vegetarian refried beans (or use our bean recipe for Smoky Bean Baked Nachos, page 100)

16 ounces (455 g) plain low-fat Greek yogurt

1 jar (16 ounces, or 455 g) high-quality prepared salsa

1¼ cups (145 g) shredded jack or high-quality Mexi-cheese combination

Lean and Classic Game Night 3-Layer Mexi-Dip

From Dr. Jonny: Mexi-dips, as Chef Jeannette likes to call them, are one of these categories like "carbs" or "movies." They range from the really good to the really, really bad. (You've got "Mexi-dips" that are the equivalent of *Citizen Kane* and "Mexi-dips" that are the equivalent of *Revenge of the Man-Eating Worms from Mars*.) Our version uses high-quality prepared ingredients for both speed and ease of preparation (after all, who wants to spend Super Bowl Sunday slaving in the kitchen?). We kept the dish lean and healthy and with a couple of simple strategic updates: grass-fed beef and vegetarian nonfat refried beans. (If grass-fed isn't an option, go for the 96 percent lean organic meat.) We made it more calorie-friendly by substituting Greek yogurt for sour cream (boosting the protein in the dish at the same time) and we used a lot less cheese. If you absolutely insist on chips instead of veggies (I know, you're rolling your eyes, but I had to say it), at least use whole-grain baked corn chips. (And for the few of you who don't insist on chips, enjoy this great dip on sticks of carrots, celery, and slices of cuke.)

Preheat the oven to 375°F (190°C, or gas mark 5).

Add the beef to a large skillet over medium heat and break it up. Add the onion and stir to combine. Cook the beef and onion for 4 minutes and then stir in the taco seasoning until well combined. Cook for 3 to 4 minutes more, or until the beef is cooked through and the onions are softened. Remove from the heat, drain any excess fat, stir in the refried beans, and mix gently until well combined.

In a medium bowl, mix together the Greek yogurt and salsa until well combined.

Spoon the meat-bean mixture into an 8 x 8-inch (20 x 20-cm) baking dish and pat it so it's smooth on the top. Spoon the yogurt-salsa mixture on top and smooth the surface for an even layer. Sprinkle the cheese evenly across the top and bake for 20 to 25 minutes, or until hot throughout and the cheese is melted.

Yield: 9 to 12 servings

Per Serving: 182.8 calories; 7 g fat (34% calories from fat); 17.6 g protein; 12.2 g carbohydrate; 2.6 g dietary fiber; 42.3 mg cholesterol; 661.6 mg sodium

Ingredients

3 tablespoons (45 g) butter, cut into
    4 pieces
1 cup (235 ml) milk (low-fat cow's, unsweet-
    ened almond, or soy)
3 eggs
4 to 8 dashes hot sauce, to taste
1 cup (125 g) whole-wheat pastry flour
½ teaspoon salt
1 teaspoon baking powder
2 packages (each 10 ounces, or 280 g)
    frozen chopped spinach, thawed and
    well drained (squeeze or press into a
    double-mesh sieve to remove excess
    moisture)
2 cups (8 ounces, or 225 g) grated sharp
    Cheddar cheese

Cheesy, Iron-Rich Spinach Squares

From Dr. Jonny: When Chef Jeannette first sent me this recipe I have to admit I didn't know what a spinach square was. (I thought she was talking about spinach pies!) But spinach squares are prevalent in many parts of the United States, such as the South, and they are typically made with flour and Cheddar cheese (unlike their spinach pie cousins, which are made with phyllo dough and feta cheese). Chef Jeannette took this classical regional spinach-based dish (the squares, not the pies) and cut back the calories from the extra butter and cheese. She also upgraded the flour from white to whole-wheat (or whole-grain) flour for additional nutrients and fiber. The eggs and milk add protein, as does the Cheddar cheese, which is also a great source of calcium. And they're as tasty as can be!

Preheat the oven to 375°F (190°C, or gas mark 5). Place the butter in a 9 x 13-inch (23 x 33-cm) pan and place the pan in the oven to melt the butter. Remove and set aside.

While the butter is heating, in a mixer beat the milk, eggs, and hot sauce, to taste, together until well combined.

In a small bowl, whisk together the flour, salt, and baking powder. Add the dry mix to the wet mix and beat until well combined. Add the spinach and beat briefly on low. Add the cheese and beat again briefly on low until incorporated. Spoon the batter into the pan and spread in an even layer. Bake for about 30 minutes, or until the edges and parts of the top are beginning to brown. Cool and cut into squares.

Yield: 15 squares
Per Serving: 147.9 calories; 9 g fat (54% calories from fat); 8 g protein; 9.5 g carbohydrate; 1.4 g dietary fiber; 65.8 mg cholesterol; 367 mg sodium

Warm and Soft Lower-Sodium Pretzels

Ingredients

3/4 cup (175 ml) water

1/2 cup (120 ml) plus 1 tablespoon (15 ml) low-fat cow's milk, divided

1 package (9 g) quick-rising yeast

2 tablespoons (28 ml) olive oil

2 tablespoons (26 g) Sucanat or brown sugar

1/2 teaspoon salt

2 cups (250 g) unbleached flour

1/3 cup (35 g) ground flaxseed

About 1 cup (125 g) whole-wheat pastry flour

Olive oil cooking spray

1 egg

Topping Options

Kosher salt, to taste

Garlic salt, to taste

Fresh-grated Parmesan cheese, to taste

From Dr. Jonny: When I was a kid in New York City, one of my favorite things to buy from street vendors was pretzels. Now they sell them at every movie refreshment stand. And while movie (or New York) pretzels might not be the worst snack ever invented, they're definitely in the top ten! Your basic movie pretzel has 483 calories, 4.5 grams of fat, and 2,008 mg of sodium (the recommended daily allowance of sodium is 2,500 mg). Add the cheese sauce, which usually comes with movie pretzels, and you're adding on another 200 calories and 10 grams of fat. Wow. But we do love our pretzels, so here's a way to make it work and still keep that warm, dense, satisfying texture and comforting, chewy taste: Use part whole-wheat pastry flour for extra fiber and add flaxseeds for healthy plant compounds called lignans (and extra fiber to boot). Use a light hand with the salt, which significantly cuts down on the sodium, and choose olive oil for a healthy fat. You'll never miss the bad stuff.

In a small pan, combine the water and 1/2 cup (120 ml) of the milk and heat over medium heat until very warm, but not steaming hot. Pour the mixture into a large bowl and stir in the yeast, oil, Sucanat, and salt, stirring until mostly dissolved. Add the flour (unbleached only, not the whole-wheat) and flaxseed and stir to combine well. Add the whole-wheat pastry flour, about 1/3 cup (42 g) at a time, stirring in between until it forms a dough (you may not need the full cup, or you may need a little more than a cup).

Turn out the dough onto a lightly floured surface and knead well for about 3 minutes, until very smooth and elastic. Return to the mixing bowl, cover with plastic, and let rest in a warm place for about 15 minutes.

Preheat the oven to 350°F (180°C, or gas mark 4) and spray 2 baking sheets with olive oil. Set aside.

From Chef Jeannette

Homemade bread products such as pretzels are nearly always significantly higher quality than anything you would buy in a store or at a stand. But because they are primarily a flour product (even with our healthy tweaks!), it's helpful to balance that carbohydrate load with the addition of one of the "time release" nutrients such as healthy fat or protein. Our version has already included a small amount of fat and fiber (another time release nutrient), so to boost the effects even further, enjoy your soft pretzel in place of the bread for lunch with a 3 to 4 ounce serving of lunch meat, such as lean and clean roast beef or sliced chicken breast. Or lay a slice of organic cheese over the top. If you do that as they come right out of the oven the cheese will melt and create a delectable hot, cheesy pretzel.

To make the classic German pretzel shape, pull off a chunk of dough about the size of a table tennis ball, and roll into a long tube (about 15 inches, or 38 cm) about the width of a thumb. Form the tube into a U shape, then cross and twist the tube ends about 3 inches (7.5 cm) from the top. Pick up the whole crossed section and flip it over, downward, so the ends of the tubes meet the bottom of the U. It should be recognizable as a pretzel now. Press the tips firmly into the lower curve so they will stay in place, and adjust the shape to your liking.

Place it on the prepared baking sheet and repeat until the dough is used up.

In a small bowl, whisk the egg and the remaining 1 tablespoon (15 ml) of milk together, and brush thoroughly over all the pretzels. Let them sit on the baking sheets for another 10 minutes to rise again.

Bake for 15 minutes and remove to brush again with the egg and milk. Sprinkle lightly with any of the suggested toppings, and return to bake for about 10 more minutes, or until they are nicely golden brown. Remove from the oven and let rest for 5 minutes.

Using a spatula, carefully remove to wire racks and let cool to desired temperature.

Yield: about 12 pretzels
Per Serving: 166.6 calories; 4.3 g fat (23% calories from fat); 5 g protein; 26.7 g carbohydrate; 1.9 g dietary fiber; 18.6 mg cholesterol; 105.4 mg sodium

Lower-Sugar Shrimp Cocktail with a Kick

Ingredients

²/₃ cup (160 g) low-sugar organic ketchup
    (to avoid high-fructose corn syrup)
2 to 3 tablespoons (30 to 45 g) prepared
    horseradish, to taste
1¹/₂ tablespoons (25 ml) organic
    Worcestershire sauce (to avoid
    high-fructose corn syrup)
2 tablespoons (28 ml) apple cider vinegar
2 tablespoons (26 g) Sucanat
2 teaspoons (10 g) Dijon mustard
¹/₂ to ³/₄ teaspoon red pepper flakes,
    optional, to taste
¹/₄ teaspoon salt
12 shelled and cooked frozen extra-large
    shrimp

From Dr. Jonny: One thing I learned when I was writing extensively about controlled carbohydrate diets was that there's sugar hiding in everything—salad dressings, breads, cereals, and sauces. So even something that looks perfectly innocent and healthy—like shrimp cocktail—frequently contains a ton of hidden sugar (or high-fructose corn syrup). Our version is still sweet, but with less sugar, and it doesn't lose a drop of tanginess. It's the perfect complement to fresh, cold shrimp. Important tip: The horseradish does a lot more than just add flavor. It's actually a medicinal food that has antimicrobial properties, and it contains glucosinolates, plant compounds that—according to research from the University of Illinois—may increase human resistance to cancer.

Combine the ketchup, horseradish, Worcestershire, vinegar, Sucanat, mustard, red pepper flakes, and salt in a small saucepan over medium heat and whisk to combine well. Bring to a simmer, reduce the heat to low, and cook for 10 minutes, stirring occasionally. Remove from the pan and chill in the refrigerator to desired temperature. When you are ready to serve the cocktail, run the frozen shrimp under cold water until just thawed and drain well. They should be very cold. Divide the cocktail sauce evenly into 4 small bowls, hook the tops of 3 shrimp over the sides of each bowl, and serve immediately.

Yield: 4 servings
Per Serving: 110 calories; 1.2 g fat (9% calories from fat); 17.2 g protein; 7.1 g carbohydrate; 0.3 g dietary fiber; 165 mg cholesterol; 1,093.6 mg sodium

Ingredients

2 cups (290 g) raw, unsalted nuts
  (try cashews, almonds, walnuts, pecans,
  or a combination)

1½ tablespoons (21 g) butter

2½ tablespoons (33 g) Sucanat (or brown
  sugar)

1½ tablespoons (25 ml) apple juice
  (or water)

About 1 teaspoon spices of your choice
  (see combo ideas)

¼ teaspoon salt

SPICE COMBO IDEAS
Curried Spice

½ teaspoon curry powder

¼ teaspoon chipotle chili powder
  (or cayenne pepper)

⅛ teaspoon allspice

Cinnamon Spice

½ teaspoon cinnamon

¼ teaspoon allspice

⅛ teaspoon ground cloves

Chocolate Spice

(use water, not juice for this combo)

1½ teaspoons (4 g) high-quality cocoa
  powder

¼ teaspoon cayenne pepper, optional

From Chef Jeannette

Time-Saver Tip: If you're in a hurry, use roasted (unsalted) nuts and skip the dry-toasting step—just add them to the spice glaze when it's hot.

Heart-Lovin' Spicy and Sweet Nuts

From Dr. Jonny: The fact that nuts are a health food is no longer in doubt. Several studies have found that eating about 5 ounces (140 g) a week reduces the risk of heart disease—by double digits! Penny Kris-Etherton, Ph.D., a distinguished professor of nutrition and lead author of a major study on nut consumption, says, "To date, five large epidemiologic studies and eleven clinical studies have demonstrated that frequent consumption of nuts decreases the risk of coronary heart disease." In addition to all kinds of healthy fats, fiber, and minerals, nuts also contain L-arginine, an amino acid that may help improve the health of your artery walls by making them more flexible and less prone to blood clots that can block blood flow. Nuts are just plain delicious, spiced nuts even more so. But spiced nuts are typically candy-coated, not to mention drowning in salt. Our versions use a combination of pungent and sweet spices to deliver on that "happy food" quality you're looking for. There's just enough sugar and butter to caramelize the whole shebang, and as long as you keep the portions small (about 1 ounce, or 28 g, at a time) you're good to go! It satisfies just like candy but gives you all the heart-healthy properties of nuts. What's not to like?

Add the nuts to a large, dry skillet over medium heat. Toast, stirring frequently, for 4 to 5 minutes, until they begin to brown and release their oils (they will become very aromatic). Pour them into a bowl and set aside.

Return the pan to the heat and add the butter, Sucanat, juice, and spices of your choice, and cook, whisking quickly to combine and prevent sticking, for about 1 minute or until the mixture caramelizes. Add the nuts to the pan and stir well, cooking for 1 or 2 more minutes, until they are evenly coated. Spread on a nonstick baking sheet in a single layer to cool. Once cool, break them up and store in the refrigerator.

Yield: 2 cups (290 g) nuts (serving size: 2 tablespoons, or 28 g)
Per Serving: 115.1 calories; 9 g fat (66% calories from fat); 3.3 g protein; 6.9 g carbohydrate; 0.7 g dietary fiber; 2.8 mg cholesterol; 4 mg sodium

Ingredients

4 fresh, sweet, cooking apples (Golden Delicious and Jonagold work well), peeled, cored, and chopped

2 tablespoons (28 ml) apple cider or water

1 tablespoon (15 ml) fresh-squeezed lemon juice

1 tablespoon (13 g) sugar, Sucanat, honey, or xylitol, optional, to taste

1½ teaspoons (4 g) ground cinnamon

From Chef Jeannette

Even Healthier: For more fiber and nutrients, leave the skins on the apples when you cook them. This will save you peeling time, but may add a minute or two on to the cooking time.

Time-Saver Tip: Omit the cooking altogether and break down the apple fibers in the freezer. Peel, core, and thickly slice the apples (I use a corer slicer tool for this), combine with the lemon juice and cinnamon only, and freeze in an airtight resealable plastic freezer bag for 6 hours to overnight. Thaw for 1 hour to overnight in the refrigerator and mash with a potato masher or immersion blender and serve.

Better-for-You Cinnamon Applesauce

From Dr. Jonny: How many people have eaten applesauce? That would be . . . let's see . . . everyone reading this book. But how many of you have tasted real applesauce, not the kind that comes in a jar, but the kind you make? Probably not as many. Well, get ready to taste what applesauce is supposed to taste like. Unlike the commercial kind, our version's not heavily sweetened with sugar, high-fructose corn syrup, or—the latest marketing ploy—"corn sugar." Our version has far less sweetener because it doesn't need it—it's got real apple taste. Choose fresh-picked apples at the height of their season to get the richest nutrient content. Remember, apples are one of the best sources of quercetin, a cancer-fighting, anti-inflammatory plant chemical from the flavonoid family. Note: If you happen to be selling your house, this is the perfect dish to have on the stove while buyers come to look around. The cinnamon gives the dish a wonderful, house-filling aroma that makes everyone within smelling distance feel good!

Place the apples, cider, lemon juice, and sweetener into a medium saucepan over medium heat and cover to bring to a simmer. When the apples are simmering, sprinkle in the cinnamon and mix well to combine. Reduce the heat to medium-low, cover, and cook, stirring periodically, until the apples have softened and broken down, usually 8 to 12 minutes depending on the type of apple. If the pan liquid evaporates before the apples have released their juices, add a little more cider to keep the mixture moist (different types of apples have different moisture contents). Stir well or use an immersion blender to obtain the desired consistency and serve warm, at room temperature, or chilled.

Yield: 4 servings

Per Serving: 91.2 calories; 0.3 g fat (<1% calories from fat); 0.4 g protein; 24.3 g carbohydrate; 3.9 g dietary fiber; 0 mg cholesterol; 1.7 mg sodium

Fiberlicious Sweet 'n Smoky Baked Beans Dip

Ingredients

1 can (15 ounces, or 425 g) low-sugar, vegetarian baked beans

1 tablespoon (15 ml) olive oil

½ small sweet onion, finely chopped

2 cloves garlic, crushed and chopped

¾ teaspoon chili powder

¼ teaspoon cumin powder

⅛ teaspoon chipotle chile pepper (or cayenne)

2 teaspoons (10.5 g) tomato paste

1 teaspoon raw apple cider vinegar

¼ teaspoon salt

4 drops liquid smoke, or to taste

From Dr. Jonny: This delicious bean dip is easy to make and a real crowd-pleaser. We've moved it a couple of notches up on the "healthy" scale by simply draining most of that sweet sauce that usually comes with conventional versions. That removes a lot of the total sugar and cuts the calories considerably, but does absolutely nothing to the flavor. Seriously! You can serve this dip with chips, if you like, but use the baked kind. Better still, serve it with vegetable crudités such as carrot and celery sticks. (You'd be surprised how well it works that way—you get all the crunchiness that comes with chips, but none of the bad stuff and a lot of vitamins and antioxidants to boot!) We use vegetarian beans because honestly, we just can't stand the way pigs are raised and farmed in the United States, and if we can avoid pork products, we'll do it. There's no loss of flavor, plus you save on the calories! And when it comes to fiber, no food beats beans. One cup (256 g) of almost any kind of beans in the world delivers between 11 and 17 grams of the stuff, dwarfing the fiber imposters, including bread (1 to 2 grams) and cereals (2 to 3 grams on average, unless you're talking about a really high-fiber cereal). Considering most Americans get a paltry 4 to 11 grams of fiber daily and most health organizations recommend 25 to 38 grams, including beans in your diet makes a lot of sense! Note: Be sure to crush the garlic before chopping . . . the health benefits of garlic (lowering blood pressure, boosting immunity) come from crushing or chopping the bulb before eating.

Let the beans drain in a colander or sieve while preparing the onion, but do not rinse.

Heat the olive oil in a medium skillet over medium heat. Add the onion and cook until just starting to brown, 3 to 4 minutes. Add the garlic, chili powder, cumin, and chipotle pepper, and cook for 1 minute, stirring the whole time. Remove the beans from the strainer and place in a food processor. Add the onion and garlic mixture, tomato paste, vinegar, salt, and liquid smoke and process until smooth, scraping down the sides as necessary. You can serve immediately, but flavors will combine and deepen over time. Store in the refrigerator and serve cold, at room temperature, or warmed.

Yield: about six ¼-cup (71-g) servings

Per Serving: 96 calories; 2.7 g fat (25% calories from fat); 3.7 g protein; 16.9 g carbohydrate; 3.3 g dietary fiber; 0 mg cholesterol; 366.4 mg sodium

Ingredients

6 extra-large eggs

2 tablespoons (30 g) plain low-fat Greek yogurt

2 teaspoons (10 g) Dijon mustard

1/2 tablespoon (7.5 ml) flaxseed oil

1 teaspoon fresh-squeezed lemon juice

1/4 teaspoon onion powder

1/4 teaspoon sea salt

Pinch cayenne pepper, optional

Sweet paprika, for sprinkling

Heavenly Omega-Boosted Deviled Eggs

From Dr. Jonny: I'll bet you're wondering where the term "deviled eggs" came from. You weren't? Oh. Well in case you ever do wonder in the future, allow me to tell you the origin of the term. Back in 1822, an Englishman named William Underwood started a condiment business on Boston's Russia Wharf. More than forty years later, his sons started fooling around with a new product made from ham mixed with all kinds of special seasonings. This led to a whole product line of seasoned meat products. The seasoning process itself was nicknamed "deviling" and the name stuck. The Underwood "red devil" was born and the rest is history. "Deviled eggs" are a snack classic, but they're often made with poor-quality mayo and eggs from factory-farmed chickens. You can upgrade: Choose eggs from free-range chickens (or even omega-3-enriched eggs) and replace the high-calorie mayo with high-protein Greek yogurt. Add flaxseed for fiber and cancer-fighting lignans (and a nice nutty taste). It's a great spin on an American classic. Mr. Underwood would have loved it.

Cover the eggs with cold water in a medium saucepan, set the timer for 15 minutes, and bring to a boil. Reduce the heat to maintain a low boil until the timer goes off. Drain and cool the hard-boiled eggs under cold water.

In a medium bowl, combine the yogurt, mustard, flaxseed oil, lemon juice, onion powder, salt, and cayenne pepper and whisk together until well blended.

Peel the eggs and slice in half lengthwise. Place the yolks in the bowl with the yogurt mixture and mix thoroughly. Using a tablespoon, scoop the yolk mixture into the egg whites and sprinkle with the paprika. Serve warm, at room temperature, or chilled.

Yield: 6 servings

Per Serving: 86.7 calories; 6.3 g fat (65% calories from fat); 6.6 g protein; 1 g carbohydrate; 0.1 g dietary fiber; 211.8 mg cholesterol; 172.8 mg sodium

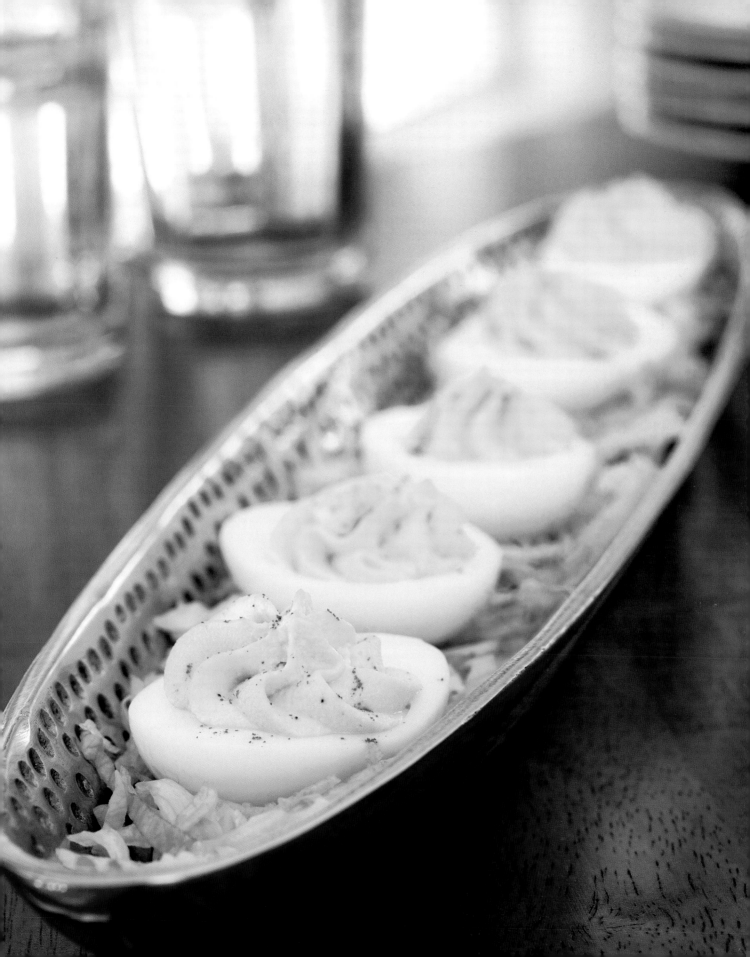

Ingredients

2 teaspoons (10 ml) olive oil

1 large Vidalia onion, halved and sliced
    lengthwise into thin strips

1/2 teaspoon Sucanat or sugar

Salt, to taste

1/4 teaspoon nutmeg

1 cup (230 g) plain low-fat Greek yogurt

Calorie-Light Caramelized Onion Dip

From Dr. Jonny: Dips are one of those foods that you never think of making from scratch, but maybe you should. It's easier than you think and you get to control the ingredients! Onion dip prepared from a package is all salt, sweeteners, and artificial flavors and often made with cream cheese or sour cream (not that there's anything wrong with either of those—they're just really high in calories). Chef Jeannette whipped this up from scratch with lots of fresh sweet onions and substituted high-protein Greek yogurt for the sour cream (fewer than half the calories, more than four times the protein!). The combination of sweet onions and tart yogurt makes the perfect party dip. Highly recommended: Try it with fresh veggie sticks. Fun fact: Onions are rich in inulin (a type of fiber) as well as quercetin, a member of the flavonoid family and one of the most anti-inflammatory and anticancer plant compounds on the planet!

Heat the oil over medium-high heat in a large, heavy-bottomed sauté pan, swirling to coat the pan. Add the onion and spread it out evenly in the pan, coating lightly with olive oil.

Cook for 10 minutes, stirring a couple of times, and sprinkle with the Sucanat, salt, and nutmeg, mixing to combine well. Decrease the heat to medium-low and continue to cook for 20 to 30 minutes, or until well browned and reduced, but not burned. When the onions begin to caramelize, stir them before they burn, but allow them to sit long enough to brown each time. Drizzle in a little additional oil if they stick too much and burn without browning. As they get darker, you will need to stir them more frequently. Once they are fully caramelized and reduced, remove them from the heat and let cool. Once cool, stir the onions into the yogurt and serve.

Yield: about 1½ cups, or 345 g (serving size: 2 tablespoons, or 30 g)
Per Serving: 24.7 calories; 1.1 g fat (39% calories from fat); 1.1 g protein; 2.7 g carbohydrate; 0.2 g dietary fiber; 1.2 mg cholesterol; 14.3 mg sodium

Ingredients

2 large, ripe heirloom tomatoes, finely diced

¼ jalapeño pepper, seeded and minced, or to taste

3 tablespoons (30 g) minced red onion

1 small clove garlic, minced

¼ cup (4 g) chopped fresh cilantro

Juice of ½ lime

Pinch of Sucanat

¼ teaspoon cumin

¼ teaspoon salt

¼ teaspoon fresh-ground black pepper

1 large ripe Hass avocado, peeled, halved, and pitted

All-Natural Spicy Salsa Guacamole

From Dr. Jonny: As many of you know, I have my own issues with late-night eating, though I'm working them out (big smile). Lately, my girlfriend, Michelle, has taken to making this fantastic guacamole with cucumber slices for dipping. It's pretty scrumptious. And it reminds me of why I'm not a huge fan of commercial guacamole—it has a lot of unnecessary preservatives to keep it bright green and too much salt (sodium) to boot. We brighten up ours with a homemade salsa, which has a ton of antioxidants (lycopene, vitamin C), plus the avocado doesn't need any artificial preservatives because the vitamin C in the juices of the tomato and lime does a fine job without the need for chemical assistance! Avocado is a real superfood—amazingly rich in potassium and surprisingly high in fiber. (Note: There's a difference between Florida and California varieties, though both are great. The Florida ones are the fiber heavyweights, with a whopping 17 grams per avocado, compared to a still-respectable 9 grams for the California variety. But the California ones are lower in calories—227 versus 365.)

In a medium bowl, combine the tomatoes, jalapeño, onion, garlic, cilantro, lime juice, Sucanat, cumin, salt, and pepper, and toss gently to combine well. Adjust the seasonings, if necessary. Finely dice the avocado just before serving and toss gently to combine (the avocado should stay in a fine dice and not become a purée).

Yield: about 4 servings

Per Serving: 92.8 calories; 6.9 g fat (62% calories from fat); 1.7 g protein; 8.6 g carbohydrate; 4.2 g dietary fiber; 0 mg cholesterol; 153.6 mg sodium

Ingredients

1 cup (235 ml) unsweetened vanilla rice
   milk, unsweetened vanilla almond milk,
   or low-fat cow's milk
1 cup (235 ml) low-fat coconut milk
2 scoops unsweetened, undenatured vanilla
   whey protein powder
1 pound (455 g) frozen mango chunks
12 ounces (340 g) frozen peaches
Juice and zest of 1 small lime, optional
2 to 3 teaspoons (13.5 to 20 g) honey,
   optional, to taste
¼ teaspoon ground cardamom, optional
4 teaspoons (7 g) toasted coconut, optional,
   for garnish

From Chef Jeannette

To toast coconut, sprinkle unsweetened,
dried, shredded coconut into a dry
skillet over medium heat. Cook, stirring
occasionally, for 3 to 4 minutes, or until
most of the coconut turns light brown.
Do not scorch! Cool and use as directed.

Lower-Cal Option: To reduce the calories
even further, omit the toasted coconut
garnish, swap the coconut milk for
another cup (235 ml) of rice or almond
milk, and add ½ teaspoon coconut
extract.

Lower-Cal Instant Tropical Frozen "Rice Cream"

From Dr. Jonny: People often ask me what my personal "sweet spots" are when it comes to foods that aren't necessarily good for me but that I crave anyway. I have two words to say about that: ice cream. To paraphrase the old saying, "Can't live with it, can't live without it." Point is that you actually can live with it (quite nicely, I might add) and that it doesn't have to be as bad for you as everyone thinks. Try the "skinnified" version below for a sweet snack that really hits the spot. (Actually, come to think of it, because of the protein blast from the whey this can even double as a meal on a hot summer's day. Seriously.) Thick, creamy, and satisfying—can you ask for anything more? Sure you can—ease of preparation. This lower-calorie, mostly fruit "rice cream" comes together in a flash.

Place the milk, coconut milk, protein powder, mango, peaches, lime zest and juice, honey, and cardamom into a powerful blender, such as Vita-Mix (if you don't have a power blender, you may have to do this in smaller batches to cream the frozen fruit). Blend until smooth but not liquefied; you should be able to scoop it with a spoon. Divide evenly into 4 dessert bowls, top each bowl with 1 teaspoon toasted coconut and serve immediately.

Yield: 4 snack servings or 2 meal servings
Per Serving: 303.4 calories; 6 g fat (17% calories from fat); 16.8 g protein; 53.4 g carbohydrate; 6 g dietary fiber; 4.9 mg cholesterol; 96.6 mg sodium

Ingredients

1 quart (946 ml) fresh-pressed apple cider,
  unsweetened

Juice of 1 orange

1 to 2 tablespoons (15 to 28 ml) ginger juice,
  to taste

2 tablespoons (40 g) mild honey, optional,
  to taste

6 cinnamon sticks

2 teaspoons (3.5 g) whole cloves

6 lightly crushed cardamom pods
  (or ¼ teaspoon ground cardamom)

8 allspice berries (or ¼ teaspoon ground
  allspice)

½ teaspoon nutmeg

4 unpeeled orange rounds (thin slices
  widthwise)

4 unpeeled lemon rounds (thin slices
  widthwise)

From Chef Jeannette

You can use prepared ginger juice, like
The Ginger People juice, or grate a good
handful of fresh ginger and squeeze
the gratings to release the juice, or put
a good chunk through a juicer. Fresh-
squeezed ginger juice is the tastiest and
most potent.

Pure and Simple Spiced Cider

From Dr. Jonny: To me, nothing says comfort like the spicy, fragrant smell of hot apple cider. Well, almost nothing. It takes me back to my childhood and reminds me of sitting around the fireplace in Woodstock, New York, where we'd sip the freshly made brew at dusk while looking out at the trees filled with beautiful autumn leaves. (No wonder they write songs about those leaves—they were gorgeous and poignant and reminded you of the impermanence of beauty and of life itself. But back to the cider.) Our version of this homey, comforting drink is lightly sweetened with a touch of (optional) honey. Plus, it's pumped up with extra citrus and a potent and fragrant blend of ginger, cardamom, nutmeg, allspice, and cloves. Interesting research on cinnamon shows that it may help with blood sugar, possibly blunting the spike in blood sugar that sometimes happens when you drink a high-carb juice. And for those of you fortunate enough to live near an orchard, get the cider directly from the folks who own it. If not, at least choose the freshest cider you can find, with the least number of additives. Then close your eyes, inhale the aroma, and start sipping!

Pour the cider, orange juice, ginger juice, and honey into a large, heavy-bottomed pot over medium-low heat and stir gently to combine. Add the spices and stir again. Float the fruit rounds on the top. Partially cover and heat for 10 to 15 minutes, until hot, but not boiling. Reduce the heat to low, cover completely, and cook for another 15 to 20 minutes, until very fragrant. Stir gently again to incorporate the honey and serve, straining the cider through a double-mesh sieve, floating a fruit round or cinnamon stick in each mug, if desired.

Yield: about 5 servings

Per Serving: 194 calories; 1.2 g fat (4% calories from fat); 1.5 g protein; 51 g carbohydrate; 11.6 g dietary fiber; 0 mg cholesterol; 13.7 mg sodium

Ingredients

1 cup (96 g) fresh mint leaves

4 limes, quartered

16 ounces (470 ml) 100 percent pineapple juice, not from concentrate

4 to 6 ounces (120 to 175 ml) coconut rum, or to taste (or substitute a few drops of coconut extract in each drink)

Ice

4 to 6 ounces (120 to 175 ml) cold seltzer

Fresh and Fruity Coconut Lime Mojito

From Dr. Jonny: Who doesn't enjoy one of those tropical drinks with the little umbrellas while relaxing at the pool in the Mediterranean? What, you say? You don't generally relax by the pool in the Mediterranean? Well, neither do I, but I do love those little umbrella drinks. Problem is, they're usually chock-full of sugars or "natural syrups" (which are basically sugar water with some chemical coloring). Our version uses no sugar at all. It's still delicious because of the natural sweetness of the magnificent pineapple, a fruit high in potassium, vitamin C, and natural enzymes. And don't discount the health benefits of even a little bit of mint—it's a potent herb that's been used medicinally for centuries, and contains potassium, calcium, and iron. The combination of flavors is so mellow and sweet it will transport you straight to Jamaica. Or St. Martin. Or the Mediterranean. Or just make wherever you are feel like that! Note: I personally don't drink alcohol so I can attest that this drink can be enjoyed "virgin"—tasty and smooth on a hot summer night!

Crush the mint leaves slightly between your fingers and divide evenly among 4 tall glasses. Using your hands, squeeze 4 quarters of 1 lime into each glass over the mint leaves and drop in the limes.

Add 4 ounces (120 ml) of pineapple juice to each glass, stir to combine, and set aside for at least 10 minutes for the flavors to release and combine.

Stir in 1 to 1½ ounces (28 to 42 ml) of the rum, to taste, fill the glass with ice, top with 1 to 1½ ounces (28 to 42 ml) of the seltzer (or more if omitting the rum), and stir gently.

Yield: 4 servings

Per Serving: 137.6 calories; 0.5 g fat (3% calories from fat); 1.7 g protein; 28 g carbohydrate; 4 g dietary fiber; 0 mg cholesterol; 18.7 mg sodium

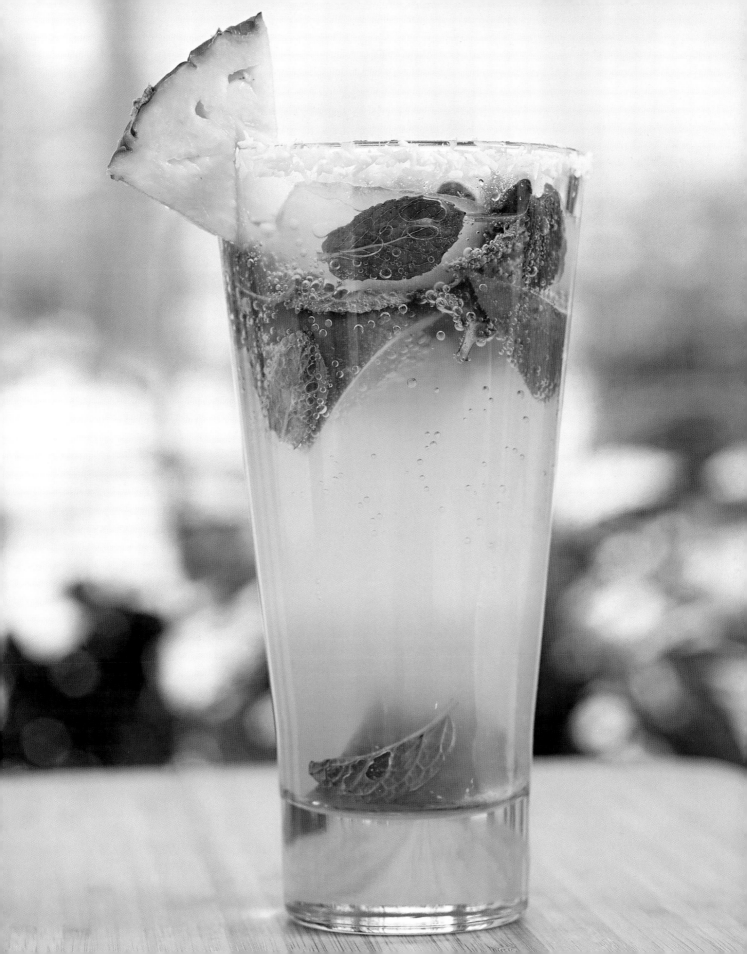

Ingredients

2 tablespoons (28 g) high-quality cocoa
powder

¼ cup (50 g) Sucanat, sugar, or xylitol, or
to taste

1 teaspoon oat flour (or wheat), optional,
for thickness

¾ teaspoon cinnamon

¼ teaspoon allspice

¼ teaspoon ground cloves

Pinch of salt

1 cup (235 ml) water

3 cups (710 ml) milk (cow's [low-fat for
fewer calories] or unsweetened vanilla
almond or soy)

½ teaspoon vanilla extract

Sweet and Spicy Antioxidant Hot Chocolate

From Dr. Jonny: Hot chocolate reminds me of childhood, specifically coming home from school in February when it was freezing cold in New York City and being welcomed with a steaming-hot cup of Nestlé's cocoa. But the packaged kind of hot chocolate has way too much sugar and too many artificial ingredients, and the wonderful health benefits of real cocoa are nowhere to be found. We make ours with real milk (personally I recommend the nut milks such as almond) and spice it up with real spices so you don't miss all that sugar. If you use real, high-quality cocoa powder, you get the extremely beneficial flavonols found in cocoa and dark chocolate, which are powerful antioxidants and have also been found to lower blood pressure.

In a small bowl, whisk together the cocoa powder, sweetener, flour, cinnamon, allspice, cloves, and salt. In a medium saucepan, combine the cocoa mix and water and whisk together over medium-high heat. Bring to a low simmer and cook, covered, for about 3 minutes, stirring frequently. Reduce the heat to medium and whisk in the milk. Cook until very hot but not boiling. Stir in the vanilla, remove from the heat, and serve.

Yield: 4 servings
Per Serving: 139.2 calories; 4.6 g fat (30% calories from fat); 7.5 g protein; 20.3 g carbohydrate; 2.7 g dietary fiber; 14.6 mg cholesterol; 77.1 mg sodium

Appendix:
The Healthy Comfort Foods Pantry

There are essentially two approaches to improving the overall quality of your diet. One is to select and combine specific foods for a high nutritional impact. Dr. Jonny is a genius at guiding healthy eating in this way.

The second approach is simpler and more fundamental: to make sure that all of the base foods and ingredients you use in your recipes are of the highest possible quality. Improving the overall quality of your foods is a straightforward and elegant way to begin the journey to improved health, and also an easy everyday method for keeping more seasoned natural eaters on track all the time.

The classic hamburger (a comfort food by almost anyone's definition) can be transformed from a poor-quality choice into a high-quality choice simply by making it yourself (as opposed to buying one at a fast food chain) using naturally lean, grass-fed beef. Conventional restaurant beef is much higher in fat calories and lower in nutrients than beef from a cow raised naturally, outside in the sun, eating grass. In addition, if you upgrade the kind of breading you keep on hand, that improves the hamburger even more: Choose a thin, whole-grain bun with no additives over the more conventional massive, starchy white roll.

Following are some tips for choosing the highest quality foods for stocking your larder. If your pantry is high quality, the comfort food dishes you make will taste like what you know and crave, but will automatically evolve into something healthier.

Brown the Whites
Simply by "browning the whites" in your pantry, you will ensure that your recipes have a higher fiber and nutrient content all the time: Choose natural, whole-grain bread, pasta, and rice over the white flour version. Keep a stock of whole-wheat flour and the finer, lighter whole-wheat pastry flour in addition to your regular unbleached. Swapping out even a portion of the white flour for whole-wheat pastry flour in your favorite recipes is a step in the right direction.

Choose Seasonal Produce
Buying fresh foods growing in season is a simple way to ensure higher quality. And the closer the source, the fresher the food, so buy from local organic farmers' markets if you can. Choosing seasonal foods is both inexpensive (foods in season are plentiful, so they tend to run lower in cost

than during the rest of the year) and healthy (foods harvested and eaten at the peak of their growing season are the richest in nutrients). Also, as a bonus, the flavors will sing on your tongue. Try it if you don't believe us!

Stock Fresh Meats from Pastured Animals and Clean, Wild-Caught Seafood

Look for high-quality, wild or grass-fed meats that are super-fresh. They should look plump and moist, with a supple firmness. Choose wild-caught, low-contaminant fish whenever possible. And fresh seafood should smell fresh, lightly briny, like the sea itself. If a piece of fish smells very fishy, it is likely past its prime. Check the freshness dates and make sure meat or seafood is sitting on top of a fresh, crisp bed of ice rather than in melted ice or pooled water.

Add Herbs and Spices for Flavor

Reduce the calories in many savory dishes by reducing the amount of cooking fats and oils you use and increasing the intensity of the flavors using herbs and spices. Choose fresh herbs when you can, and keep a good stock of potent dried herbs and spices on hand for times when it's not convenient to use fresh.

Wash fresh herbs well to remove any grit, then chop and add them to your dish toward the end of the cook time. If using dried herbs, the general rule of thumb is to use about one-third the amount of dried herb as fresh, so 1 teaspoon dried oregano to 1 tablespoon of fresh. Organic dried herbs tend to be more potent than most conventional herbs because they are harvested in smaller quantities and require less processing time before they actually reach the shelves.

Most spices are dried, and you can buy them whole or ground. Whole spices retain their potency for longer than ground, so they can be more economical in the long run. Simply grind or grate the amount you need right before cook time. I keep a mortar and pestle for grinding small amounts, and a designated coffee grinder for larger amounts. If you toast the spices for a couple of minutes in a dry skillet or in a very small amount of butter or oil before grinding, that will boost their flavors even more.

Use the following chart as a general pantry list for the recipes you will find in this book. We did not include the fresh ingredients such as produce, meats, and dairy, but rather the dried and refrigerated or frozen goods that have a long shelf life. With a ready stock of the highest quality pantry staples, you will be well on your way to preparing the healthiest possible comfort food dishes.

HERBS, SPICES, AND CONDIMENTS

Apple cider vinegar, raw	Dry mustard	Red pepper flakes
Balsamic vinegar	Garlic	Red wine vinegar
Blackstrap molasses	Ginger, fresh and ground	Rice wine vinegar
Capers	High-heat cooking spray	Sucanat
Cayenne pepper	Honey, raw	Sundried tomato paste
Chives	Ketchup, low sugar	Sundried tomato strips (dried and in oil)
Cilantro	Maple syrup, 100 percent, preferably grade B	Tamari, low sodium
Cinnamon	Mayonnaise, natural or vegan	Turmeric
Coriander	Miso paste	Vanilla extract
Cumin	Nutmeg	Worcestershire sauce (organic, to avoid high-fructose corn syrup)
Curry powder	Olives	Xylitol
Dijon mustard	Paprika	Zest, orange and lemon

(continued on page 238)

GRAINS, NUTS, AND SEEDS

Almonds	Oats	Sunflower seeds
Barley	Sesame seeds	Wheat germ
Brown basmati rice	Pasta, preferably Barilla Plus	Whole-wheat flour
Cashews	Peanuts	Whole-wheat panko bread crumbs
Flaxseed	Pecans	Whole-wheat pastry flour
Macadamia nuts	Quinoa	

OILS AND FATS

Almond oil	Macadamia nut oil	Peanut oil
Coconut oil, unsweetened	Olive oil, extra virgin	Sesame oil
Ghee, melted (or organic butter)		

MISCELLANEOUS

Apple juice concentrate, frozen	High-quality cocoa powder	Neufchâtel cheese
Applesauce, natural	Kudzu	

ACKNOWLEDGMENTS
From Jonny and Jeannette:

Jonny and Jeannette would like to extend our deep gratitude to the tireless team at Fair Winds, especially editor extraordinaire Cara Connors, organizational queen Tiffany Hill, and idea mastermind Will Kiester. Thanks also to Bill Bettencourt and Jenna Van Growski for the beautiful images. Special thanks as always to our friend and fabulous agent, Coleen O'Shea.

In addition, Jeannette would like to extend a warm-thank you to her testers, tasters, and clients for their indispensable feedback and ideas for the recipes, including Frank and Karen Knapp, Jodi Bass, Jeff and Lisa Kerr, Charles Hripak, Judie Porter (thanks, Mom!), Pam Goff, and especially fellow Real Food Mom, Tracee Yablon Brenner, and my beloveds, Jay, Jesse, and Julian.

ABOUT THE AUTHORS

Jonny Bowden, Ph.D., C.N.S., a board-certified nutritionist with a master's degree in psychology, is a nationally known expert on nutrition, weight loss, and health. A member of the Editorial Advisory Board of *Men's Health* magazine and a health columnist for America Online, he's also written or contributed to articles for dozens of national publications (print and online), including the *New York Times, The Wall Street Journal, Forbes, Time, Oxygen, Marie Claire, W, Remedy, Diabetes Focus, US Weekly, Cosmopolitan, Family Circle, Self, Fitness, Allure, Essence, Men's Health, Weight Watchers, Pilates Style, Prevention, Woman's World, InStyle, Fitness, Natural Health,* and *Shape.* He is the author of *The Most Effective Ways to Live Longer, The 150 Most Effective Ways to Boost Your Energy,* and *The 100 Healthiest Foods to Eat During Pregnancy* (with Allison Tannis, R.D.).

In addition to the above, he is the author of the award-winning *Living Low Carb: Controlled Carbohydrate Eating for Long-Term Weight Loss, The Most Effective Natural Cures on Earth, The Healthiest Meals on Earth* (with Jeannette Bessinger), and his acclaimed signature best seller, *The 150 Healthiest Foods on Earth.*

A popular, dynamic, and much sought-after speaker, he's appeared on CNN, Fox News, MSNBC, ABC, NBC, and CBS, and speaks frequently around the country.

You can find his DVDs, *The Truth about Weight Loss* and *The 7 Pillars of Longevity,* his popular motivational CDs, free newsletter, free audio programs, and many of the supplements and foods recommended in this book on his website, www.jonnybowden.com.

He lives in Southern California with his beloved animal companions Emily (a pit bull) and Lucy (an Argentine Dogo).

Jeannette Bessinger, ww.cleanfoodcoach.com, owner of Balance for Life, LLC, is a board-certified health counselor and award-winning lifestyle and nutrition educator. She is the author and coauthor of seven books featuring healthy eating, including *The Healthiest Meals on Earth*, *The Healthiest 15-Minute Recipes on Earth*, *Simple Food for Busy Families*, and *Great Expectations: Best Food for Your Baby and Toddler*. She has written or contributed to articles for multiple magazines, including *Better Nutrition*, *Better Homes and Gardens*, *Clean Eating*, *Consumer Reports*, and *Parenting*.

Designer and lead facilitator of a successful hospital-based lifestyle change program, she acts as a consultant and speaker to public and private groups and coalitions working to improve the health of schools and cities in the U.S. Jeanette is known as the Clean Food Coach, and her simple, practical approach has helped hundreds of women successfully meet the challenges of imbalanced health and nutrition with hope and grace.

She lives in Portsmouth, Rhode Island, with her patient husband, two awesome teenagers, three dogs, and their pesky cat.

INDEX

Best-selling Books by Acclaimed Nutritionist JONNY BOWDEN, Ph.D., C.N.S.

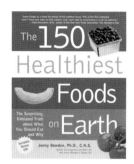

The 150 Healthiest Foods on Earth

The Surprising, Unbiased Truth about What You Should Eat and Why

"*The 150 Healthiest Foods on Earth* is simply delightful! The information is accurate; the presentation is a visual feast. All in all, reading this book is a very satisfying experience."

—Christiane Northrup, M.D., author of
Mother-Daughter Wisdom, The Wisdom of Menopause, and
Women's Bodies, Women's Wisdom

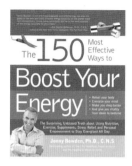

The Most Effective Ways to Boost Your Energy

The Surprising, Unbiased Truth about Using Nutrition, Exercise, Supplements, Stress Relief, and Personal Empowerment to Stay Energized All Day

"Get everyone you love to read my friend Dr. Jonny's brilliance!"

—Mark Victor Hansen, coauthor of
Chicken Soup for the Soul

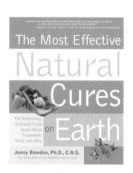

The Most Effective Natural Cures on Earth

The Surprising, Unbiased Truth about What Treatments Work and Why

"I reference this beautifully written and illustrated review of the best cures on the planet so often that it lives on my desk rather than the bookshelf."

—Mehmet C. Oz, M.D., coauthor of
You: The Owner's Manual

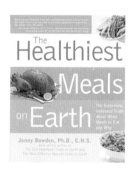

The Healthiest Meals on Earth

The Surprising, Unbiased Truth about What Meals to Eat and Why

"What a simply irresistible book with mouthwatering recipes from all around the world! I plan to use this book as a resource guide and as a gift for all the people I truly care about."

—Ann Louise Gittleman, Ph.D., C.N.S., *New York Times* best-selling author of *The Fat Flush Plan, Zapped,* and *Before the Change*

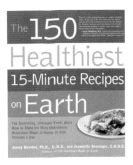

The 150 Healthiest 15-Minute Recipes on Earth

The Surprising, Unbiased Truth about How to Make the Most Deliciously Nutritious Meals at Home in Just Minutes a Day

"A gem of a book and a collector's piece for all of Dr. Jonny's fans!"

—Ann Louise Gittleman, Ph.D., C.N.S., *New York Times* best-selling author of *The Fat Flush Plan*, *Zapped*, and *Before the Change*

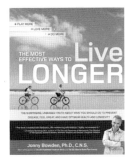

The Most Effective Ways to Live Longer

The Surprising, Unbiased Truth about What You Should Do to Prevent Disease, Feel Great, and Have Optimum Health and Longevity

"A must-read for anyone who wants to live longer! Jonny Bowden takes the lessons we've learned from the world's longest-lived people and offers a research-backed formula for the rest of us to get the most good years out of our lives."

—Dan Buettner, author of *The Blue Zones: Lessons on Living Longer from the People Who've Lived the Longest*

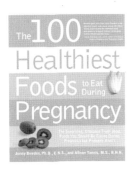

The 100 Healthiest Foods to Eat During Pregnancy

The Surprising, Unbiased Truth about Foods You Should Be Eating During Pregnancy but Probably Aren't

"Another great book from Jonny Bowden! In his signature expert style, Jonny, along with Allison Tannis, recommends the healthiest foods and spices for pregnant women … all pregnant women should read this book."

—Dean Raffleock, D.C., C.C.N., author of *A Natural Guide to Pregnancy and Postpartum Health*

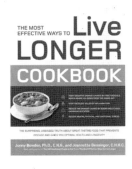

The Most Effective Ways to Live Longer Cookbook

The Surprising, Unbiased Truth about Great-Tasting Food That Prevents Disease and Gives You Optimal Health and Longevity

"Lusciously healthy and mouthwatering recipes—all beautifully organized into five key body systems. Another nutritional masterpiece from Dr. Jonny Bowden!"

—Deirdre Rawlings, Ph.D., author of *Foods That Help Win the Battle Against Fibromyalgia*

Hundreds of hours of my personal nutritional research reveals...

7 SUPER FOODS

That Could Change Your Life!

Dr. Jonny Bowden says...

"Do you want to know the best foods to eat to live a longer, healthier, happier, and more energized life?

If so then follow the instructions below and I'll send you the 7 Super Foods audio course...for free!"

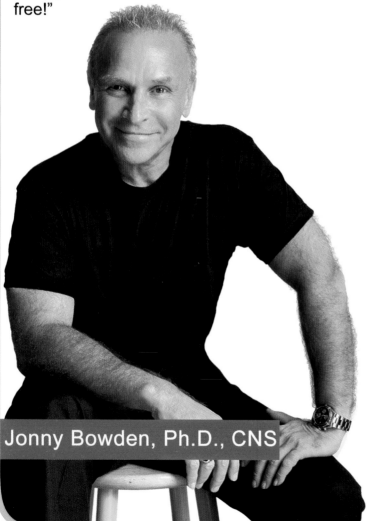

Jonny Bowden, Ph.D., CNS

This **FREE AUDIO COURSE** reveals the best foods to help you...

- **control weight**
- **look & feel younger**
- **prevent disease**
- **extend your life**
- **increase energy levels**

FREE!

Get started by signing up online now!

Simply go to

http://feelyourpower.com

NOW and enter your name and email address.

It's that easy! And you can rest assured that we will keep your email address private. We will NEVER sell or rent your information.

Change your body. Change your life...with Dr. Jonny Bowden!